A FESTIVAL OF FACTS—

For people who are concerned with the damaging effects of too much sodium in their diet. *Barbara Kraus Complete Guide to Sodium* lists the actual sodium count for thousands of basic and ready-to-eat foods, from appetizers to desserts, soups to main dishes. This is the essential handbook to good health through good nutrition. Take it to the supermarket, to the restaurant, to the coffee cart, and on trips.

Whether you're enjoying Chicken McNuggets at *McDonald's* or lounging around the pool sipping *Holland House* strawberry daiquiris, this extraordinary guide makes it easy to learn the sodium count of your favorite foods and drinks.

BARBARA KRAUS
COMPLETE GUIDE TO SODIUM

Barbara Kraus Complete Guide to Sodium

FIFTH EXPANDED EDITION

With *A Note on Sodium* by
Reva T. Frankle, Ed.D., R.D.,
Former Director of Nutrition,
Weight Watchers® International, Inc.

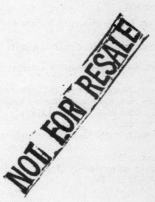

A PLUME BOOK

PLUME
Published by the Penguin Group
Penguin Books USA Inc., 375 Hudson Street,
New York, New York 10014, U.S.A.
Penguin Books Ltd, 27 Wrights Lane,
London W8 5TZ, England
Penguin Books Australia Ltd, Ringwood,
Victoria, Australia
Penguin Books Canada Ltd, 10 Alcorn Avenue,
Toronto, Ontario, Canada M4V 3B2
Penguin Books (N.Z.) Ltd, 182–190 Wairau Road,
Auckland 10, New Zealand

Penguin Books Ltd, Registered Offices:
Harmondsworth, Middlesex, England

First published by Plume, an imprint of New American Library,
a division of Penguin Books USA Inc.

First Printing, February, 1992
10 9 8 7 6 5 4 3 2 1

Excerpted from *The Dictionary of Sodium, Fats, and Cholesterol*

Ⓟ REGISTERED TRADEMARK—MARCA REGISTRADA

LIBRARY OF CONGRESS CATALOGING-IN-PUBLICATION DATA:
Kraus, Barbara.
   [Dictionary of sodium, fats, and cholesterol. Selections]
   Complete guide to sodium / Barbara Kraus : with a note on sodium
by Reva T. Frankle.—5th expanded ed.
        p.   cm.
   "Excerpted from the Dictionary of sodium, fats, and cholesterol"—
T.p.verso.
   ISBN 0-452-26760-9
   1. Food—Sodium content—Tables.   I. Title.
   TX553.S65K7425   1992
641.1'7—dc20   91-28540
                                                                  CIP
Printed in the United States of America

Donna Nelson
and
Farah Jeudy

Contents

vii

A Note on Sodium

by Reva T. Frankle, Ed.D., R.D.
Former Director of Nutrition,
Weight Watchers® International, Inc.

> "Excess of salty flavor hardens the pulse."
> *The Yellow Emperor's Classic*
> *of Internal Medicine,* circa 1000 B.C.

Salt has always been considered the king of seasonings. Historically, it has been associated with social status and wealth. In previous centuries, the most important guests at the table were seated "above the salt," and salt provided the root for the word "salary" (literally, money earned for the purchase of salt).

Today, however, salt's age-old preeminence is being challenged. Research has linked excessive salt consumption with hypertension (high blood pressure), an important risk factor in cardiovascular disease. For this reason, the government's "Dietary Guidelines for Americans," published by the Department of Agriculture in 1980, recommends avoiding too much sodium.

It has been estimated that Americans consume about 10 to 12 grams of salt daily, which amounts to about 2 to 2½ teaspoons. Since salt (sodium chloride) is about 40 percent sodium, this level of salt intake is equal to between 4 and 4½ grams of sodium per day. Where does this salt come from? Of the 10 to 12 grams of salt consumed daily, approximately one-third occurs naturally in foods, one-third comes from salt-containing ingredients added to foods during processing, and one-third represents discretionary salt added by the consumer (from the salt shaker during cooking and at the table). Drinking water also contains sodium, the amount varying from locale to locale.

Though there has been much discussion recently about the dangers of salt, let's not lose sight of the fact that sodium, a naturally occurring constituent of all foods, is an essential nutrient. Sodium is a key element in the regulation of body water and plays a vital role in the acid-base balance of the body. In fact, sodium, like chloride, is indispensable for many body processes, including the conduction of nerve impulses, heart action, and the function of certain enzyme systems. It's the *excessive* intake of salt that is being questioned.

Today, about 20 percent of the American population has high blood pressure—a primary cause of the 500,000 cases of stroke and the 1.2 million heart attacks that occur each year. High blood pressure is painless, "silent," and therefore often ignored until a complicating event causes it to manifest itself. Yet with proper diet and medical treatment, high blood pressure can be controlled and its complications prevented. For many Americans who suffer this silent disease, a reduced sodium intake is critical. In addition, those people who tend to retain body fluids due to kidney, heart, and liver conditions may want to check with their physicians about a decreased sodium intake. Available evidence indicates that restricting sodium to approximately 3.5 grams of salt per day will effect a slight reduction in blood pressure among moderately hypertensive adults. Several very carefully controlled studies of severely hypertensive adults have shown that sodium must be restricted to 200 milligrams (0.5 grams of salt) per day in order to achieve a significant reduction in blood pressure.

Although efforts to correlate salt intake with the incidence of hypertension have not provided definitive evidence of a causal relationship, nonetheless, evidence seems to indicate there is no risk in lowering present intakes of dietary sodium. The possible link between sodium intake and hypertension has become an issue of increased concern in the United States. Since hypertension is a potent risk factor for coronary heart disease and stroke, its control is a major health concern. Current treatment of hypertension requires a change in lifestyle—particularly in terms of dietary habits.

A discussion of dietary sodium is complicated. As you will learn as you use this book, some high-sodium foods do not taste salty or are not thought of as salty. For example, an analysis of a serving of fast-food french fries shows about 115 milligrams of sodium per serving, whereas a serving of cherry pie has nearly four times this amount, or about 450 milligrams.

As a public health nutritionist and a clinical dietitian, may I suggest that in place of salt you try seasoning foods with some of the following condiments and spices. Onion, garlic, lemon, lime, and vinegar are particularly useful, as are herbs and spices like allspice, aniseed, basil, bay leaf, caraway seed, cardamom, cayenne pepper, celery seed, chili powder, cinnamon, cloves, curry powder, dill seed, fennel seed, garlic, ginger, mace, marjoram, mint, mustard (dry), mustard seed, nutmeg, onion powder, oregano, parsley, pepper, poppy seed, poultry seasoning, rosemary, saffron, sage, sesame seed, tarragon, thyme, turmeric, and vanilla.

Agreed, the sodium intake of Americans is excessive. Since there is no reason to believe that reducing sodium chloride intake would be harmful for healthy persons, and it may even help prevent hypertension in some people, it is time to evaluate our sodium intake. The consumer can meet the challenge of decreasing sodium intake by being aware of the sodium content of foods and using discretion with the salt shaker. There is no specific recommended amount or safety level, but the National Research Council suggests that the estimated safe and adequate daily dietary intake of sodium is about 1100 to 3300 milligrams (1.1 to 3.3 grams). Limiting salt intake to 3 grams per day would allow for some salt to be used in cooking but none at the table.

Industry is responding. Sodium-containing substances such as salt are added to foods for three basic reasons: 1) to provide and enhance flavors in foods, 2) to develop and maintain expected characteristics of foods such as texture and freshness, and 3) as a preservative. Gradual reduction, appropriate for some foods, is taking place. Industry is experimenting with safe new processes for the use of salt, with reduced sodium formulas, and with the use of alternatives to sodium-containing ingredients. Gradual reduction will allow time for industry to determine the microbiologic safety of certain reduced-sodium products.

The FDA is working with the processed-food industry on a voluntary basis to lower the sodium content of foods they produce. (Sodium is used almost universally in the preserving and processing of food.) The Department of Health and Human

Services is working to give consumers more information about the sodium content of foods they buy and has said it "would like to see more public awareness in general about sodium and health."

Dietary change is the cornerstone of safe, effective, long-term blood pressure control. How fortunate that we now have the *Barbara Kraus Complete Guide to Sodium*, a comprehensive and easy-to-use book that enables readers to estimate their daily salt intake and to plan a diet that is lower in sodium.

Introduction

ARRANGEMENT OF THIS BOOK

This guide lists several thousand brand-name products and basic foods with their sodium counts. Foods are listed alphabetically by brand name or by the name of the food. The singular form is used for entries; that is, blackberry instead of blackberries. Most items are listed individually although a few are grouped. For example, all candies are listed together so that if you are looking for *Mars Bar*, you look first under *Candy*, then under *M* in alphabetical order. But, if you are looking for a breakfast food such as *Oatmeal*, you will find it under *O* in the main alphabet. Many cross references are included to assist you in finding items known by different names.

Under the main headings, it was often not possible nor even desirable to follow an alphabetical arrangement. For basic foods, such as apricots, the first entries are for the fresh product weighed with seeds as it is purchased from the store, then the fruit in small portions as they may be eaten or measured. These entries are followed by the processed products, canned (although it may actually be a bottle or a jar), dehydrated, dried, and frozen items. This basic plan, with adaptations where necessary, was followed for fruits, vegetables, and meats.

In almost all entries, where data were available, the U.S. Department of Agriculture figures are shown first. The Department values represent averages from several manufacturers and are shown for comparison with the values from individual companies or for use where particular brands are not available.

All brand-name products have been italicized and company names appear in parentheses.

Portions Used

The Measure or Quantity column is a most important one to read and note. Common household measures are used wherever possible. For some items, the amounts given are those commonly purchased in the store, such as one pound of meat, or a 15-ounce package of cake mix. These quantities can be divided into the number of servings used in the home and the nutritive values in each portion can then be readily determined. Any ingredients added in preparing such products must also be taken into account.

The smaller portions given are for foods as served or measured in moderate amounts, such as one-half cup of reconstituted juice, or four ounces of meat. Be sure to adjust the amount of the nutrients to the actual portions you use. For example, if you serve one cup of juice instead of one-half cup, multiply the amount of nutrients shown for the smaller amount by two.

The size of portions you use is extremely important in controlling the intake of any nutrient. The amount of a nutrient is directly related to the weight of the food served. The weight of a volumetric measure, such as a cup or a pint, may vary considerably depending on many factors; four ounces by weight may be very different from one-half cup or four fluid ounces. Ounces in the tables are always ounces by weight unless specified as fluid ounces, fractions of a cup, or other volumetric measure. Foods that are fluffy in texture such as flaked coconut and bean sprouts vary greatly in weight per cup, depending on how tightly they are packed. Such foods as canned green beans also vary when measured with and without liquid; for instance, canned beans with liquid weigh 4.2 ounces for one-half cup, but drained beans weigh 2.5 ounces for the same half cup. Check the weights of your serving portions regularly. Bear in mind that you can reduce or increase the intake of any nutrient by changing the serving size.

It was impossible to convert all the portions to a uniform

basis. Some sources were able to report data only in terms of weights with no information on cup or other volumetric measures. We have shown small portions in quantities that might reasonably be expected to be served or measured in the home or institution.

You will find in the Measure or Quantity column the phrases "weighed with bone," and "weighed with skin and seeds." These descriptions apply to the products as you purchase them in the markets, but the nutritive values as shown are for the amount of edible foods after you discard the bone, skin, seed, or other inedible part. The weight given in the "measure" or "quantity" column is to the nearest gram or fraction of an ounce.

Data on the composition of foods are constantly changing for many reasons. Better sampling and analytical methods, improvements in marketing procedures, and changes in formulas of mixed products may alter values for all of the nutrients. Weights of packaged foods are frequently changed. It is essential to read label information in order to be knowledgeable about these matters and to make intelligent use of food tables.

Sources of Data

Values in this guide are based on publications issued by the U.S. Department of Agriculture and on data submitted by manufacturers and processors. The U.S. Department of Agriculture issues basic tables on food composition for use in the United States. The commercial products from USDA publications represent average values obtained on products of more than one company. The figures designated as "home recipe" are based on recipes on file with the Department of Agriculture. Data on commercial products listed by brand name in this publication are based on values supplied by manufacturers and processors for their own individual products. Supermarket brand names, such as the A & P's *Ann Page*, or private labels could not be included in this guide inasmuch as they are not usually analyzed under these trade names. Every care has been taken to interpret the data and the descriptions supplied by the companies as fully and as accurately as possible. Many values have been recalculated to different portions from those submitted, in order to bring about greater uniformity among similar items.

Analyses of foods to provide information on nutritive values are extremely expensive to conduct. Many small companies cannot afford to have their products analyzed and were unable to provide data. Other companies have simply never gotten around to having the analyses done. New requirements for labeling nutritive values for products may provide information on additional items in the future.

Foods Listed by Groups

Foods in the following classes are reported together rather than as individual items in the main alphabet: baby food, bread, cake, cake mix, cake icing, cake icing mix, candy, cheese, cookies, cookie mix, crackers, gravy, ice cream, pie, pie filling, salad dressing, sauce, soft drinks, soup, and yogurt.

BARBARA KRAUS

Abbreviations and Symbols

(USDA) = United States Department of Agriculture

(HHS/FAO) = Health and Human Services (formerly Health, Education and Welfare)/Food and Agriculture Organization

* = prepared as package directs[1]
< = less than
& = and
" = inch
canned = bottles or jars as well as cans
dia. = diameter
fl. = fluid

g. = gram
liq. = liquid
lb. = pound
med. = medium
oz. = ounce
pkg. = package
pt. = pint
qt. = quart
sq. = square
T. = tablespoon
Tr. = trace
tsp. = teaspoon
wt. = weight

italics or name in parentheses = registered trademark™
The letters DNA indicate that no data are available.

[1] If the package directions call for whole or skim milk, the data given here are for whole milk, unless otherwise stated.

Equivalents

By Weight
1 pound = 16 ounces
1 ounce = 28.35 grams
3.52 ounces = 100 grams
1 gram = 1,000 milligrams

By Volume
1 quart = 4 cups
1 cup = 8 fluid ounces
1 cup = ½ pint
1 cup = 16 tablespoons
2 tablespoons = 1 fluid ounce
1 tablespoon = 3 teaspoons

Food and Description	Measure or Quantity	Sodium (milligrams)

A

AC'CENT	¼ tsp. (1 g.)	129
ACEROLA, fresh (USDA)	½ lb. (weighed with seeds)	15
AGNELOTTI, frozen (Buitoni)		
Cheese filling	2 oz.	158
Meat filling	2 oz.	237
ALBACORE, raw, meat only (USDA)	4 oz.	45
ALCOHOLIC BEVERAGES (See individual listings)		
ALE (See **BEER**)		
ALLSPICE (French's)	1 tsp. (1.7 g.)	1
ALMOND:		
Shelled (USDA):		
Whole	½ cup (2½ oz.)	3
Whole	1 oz.	Tr.
Whole	13–15 almonds (.6 oz.)	Tr.
Chopped	1 cup (4½ oz.)	5
Blanched (USDA) salted	½ cup	155
Chocolate-covered (See **CANDY**)		
Roasted:		
(USDA) salted	½ cup (2.8 oz.)	155
(Blue Diamond) diced	1 oz.	56
(Fisher):		
Dry, smoked	1 oz.	220
Honey roasted	1 oz.	75
(Planters) dry roasted, salted	1 oz.	200
(Tom's) salted	1 oz.	120
ALMOND BUTTER (Hain)	1 T.	2

Food and Description	Measure or Quantity	Sodium (milligrams)
ALMOND DELIGHT, cereal (Ralston Purina)	¾ cup	200
ALMOND EXTRACT, pure (Durkee or Virginia Dare)	1 tsp.	0
ALPHA-BITS, cereal (Post) regular	1 cup (1 oz.)	176
ANCHOVY, PICKLED (Granadaisa)	1 oz.	1587
ANISE EXTRACT, imitation (Durkee)	1 tsp.	0
APPLE, any variety:		
Fresh (USDA):		
Eaten with skin	1 lb. (weighed with skin & core)	4
Eaten with skin	1 med., 2½″ dia. (about 4 per lb.)	1
Eaten without skin	1 lb. (weighed with skin & core)	4
Eaten without skin	1 med., 2½″ dia. (about 4 per lb.)	1
Pared, diced or sliced	1 cup (3.9 oz.)	1
Pared, quartered	1 cup (4.4 oz.)	1
Canned:		
(Comstock) rings, drained	1 ring (1.1. oz.)	8
(White House):		
Rings, spiced, drained	1 ring (.5 oz.)	5
Sliced	½ cup (4 oz.)	10
Dehydrated (USDA):		
Uncooked	1 oz.	2
Cooked, sweetened	½ cup (4½ oz.)	1
Dried:		
(USDA)		
Uncooked	1 cup (3 oz.)	4
Cooked, unsweetened	½ cup (4½ oz.)	1
Cooked, sweetened	½ cup (4.9 oz.)	1
(Del Monte) uncooked	1 cup (2 oz.)	57
Frozen, sweetened, slices, not thawed (USDA)	10-oz. pkg.	40

Food and Description	Measure or Quantity	Sodium (milligrams)
APPLE BROWN BETTY, home recipe (USDA)	1 cup (7.6 oz.)	330
APPLE BUTTER:		
(USDA)	1 T. (.6 oz.)	<1
(Bama)	1 T.	7
(Home Brands)	1 T.	8
(White House)	1 T.	7
APPLE CHERRY BERRY DRINK, canned (Lincoln)	6 fl. oz.	30
APPLE CHERRY JUICE, canned (Red Cheek)	6 fl. oz.	11
APPLE CIDER:		
(USDA)	½ cup (4.4 oz)	1
Canned:		
(Johanna Farms) sweet	½ cup	1
(Tree Top)	6 fl. oz.	10
*Frozen (Tree Top)	6 fl. oz.	90
APPLE-CRANBERRY DRINK:		
Canned:		
(Hi-C)	6 fl. oz.	23
(Mott's)	8.45-fl. oz. container	24
(Smucker's)	8 fl. oz.	10
(Tree Top)	6 fl. oz.	10
*Frozen (Tree Top)	6 fl.oz.	10
APPLE DRINK, canned:		
Capri Sun, natural	6¾ fl. oz.	2
Ssips (Johanna Farms)	8.45-fl.-oz. container	<10
APPLE DUMPLING, frozen (Pepperidge Farm)	1 dumpling	240
APPLE, ESCALLOPED:		
Canned (White House)	½ cup (4.5 oz.)	59
Frozen (Stouffer's)	4 oz.	15
APPLE-GRAPE JUICE:		
Canned:		
(Mott's)	9.5-oz. can	27
(Red Cheek)	6 fl. oz.	9
(Tree Top)	6 fl. oz.	10

Food and Description	Measure or Quantity	Sodium (milligrams)
*Frozen (Tree Top)	6 fl. oz.	10
APPLE JACKS, cereal		
(Kellogg's)	1 cup (1 oz.)	125
APPLE JELLY:		
Sweetened:		
(Bama)	1 T.	7
(Home Brands)	1 T.	8
(Smucker's)	1 T.	2
Dietetic (See **APPLE SPREAD**)		
APPLE JUICE:		
Canned:		
(USDA)	1 cup (8.7 oz.)	2
(Ardmore Farms)	6 fl. oz.	Tr.
(Borden) *Sippin' Pak*	8.45-fl.-oz. container	25
(Johanna Farms):		
Florida citrus	6 fl. oz.	3
Tree Ripe	8.45-fl.-oz. container	2
(Land O'Lakes)	6 fl. oz.	15
(Libby's)	6 fl. oz.	6
(Minute Maid)	6 fl. oz.	2
(Mott's) regular or McIntosh	6 fl. oz.	13
(Ocean Spray)	6 fl. oz.	7
(Red Cheek)	6 fl. oz.	2
(Tree Top) regular or unfiltered	6 fl. oz.	10
(White House)	6 fl. oz.	Tr.
Chilled (Minute Maid)	6 fl. oz.	2
*Frozen:		
(Minute Maid)	6 fl. oz.	23
(Sunkist)	6 fl. oz.	59
(Tree Top)	6 fl. oz.	10
APPLE JUICE DRINK, canned		
Squeezit (General Mills)	6.¾ oz. bottle	5
APPLE NECTAR, canned		
(Libby's)	6 fl. oz.	25
APPLE-PEAR JUICE, canned		
(Tree Top)	6 fl. oz.	10

Food and Description	Measure or Quantity	Sodium (milligrams)
APPLE PUNCH DRINK,		
canned (Red Cheek)	6 fl. oz.	7
APPLE RAISIN CRISP, cereal		
(Kellogg's)	⅔ cup (1 oz.)	230
APPLE-RASPBERRY DRINK,		
canned (Mott's)	10-fl.-oz. container	17
APPLE-RASPBERRY JUICE:		
Canned:		
(Mott's)	8.45-fl.-oz. container	67
(Mott's)	9½-oz. can	76
(Red Cheek)	6 fl. oz.	8
(Tree Top)	6 fl. oz.	10
*Frozen (Tree Top)	6 fl. oz.	10
APPLESAUCE, canned:		
Sweetened:		
(USDA)	½ cup (4.5 oz.)	3
(Comstock)	½ cup (4.4 oz.)	90
(Del Monte)	½ cup (4.0 oz.)	1
(Hunt's) any flavor	4¼ oz.	0
(Mott's):		
Regular, jarred:		
Plain or cinnamon	6 oz.	<1
Chunky	6 oz.	11
Single-serve cups:		
Plain or cinnamon	4-oz. container	<1
Cherry	3¾-oz. container	8
Peach	3¾-oz. container	7
Strawberry	3¾-oz. container	10
(Tree Top)	½ cup	0
(White House) regular or chunky	½ cup (5 oz.)	5
Unsweetened, dietetic or low calorie:		
(USDA)	½ cup (4.3 oz.)	2
(Mott's):		
Jarred	6 oz.	3
Single-serve cups	4-oz. container	2

Food and Description	Measure or Quantity	Sodium (milligrams)
(Thank You Brand)	½ cup (4.3 oz.)	12
(White House) regular or with added apple juice	½ cup (4.7 oz.)	5
APPLE SPREAD, low sugar:		
(Estee)	1 T. (.6 oz.)	<3
(Slenderella)	1 T. (.6 oz.)	19
(Smucker's)	1 T. (.6 oz.)	19
APRICOT:		
Fresh (USDA):		
Whole	1 lb. (weighed with pits)	4
Whole	3 apricots (about 12 per lb.)	1
Halves	1 cup (5½ oz.)	2
Canned, regular pack, solids & liq.:		
(USDA):		
Juice pack	4 oz.	1
Light syrup	4 oz.	1
Heavy syrup, halves	½ cup (4.6 oz.)	1
Heavy syrup, halves	3 med. halves with 1¾ T. syrup (3 oz.)	1
Extra heavy syrup	4 oz.	1
(Del Monte):		
Halves, unpeeled	½ cup (4¼ oz.)	7
Whole, peeled	½ cup (4¼ oz.)	18
(Libby's) heavy syrup, halves	½ cup (4½ oz.)	7
(Stokely-Van Camp)	½ cup (4.6 oz.)	22
Canned, unsweetened or dietetic, solids & liq.:		
(USDA) water pack, halves	½ cup (4.4. oz.)	1
(Del Monte) *Lite*, unpeeled, extra light syrup	½ cup (4.3 oz.)	2
(Diet Delight) juice pack	½ cup (4.4 oz.)	5
(Featherweight):		
Juice pack	½ cup	<10
Water pack	½ cup	<10

Food and Description	Measure or Quantity	Sodium (milligrams)
Dehydrated (USDA):		
Uncooked, sulfured	4 oz.	37
Cooked, sugar added, solids & liq.	4 oz.	9
Dried:		
(USDA):		
Uncooked	1 cup (4.6 oz.)	34
Uncooked	10 large halves (¼ cup or 1.7 oz.)	13
Cooked, sweetened	½ cup with liq. (4.7 oz.)	9
Cooked, unsweetened	½ cup with liq. (4.4 oz.)	10
(Del Monte)	½ cup (2.3 oz.)	4
(Sun-Maid)	½ cup (3.5 oz.)	52
(Sunsweet)	½ cup (3½ oz.)	52
Frozen, unthawed, sweetened (USDA)	10-oz. pkg.	11
APRICOT NECTAR, canned, sweetened:		
(USDA)	½ cup (4.4 oz.)	Tr.
(Del Monte)	6 fl. oz. (6.6 oz.)	<10
APRICOT & PINEAPPLE PRESERVE, sweetened (Smucker's)	1 T. (.7 oz.)	3
APRICOT PRESERVE:		
Sweetened (Home Brands)	1 T.	7
Dietetic:		
(Estee)	1 T.	<3
(Featherweight)	1 T.	40–50
(Louis Sherry)	1 T.	Tr.
ARBY'S:		
Bac'n Cheddar Deluxe	7.8-oz. sandwich	1385
Beef'n Cheddar	6-oz. sandwich	1520
Chicken breast sandwich	7¼-oz. sandwich	1340
Croissant:		
Bacon & egg	4.5-oz. croissant	550
Butter	2-oz. croissant	225
Chicken salad	5-oz. croissant	725

Food and Description	Measure or Quantity	Sodium (milligrams)
Ham & Swiss	4-oz. croissant	995
Mushroom & Swiss	4-oz. croissant	630
Sausage & egg	5¾-oz. croissant	745
Ham & cheese	1 sandwich	1655
Potato:		
Cake	3-oz. serving	425
French fries	2½-oz. serving	30
Stuffed:		
Broccoli & cheese	12-oz. potato	475
Deluxe	11.1-oz. potato	475
Mushroom & cheese	10.6-oz. potato	635
Taco	15-oz. potato	1065
Roast beef sandwich:		
Regular	5.2-oz. sandwich	590
Junior	3-oz. sandwich	345
Super	8.3-oz. sandwich	800
Shake:		
Chocolate	10.6-oz. shake	300
Jamocha	10.6-oz. shake	280
Vanilla	8.8-oz. shake	245
ARTICHOKE, Globe or French:		
Raw (USDA) whole	1 lb. (weighed untrimmed)	78
Boiled (USDA) without salt, drained	4 oz.	34
Canned (Cara Mia) marinated, drained	6-oz. jar	94
Frozen (Birds Eye) deluxe hearts	⅓ of 9-oz. pkg.	40
ASPARAGUS:		
Raw (USDA) whole spears	1 lb. (weighed untrimmed)	5
Boiled (USDA) without salt, drained:		
Whole spears	4 spears (½″ at base, 2.1 oz.)	<1
Cut spears, 1½″-2″ pieces	1 cup (5.1 oz.)	1
Canned, regular pack: (USDA):		

Food and Description	Measure or Quantity	Sodium (milligrams)
Green spears, solids & liq.	1 cup (8.6 oz.)	576
Green spears, drained	1 cup (8.3 oz.)	536
Green spears only	4 med. spears (2.8 oz.)	188
Green, liquid only	2 T. liquid	71
White spears, solids & liq.	1 cup (8.6 oz.)	577
White spears only	4 med. spears (2.8 oz.)	188
White, liquid only	2 T. liquid	71
(Del Monte):		
Green tips & spears, solids & liq.	½ cup	355
Green or white spears, solids & liq.	½ cup	355
(Green Giant) green, cut spears, solids & liq.	½ of 8-oz. can	420
(Lindy) green, cut spears, solids & liq.	⅓ of 10½-oz. can	360
(Stokely-Van Camp):		
Green, spears, solids & liq.	1 cup (8.4 oz.)	896
Green, cut spears, solids & liq.	1 cup (8.4 oz.)	896
Canned, dietetic or low calorie:		
(USDA):		
Green, spears, solids & liq.	4 oz.	3
Green, spears, drained solids	4 oz.	3
Green, liquid only	4 oz. liquid	3
White, spears, drained solids	4 oz.	5
(Diet Delight) solids & liq.	½ cup (4.2 oz.)	5
(S&W) *Nutradiet*, green spears, solids & liq.	½ cup	<10
Frozen:		
(USDA):		
Cuts & tips, boiled, drained	½ cup (3.2 oz.)	<1

Food and Description	Measure or Quantity	Sodium (milligrams)
Spears, unthawed	4 oz.	2
Spears, boiled, drained	4 oz.	1
(Birds Eye):		
Cuts	⅓ of 10-oz. pkg.	6
Spears	⅓ of 10-oz. pkg.	4
(Frosty Acres) cuts & tips		
or spears	3.3 oz.	4
(McKenzie) spears	3⅓-oz. serving	19
ASPARAGUS PILAF, frozen		
(Green Giant)	9½-oz. pkg.	610
ASPARAGUS PUREE, canned		
(Larsen) no salt added	½ cup (4.4 oz.)	6
AUNT JEMIMA SYRUP (See **SYRUP**)		
AVOCADO, peeled, pitted, all commercial varieties (USDA):		
Whole	1 fruit (10.7 oz., weighed with seed & skin)	12
Cubed	1 cup (5.3 oz.)	6
Puree	1 cup (8.1 oz.)	9
AWAKE (Birds Eye)	6 fl. oz.	14

Food and Description	Measure or Quantity	Sodium (milligrams)

B

BABY FOOD:

Advance (Similac)	1 fl. oz.	Tr.
Apple-banana juice (Gerber) strained	4.2 fl. oz.	4
Apple betty (Beech-Nut):		
Junior	7¾-oz. jar	1
Strained	4¾-oz. jar	<1
Apple-blueberry (Gerber):		
Junior	7½-oz. jar	6
Strained	4½-oz. jar	4
Apple-cherry juice:		
Strained:		
(Beech-Nut)	4⅕ fl. oz.	6
(Gerber)	4.2 fl. oz.	Tr.
Toddler (Gerber)	4 fl. oz.	2
Apple-cranberry juice (Beech-Nut) strained	4½ fl. oz.	6
Apple dessert, Dutch (Gerber):		
Junior	7¾-oz. jar	46
Strained	4¾-oz. jar	27
Apple-grape juice:		
Strained:		
(Beech-Nut)	4⅕ fl. oz.	6
(Gerber)	4.2 fl. oz.	2
Toddler (Gerber)	4 fl. oz.	2
Apple juice:		
Strained:		
(Beech-Nut)	4.2 fl. oz.	5
(Gerber)	4.2 fl. oz.	2
Toddler (Gerber)	4 fl. oz.	1

Food and Description	Measure or Quantity	Sodium (milligrams)
Apple-peach juice, strained:		
(Beech-Nut)	4⅕ fl. oz.	6
(Gerber)	4.2 fl. oz.	4
Apple-plum juice (Gerber)		
strained	4.2 fl. oz.	4
Apple-prune juice (Gerber)		
strained	4.2 fl. oz.	5
Applesauce:		
Junior:		
(Beech-Nut)	7¾-oz. jar	5
(Gerber)	7½-oz. jar	2
Strained:		
(Beech-Nut)	4¾-oz. jar	0
(Gerber)	4½-oz. jar	3
Applesauce & apricots (Gerber):		
Junior	7½-oz. jar	6
Strained	4½-oz. jar	3
Applesauce & bananas (Beech-Nut) strained	4¾-oz. jar	<1
Applesauce & cherries (Beech-Nut):		
Junior	7¾-oz. jar	5
Strained	4¾-oz. jar	3
Applesauce with pineapple (Gerber) strained	4½-oz. jar	3
Applesauce & raspberries (Beech-Nut):		
Junior	7¾-oz. jar	5
Strained	4¾-oz. jar	3
Apple & yogurt (Gerber) strained	4½-oz. jar	22
Apricot with tapioca:		
Junior:		
(Beech-Nut)	7½-oz. jar	15
(Gerber)	7¾-oz. jar	22
Strained (Gerber)	4¾-oz. jar	8
Apricot with tapioca & apple juice (Beech-Nut) strained	4¾-oz. jar	9
Banana-apple dessert (Gerber):		

Food and Description	Measure or Quantity	Sodium (milligrams)
Junior	7¾-oz. jar	9
Strained	4¾-oz. jar	3
Banana dessert (Beech-Nut) junior	7½-oz. jar	10
Banana with pineapple & tapioca (Gerber):		
Junior	7½-oz. jar	8
Strained	4½-oz. jar	6
Banana & pineapple with tapioca & apple juice (Beech-Nut):		
Junior	7¾-oz. jar	20
Strained	4¾-oz. jar	12
Banana with tapioca:		
Junior:		
(Beech-Nut)	7¾-oz. jar	10
(Gerber)	7½-oz. jar	8
Strained:		
(Beech-Nut)	4¾-oz. jar	6
(Gerber)	7½-oz. jar	9
Banana & yogurt (Gerber) strained	4½-oz. jar	22
Bean, green:		
Junior (Beech-Nut)	7¼-oz. jar	5
Strained:		
(Beech-Nut)	4½-oz. jar	3
(Gerber)	4½-oz. jar	4
Bean, green, creamed (Gerber) junior	7½-oz. jar	19
Bean, green, potatoes & ham casserole (Gerber) toddler	6¼-oz. jar	538
Beef (Gerber):		
Junior	3½-oz. jar	52
Strained	3½-oz. jar	52
Beef & beef broth (Beech-Nut):		
Junior	7½-oz. jar	162
Strained	4½-oz. jar	88
Beef with beef heart (Gerber) strained	3½-oz. jar	58

Food and Description	Measure or Quantity	Sodium (milligrams)
Beef dinner, high meat, with vegetables (Gerber):		
Junior	4½-oz. jar	36
Strained	4½-oz. jar	31
Beef & egg noodle (Beech-Nut):		
Junior	7½-oz. jar	54
Strained	4½-oz. jar	32
Beef & egg noodles with vegetables (Gerber):		
Junior	7½-oz. jar	36
Strained	4½-oz. jar	19
Beef lasagna (Gerber) toddler	6¼-oz. jar	685
Beef liver (Gerber) strained	3½-oz. jar	47
Beef & rice with tomato sauce (Gerber) toddler	6¼-oz. jar	680
Beef stew (Gerber) toddler	6-oz. jar	593
Beef with vegetables & cereal, high meat (Beech-Nut):		
Junior	4½-oz. jar	38
Strained	4½-oz. jar	38
Beet (Gerber) strained	4½-oz. jar	119
Biscuit (Gerber)	11-gram piece	30
Carrot:		
Junior:		
(Beech-Nut)	7½-oz. jar	147
(Gerber)	7½-oz. jar	111
Strained:		
(Beech-Nut)	4½-oz. jar	88
(Gerber)	4½-oz. jar	47
Cereal, dry:		
Barley:		
(Beech-Nut)	½-oz. serving	4
(Gerber)	4 T. (½ oz.)	4
High protein:		
(Beech-Nut)	½-oz. serving	<20
(Gerber)	4 T. (½ oz.)	3
High protein with apple & orange (Gerber)	4 T. (½ oz.)	15
Mixed:		

Food and Description	Measure or Quantity	Sodium (milligrams)
(Beech-Nut)	½-oz. serving	<20
(Gerber)	4 T. (½ oz.)	4
Mixed with banana (Gerber)	4 T. (½ oz.)	13
Oatmeal:		
(Beech-Nut)	½-oz. serving	<20
(Gerber)	4 T. (½ oz.)	4
Oatmeal & banana (Gerber)	4 T. (½ oz.)	14
Rice:		
(Beech-Nut)	½-oz. serving	<20
(Gerber)	4 T. (½ oz.)	4
Rice with banana (Gerber)	4 T. (½ oz.)	11
Cereal or mixed cereal:		
With applesauce & banana:		
Junior (Gerber)	7½-oz. jar	8
(Beech-Nut)	4½-oz. jar	27
(Gerber)	4½-oz. jar	3
& egg yolk (Gerber):		
Junior	7½-oz. jar	26
Strained	4½-oz. jar	17
With egg yolks & bacon (Beech-Nut):		
Junior	7½-oz. jar	168
Strained	4½-oz. jar	88
Oatmeal with applesauce & banana (Gerber):		
Junior	7½-oz. jar	4
Strained	4½-oz. jar	3
Rice with applesauce & banana, strained:		
(Beech-Nut)	4¾-oz. jar	34
(Gerber)	4¾-oz. jar	34
Rice with mixed fruit (Gerber) junior	7¾-oz. jar	8
Cherry vanilla pudding (Gerber):		
Junior	7½-oz. jar	18
Strained	4½-oz. jar	17
Chicken (Gerber):		
Junior	3½-oz. jar	39
Strained	3½-oz. jar	39

Food and Description	Measure or Quantity	Sodium (milligrams)
Chicken & chicken broth (Beech-Nut):		
Junior	7½-oz. jar	147
Strained	4½-oz. jar	88
Chicken & noodles:		
Junior:		
(Beech-Nut)	7½-oz. jar	44
(Gerber)	7½-oz. jar	28
Strained:		
(Beech-Nut)	4½-oz. jar	26
(Gerber)	4½-oz. jar	20
Chicken & rice (Beech-Nut) strained	4½-oz. jar	20
Chicken with vegetables, high meat (Gerber) junior	4½-oz. jar	33
Chicken with vegetables & cereal (Beech-Nut):		
Junior	7½-oz. jar	61
Strained	4½-oz. jar	38
Chicken soup, cream of (Gerber) strained	4½-oz. jar	29
Chicken stew (Gerber) toddler	6-oz. jar	651
Chicken sticks (Gerber) junior	2½-oz. jar	323
Cookie (Gerber):		
Animal-shaped	6½-g. piece	13
Arrowroot	5½-g. piece	20
Corn, creamed:		
Junior:		
(Beech-Nut)	7½-oz. jar	34
(Gerber)	7½-oz. jar	21
Strained:		
(Beech-Nut)	4½-oz. jar	20
(Gerber)	4½-oz. jar	11
Cottage cheese with pineapple juice (Beech-Nut):		
Junior	7¾-oz. jar	46
Strained	4¾-oz. jar	28
Custard:		
Apple (Beech-Nut):		

Food and Description	Measure or Quantity	Sodium (milligrams)
Junior	7½-oz. jar	54
Strained	4½-oz. jar	32
Chocolate (Gerber) strained	4½-oz. jar	30
Vanilla:		
Junior:		
(Beech-Nut)	7½-oz. jar	69
(Gerber)	7¾-oz. jar	51
Strained:		
(Beech-Nut)	4½-oz. jar	41
(Gerber)	4½-oz. jar	31
Egg yolk (Gerber):		
Junior	3⅓-oz. jar	57
Strained	3⅓-oz. jar	45
Fruit dessert:		
Junior:		
(Beech-Nut):		
Regular	7¾-oz. jar	46
Tropical	7¾-oz. jar	35
(Gerber)	7¾-oz. jar	18
Strained:		
(Beech-Nut)	4½-oz. jar	26
(Gerber)	4¾-oz. jar	13
Fruit juice, mixed:		
Strained:		
(Beech-Nut)	4⅕ fl. oz.	6
(Gerber)	4.2 fl. oz.	2
Toddler (Gerber)	4 fl. oz.	1
Fruit, mixed, with yogurt:		
Junior (Beech-Nut)	7½-oz. jar	54
Strained:		
(Beech-Nut)	4¾-oz. jar	34
(Gerber)	4½-oz. jar	23
Guava (Gerber) strained	4½-oz. jar	.5
Guava & papaya (Gerber) strained	4½-oz. jar	.6
Ham (Gerber):		
Junior	3½-oz. jar	39
Strained	3½-oz. jar	40

Food and Description	Measure or Quantity	Sodium (milligrams)
Ham & ham broth (Beech-Nut) strained	4½-oz. jar	76
Ham with vegetables, high meat (Gerber):		
Junior	4½-oz. jar	24
Strained	4½-oz. jar	22
Ham with vegetable & cereal (Beech-Nut):		
Junior	4½-oz. jar	44
Strained	4½-oz. jar	44
Hawaiian Delight (Gerber):		
Junior	7¾-oz. jar	40
Strained	4½-oz. jar	23
Isomil (Similac) ready-to-feed	1 fl. oz.	Tr.
Lamb (Gerber):		
Junior	3½-oz. jar	53
Strained	3½-oz. jar	51
Lamb & lamb broth (Beech-Nut):		
Junior	7½-oz. jar	172
Strained	4½-oz. jar	97
Macaroni & cheese (Gerber):		
Junior	7½-oz. jar	168
Strained	4½-oz. jar	102
Macaroni & tomato with beef:		
Junior:		
(Beech-Nut)	7½-oz. jar	64
(Gerber)	7½-oz. jar	34
Strained:		
(Beech-Nut)	4½-oz. jar	32
(Gerber)	4½-oz. jar	38
Mango (Gerber) strained	4¾-oz. jar	5
MBF (Gerber)		
Concentrate	1 fl. oz. (2 T.)	16
Concentrate	15-fl.-oz. can	248
*Diluted, 1 to 1	1 fl. oz. (2 T.)	8
Meat sticks (Gerber) junior	2½-oz. jar	325
Orange-apple juice, strained:		
(Beech-Nut)	4½ fl. oz.	3
(Gerber)	4.2 fl. oz.	5

Food and Description	Measure or Quantity	Sodium (milligrams)
Orange-apricot juice (Beech-Nut) strained	4.2 fl. oz.	7
Orange-banana juice (Beech-Nut) strained	4⅕ fl. oz.	3
Orange juice, strained:		
(Beech-Nut)	4⅕ fl. oz.	3
(Gerber)	4.2 fl. oz.	4
Orange-pineapple dessert (Beech-Nut) strained	4¾-oz. jar	28
Orange-pineapple juice, strained:		
(Beech-Nut)	4⅕ fl. oz.	3
(Gerber)	4.2 fl. oz.	1
Orange pudding (Gerber) strained	4¾-oz. jar	28
Papaya & applesauce (Gerber) strained	4½-oz. jar	6
Pea:		
Junior:		
(Beech-Nut)	7¼-oz. jar	5
(Gerber)	7½-oz. jar	11
Strained:		
(Beech-Nut)	4½-oz. jar	3
(Gerber)	4½-oz. jar	11
Pea & carrot (Beech-Nut) strained	4½-oz. jar	50
Peach:		
Junior:		
(Beech-Nut)	7¾-oz. jar	15
(Gerber)	7½-oz. jar	6
Strained:		
(Beech-Nut)	4¾-oz. jar	0
(Gerber)	4½-oz. jar	4
Peach & apple with yogurt (Beech-Nut):		
Junior	7½-oz. jar	54
Strained	4½-oz. jar	32
Peach cobbler (Gerber):		
Junior	7¾-oz. jar	20
Strained	4¾-oz. jar	9

Food and Description	Measure or Quantity	Sodium (milligrams)
Peach melba (Beech-Nut):		
Junior	7¾-oz. jar	20
Strained	4¾-oz. jar	12
Pear:		
Junior:		
(Beech-Nut)	7½-oz. jar	5
(Gerber)	7½-oz. jar	6
Strained:		
(Beech-Nut)	4½-oz. jar	0
(Gerber)	7½-oz. jar	4
Pear & pineapple:		
Junior:		
(Beech-Nut)	7½-oz. jar	10
(Gerber)	7½-oz. jar	4
Strained:		
(Beech-Nut)	4½-oz. serving	6
(Gerber)	4½-oz. jar	3
Pineapple dessert (Beech-Nut) strained	4¾-oz. jar	12
Pineapple with yogurt (Beech-Nut):		
Junior	7½-oz. jar	64
Strained	4¾-oz. jar	40
Plum with tapioca (Gerber):		
Junior	7¾-oz. jar	11
Strained	4¾-oz. jar	5
Plum with tapioca & apple juice (Beech-Nut):		
Junior	7¾-oz. jar	15
Strained	4¾-oz. jar	9
Pork (Gerber) strained	3½-oz. jar	38
Pretzel (Gerber)	6-g. piece	15
Prune-orange juice (Beech-Nut) strained	4⅕ fl. oz.	6
Prune with tapioca:		
Junior:		
(Beech-Nut)	7¾-oz. jar	10
(Gerber)	7¾-oz. jar	20
Strained:		

Food and Description	Measure or Quantity	Sodium (milligrams)
(Beech-Nut)	4¾-oz. jar	6
(Gerber)	4¾-oz. jar	13
Similac:		
Ready-to-feed or concentrated liquid, with or without added iron	1 fl. oz.	9
*Powder, regular or with iron	1 fl. oz.	11
Spaghetti & meatballs (Gerber) toddler	6½-oz. jar	63
Spaghetti, tomato & beef (Beech-Nut) junior	7½-oz. jar	74
Spaghetti with tomato sauce & beef (Gerber) junior	7½-oz. jar	58
Spinach, creamed (Gerber) strained	4½-oz. jar	49
Split pea & ham, junior:		
(Beech-Nut)	7½-oz. jar	55
(Gerber)	7½-oz. jar	36
Squash:		
Junior:		
(Beech-Nut)	7½-oz. jar	5
(Gerber)	7½-oz. jar	4
Strained:		
(Beech-Nut)	4½-oz. jar	3
(Gerber)	4½-oz. jar	5
Sweet potato:		
Junior:		
(Beech-Nut)	7¾-oz. jar	111
(Gerber)	7¾-oz. jar	51
Strained (Gerber)	4¾-oz. jar	24
Turkey (Gerber):		
Junior	3½-oz. jar	50
Strained	3½-oz. jar	56
Turkey & rice (Beech-Nut):		
Junior	7½-oz. jar	55
Strained	4½-oz. jar	33
Turkey & rice with vegetables (Gerber):		

Food and Description	Measure or Quantity	Sodium (milligrams)
Junior	7½-oz. jar	36
Strained	4½-oz. jar	23
Turkey & vegetables, high meat (Gerber):		
Junior	4½-oz. jar	40
Strained	4½-oz. jar	37
Turkey with vegetables & cereal (Beech-Nut) high meat:		
Junior	4½-oz. jar	65
Strained	4½-oz. jar	65
Turkey sticks (Gerber) junior	2½-oz. jar	33
Turkey & turkey broth (Beech-Nut) strained	4½-oz. jar	76
Veal (Gerber):		
Junior	3½-oz. jar	55
Strained	3½-oz. jar	52
Veal & veal broth (Beech-Nut) strained	4½-oz. jar	88
Veal & vegetables (Gerber):		
Junior	4½-oz. jar	31
Strained	4½-oz. jar	27
Veal with vegetables & cereal, high meat (Beech-Nut) junior or strained	4½-oz. jar	44
Vegetable & bacon:		
Junior (Gerber)	7½-oz. jar	121
Strained:		
(Beech-Nut)	4½-oz. jar	141
(Gerber)	4½-oz. jar	79
Vegetable & beef:		
Junior:		
(Beech-Nut)	7½-oz. jar	55
(Gerber)	7½-oz. jar	26
Strained:		
(Beech-Nut)	4½-oz. jar	33
(Gerber)	4½-oz. jar	17
Vegetable & chicken:		
Junior:		
(Beech-Nut)	7½-oz. jar	44

Food and Description	Measure or Quantity	Sodium (milligrams)
(Gerber)	7½-oz. jar	21
Strained:		
(Beech-Nut)	4½-oz. jar	38
(Gerber)	4½-oz. jar	14
Vegetable & ham:		
Junior (Gerber)	7½-oz. jar	30
Strained:		
(Beech-Nut)	4½-oz. jar	33
(Gerber)	4½-oz. jar	15
Vegetable & lamb (Gerber):		
Junior	7½-oz. jar	26
Strained	4½-oz. jar	15
Vegetable & lamb with rice & barley (Beech-Nut):		
Junior	7½-oz. jar	44
Strained	4½-oz. jar	26
Vegetable & liver (Gerber):		
Junior	7½-oz. jar	28
Strained	4½-oz. jar	19
Vegetable & liver with rice & barley (Beech-Nut):		
Junior	7½-oz. jar	44
Strained	4½-oz. jar	26
Vegetable, mixed:		
Junior:		
(Beech-Nut)	7½-oz. jar	64
(Gerber)	7½-oz. jar	77
(Gerber):		
Regular	4½-oz. jar	38
Garden	4½-oz. jar	50
Strained:		
Regular	4½-oz. jar	27
Garden	4½-oz. jar	28
Vegetable & turkey:		
Junior (Gerber)	7½-oz. jar	32
Strained:		
(Beech-Nut)	4½-oz. jar	26
(Gerber)	4½-oz. jar	20

Food and Description	Measure or Quantity	Sodium (milligrams)
Vegetable & turkey casserole (Gerber) toddler	6¼-oz. jar	58
BACON, cured:		
Raw (USDA):		
Slab	1 oz. (weighed with rind)	181
Sliced	1 oz.	193
Broiled or fried crisp, drained:		
(USDA):		
Medium slice	1 slice (7½ g.)	77
Thick slice	1 slice (12 g.)	123
Thin slice	1 slice (5 g.)	51
(Hormel):		
Black Label	1 slice	149
Range Brand	1 slice	186
(Oscar Mayer):		
Regular	.2-oz. slice	118
Center cut	.2-oz. slice	112
Lower salt	.2-oz. slice	86
Thick slice	.4-oz. slice	208
BACON BITS:		
(Estee) imitation	1 tsp.	30
(French's) imitation, crumbles	1 tsp. (2 g.)	55
(General Mills) *Bac*Os*	1 T. (7.6 g.)	135
(Oscar Mayer) real	1 tsp. (.1 oz.)	52
BACON, CANADIAN:		
Unheated:		
(USDA)	1 oz. (3⅜" dia., ³⁄₁₆" thick)	536
(Eckrich)	1-oz. slice	460
(Hormel) regular	1 oz.	315
(Oscar Mayer) 93% fat free:		
Sliced	.7-oz. slice	272
Sliced	.8-oz. slice	311
Sliced	1-oz. slice	389
Broiled or fried (USDA) drained	1 oz.	726
BACON, SIMULATED (See also **TEXTURED VEGETABLE PROTEIN**) cooked:		

Food and Description	Measure or Quantity	Sodium (milligrams)
(Oscar Mayer) *Lean 'N Tasty*		
Beef or pork	1 strip	197
(Swift) *Sizzlean*, pork	.4-oz. strip	159
BAGEL:		
(USDA):		
Egg	3" dia. (1.9 oz.)	245
Water	3" dia. (1.9 oz.)	205
(Lender's):		
Plain:		
Regular	2-oz. piece	350
Bagelettes	.9-oz. piece	Tr.
Onion	1 bagel	290
Raisin & honey or wheat & raisin with honey	2½-oz. bagel	310
BAKING POWDER:		
(USDA):		
Low sodium	1 tsp (3.7 g.)	<1
Phosphate	1 tsp. (3.8 g.)	312
SAS	1 tsp. (3 g.)	329
Tartrate	1 tsp. (2.8 g.)	204
(Calumet)	1 tsp. (3.8 g.)	396
(Davis)	1 tsp. (.1 oz.)	326
(Featherweight) low sodium	1 tsp.	2
BALSAMPEAR, fresh		
(HEW/FAO):		
Whole	1 lb. (weighed with cavity contents)	7
Flesh only	4 oz.	2
BAMBOO SHOOT, canned:		
(Chun King) drained	8½-oz. can	0
(La Choy) drained	¼ cup (1½ oz.)	0
BANANA (USDA):		
Common yellow:		
Fresh:		
Whole	1 lb. (weighed with skin)	3
Small size	5.9-oz. banana (7¾" × ¹¹/₃₂")	1

Food and Description	Measure or Quantity	Sodium (milligrams)
Medium size	6.2-oz. banana (8 ¾" × 1 ¹³⁄₃₂")	1
Large size	7-oz. banana (9¾" × 1⁷⁄₁₆")	1
Mashed	1 cup (about 2 med.)	2
Sliced	1 cup (about 1¼ med.)	1
Dehydrated flakes	½ cup (1.8 oz.)	2
Red, fresh, whole	1 lb. (weighed with skin)	3
BANANA NECTAR, canned (Libby's)	6 fl. oz.	15
BARBECUE SEASONING (French's)	1 tsp. (2½ g.)	70
BARLEY, pearl, dry:		
Light (USDA)	¼ cup (1.8 oz.)	2
Pot or Scotch (Quaker)	¼ cup (1.7 oz.)	5
BASIL:		
Fresh (HEW/FAO) sweet, leaves	½ oz.	2
Dried (French's) leaves	1 tsp. (1.1 g.)	Tr.
BASS (USDA) Black Sea, raw, whole	1 lb. (weighed whole)	120
BATMAN, cereal (Ralston-Purina)	1 cup (1 oz.)	140
BAY LEAF (French's) dried	1 tsp. (1.3 g.)	Tr.
BEAN, BAKED, canned:	(USDA):	
With pork & molasses sauce	1 cup (9 oz.)	969
With pork & tomato sauce	1 cup (9 oz.)	1181
With tomato sauce	1 cup (9 oz.)	862
(Allen's) & pork, *Wagon Master*	1 cup (8 oz.)	1200
(B&M) *Brick Oven:*		
Pea bean with pork in brown sugar sauce	8-oz. serving	750
Red kidney in brown sugar sauce	½ of 16-oz. can	640

Food and Description	Measure or Quantity	Sodium (milligrams)
Yellow eye bean in brown sugar sauce	½ of 16-oz. can	770
(Campbell):		
Home style	8-oz. can	1130
Old fashioned, in molasses & brown sugar sauce	8-oz. can	1060
With pork & tomato sauce	8-oz. can	820
(Friend's):		
Pea	9-oz. can	1270
Red kidney	9-oz. can	1320
Yellow eye	9-oz. can	1470
(Furman's) & pork, in tomato sauce	8 oz.	718
(Hormel) *Short Orders:*		
With bacon	7½-oz. can	813
With ham	7½-oz. can	1182
(Hunt's) & pork	8 oz.	800
BEAN, BARBECUE (Campbell)	7⅞-oz. can	1110
BEAN, BAYO, black or brown (USDA) dry	4 oz.	28
BEAN, BLACK:		
Dry (USDA)	4 oz.	28
Canned:		
(Goya)	1 cup	810
(Progresso)	½ cup	480
BEAN, BROWN (USDA) dry	4 oz.	28
BEAN, CALICO (USDA) dry	4 oz.	11
BEAN, CANNELLINI, canned (Progresso)	½ cup	390
BEAN, CHILI (See **CHILI**)		
BEAN & FRANKFURTER, canned:		
(USDA)	1 cup (9 oz.)	1374
(Campbell) in tomato & molasses sauce	7⅞-oz. serving	1140
(Hormel) & weiners, *Short Orders*	7½-oz. can	1342
BEAN & FRANKFURTER DINNER, frozen:		
(Banquet)	10-oz. dinner	1230

Food and Description	Measure or Quantity	Sodium (milligrams)
(Morton)	10-oz. dinner	1490
(Swanson)	12½-oz. dinner	1100
BEAN, GARBANZO, canned:		
Regular (Old El Paso) solids & liq.	½ cup	250
Dietetic (S&W) *Nutradiet*, solids & liq.	½ cup	<10
BEAN, GREEN or SNAP:		
Fresh (USDA):		
Whole	1 lb. (weighed untrimmed)	28
French style	½ cup (1.4 oz.)	3
Boiled (USDA):		
Whole, drained	½ cup (2.2 oz.)	2
Pieces, 1½″ to 2″, drained	½ cup (2.4 oz.)	3
Canned, regular pack:		
(USDA):		
Whole, solids & liq.	½ cup (4.2 oz.)	283
Whole, drained solids	4 oz.	268
Cut, drained solids	½ cup (2.5 oz.)	165
Drained, liquid only	4 oz.	268
(Allen's) solids & liq.:		
Regular, cut, French or whole	½ cup	350
Cut with dry, shelled beans	½ cup	230
(Comstock) cut or French style, solids & liq.	½ cup (4.2 oz.)	400
(Green Giant) solids & liq.:		
Cut:	½ cup (4 oz.)	300
French style	½ cup (4 oz.)	330
Kitchen sliced	½ cup (4.1 oz.)	280
(Larsen) any style, *Freshlike*, solids & liq.	½ cup	340
(Stokely-Van Camp) cut, sliced or whole, solids & liq.	½ cup (4.2 oz.)	103
(Sunshine) solids & liq.	½ cup (4.2 oz.)	312
Canned, dietetic or low calorie:		
(USDA):		

Food and Description	Measure or Quantity	Sodium (milligrams)
Solids & liq.	4 oz.	2
Drained solids	4 oz.	2
(Del Monte) no salt added, solids & liq.	½ cup	<10
(Diet Delight) solids & liq.	½ cup (4.2 oz.)	5
(Featherweight) cut or French style, solids & liq.	½ cup (4 oz.)	<10
(Larsen) *Fresh-Lite*, solids & liq.	½ cup	6
Frozen:		
(USDA):		
Cut or French style, unthawed	10-oz. pkg.	3
Cut or French style, boiled, drained	½ cup (2.8 oz.)	<1
(Birds Eye):		
Cut:		
Plain	3 oz.	3
With mushrooms	5 oz.	789
French style:		
Plain	3 oz.	3
With toasted almonds	3 oz.	335
Petite, deluxe	⅓ of 8-oz. pkg.	3
Whole	3 oz.	4
(Frosty Acres)	3 oz.	0
(Green Giant):		
In butter sauce:		
Regular, cut	3 oz.	230
One Serving style	5½-oz. pkg.	360
Harvest Fresh, cut	⅓ of 8-oz. pkg.	150
Polybag	2½ oz.	10
(Larsen) any style	3 oz.	5
(Southland)	⅕ of 16-oz. pkg.	0
BEAN, GREEN, & MUSHROOM CASSEROLE, frozen (Stouffer's)	4¾ oz.	680
BEAN, ITALIAN, frozen:		
(Birds Eye)	3 oz.	<1
(Frosty Acres)	3 oz.	0

Food and Description	Measure or Quantity	Sodium (milligrams)
(Larsen)	3 oz.	5
BEAN, KIDNEY or RED:		
(USDA):		
Dry	1 lb.	45
Dry	½ cup (3.3. oz.)	9
Cooked	½ cup (3.3. oz.)	6
Canned, solids & liq.:		
Regular:		
(Allen's) dark or light	½ cup	290
(Comstock)	½ cup	410
(Goya):		
Red	½ cup	390
White	½ cup	340
(Hunt's):		
Regular	4 oz.	400
Small	½ cup (3½ oz.)	500
(Van Camp):		
Dark	8 oz.	732
Light	8 oz.	680
New Orleans style	8 oz.	793
Red	8 oz.	930
(Progresso) red	½ cup	400
Dietetic (S&W)		
Nutradiet	½ cup	<10
BEAN, LIMA:		
Raw (USDA):		
Young, whole	1 lb. (weighed in pod)	4
Mature, dry	½ cup (3.4 oz.)	4
Young, without shell	1 lb. (weighed shelled)	9
Boiled (USDA) mature, drained	½ cup (3.4 oz.)	2
Canned, regular pack:		
(USDA) drained solids	½ cup (3 oz.)	201
(Allen's) solids & liq.:		
Regular	½ cup (4 oz.)	370
Large butter	½ cup (4 oz.)	330
(Comstock) solids & liq.:		
Regular	½ cup	400

Food and Description	Measure or Quantity	Sodium (milligrams)
Butter	½ cup	500
(Del Monte) solids & liq.	½ cup (4 oz.)	355
(Furman's) butter, solids & liq.	½ cup (3.9 oz.)	459
(Larsens) *Freshlike*, solids & liq.	½ cup (4 oz.)	320
Canned, dietetic or low calorie: (USDA):		
Low sodium, solids & liq.	4 oz.	5
Low sodium, drained solids	4 oz.	5
(Featherweight) solids & liq.	½ cup	25
(Larsen) *Fresh-Lite*, solids & liq.	½ cup	6
Frozen:		
(USDA):		
Baby, unthawed	4 oz.	167
Fordhook, unthawed	4 oz.	115
Boiled, drained solids	½ cup (3.1 oz.)	114
Boiled, Fordhook, drained	½ cup (3 oz.)	86
(Birds Eye):		
Baby	⅓ of 10-oz. pkg.	114
Fordhook	⅓ of 10-oz. pkg.	101
(Frosty Acres):		
Baby	3.3 oz.	125
Butter	3.2 oz.	213
Fordhook	3.3 oz.	70
(Green Giant):		
Baby, in butter sauce	3.3 oz.	468
Harvest Fresh	3 oz.	180
Polybag	½ cup	30
(Larsen) baby	3.3 oz.	100
(McKenzie):		
Baby	3.3 oz.	117
Fordhook	3.3 oz.	94
Speckled butter	3.3 oz.	28
BEAN, MUNG (USDA) dry	½ cup (3.7 oz.)	6
BEAN, PINK, canned (Goya) solids & liq.	½ cup	400

Food and Description	Measure or Quantity	Sodium (milligrams)
BEAN, PINTO:		
Dry (USDA)	½ cup (3.4 oz.)	10
Canned, solids & liq.:		
(Gebhardt)	¼ of 15-oz. can	570
(Goya):		
Regular	½ cup (4 oz.)	267
Butter	½ cup	390
(Green Giant) picante style	½ cup (5 oz.)	580
(Old El Paso)	½ cup	320
(Progresso)	½ cup	410
BEAN, RED MEXICAN, dry		
(USDA)	4 oz.	11
BEAN, REFRIED, canned:		
(Gebhardt):		
Regular	4 oz.	490
Jalapeño	4 oz.	320
Little Pancho	½ cup	330
(Old El Paso):		
Plain	½ cup	400
With bacon	½ cup	380
With cheese or spicy	½ cup	560
With green chiles	½ cup	504
With jalapeños	½ cup	530
With sausage	½ cup	600
Vegetarian	½ cup	1180
(Rosarita):		
Plain	4 oz.	460
With bacon	4 oz.	508
With green chiles	4 oz.	438
With nacho cheese & onion	4 oz.	497
Spicy	4 oz.	468
Vegetarian	4 oz.	466
BEAN, ROMAN, canned		
solids & liq.:		
(Goya)	½ cup (2.3 oz.)	380
(Progresso)	½ cup	420
BEAN SALAD, canned		
(Green Giant)	½ cup	410

Food and Description	Measure or Quantity	Sodium (milligrams)
BEANS 'N FIXIN'S		
(Hunt's) canned, *Big John's:*		
Beans	3 oz.	370
Fixin's	1 oz.	125
BEAN SPROUT:		
Fresh (USDA) Mung:		
Raw	½ lb.	11
Raw	½ cup (1.6 oz.)	2
Boiled, drained	½ cup (2.2. oz.)	2
Canned (La Choy) drained	⅔ cup (2 oz.)	18
BEAN, WAX (See **BEAN, YELLOW**)		
BEAN, WHITE (USDA):		
Raw:		
Great Northern	½ cup (3.1 oz.)	17
Navy or pea	½ cup	20
White	1 oz.	5
Cooked:		
Great Northern	½ cup (3 oz.)	6
Navy or pea	½ cup (3.4 oz.)	7
All other white	4-oz. serving	8
BEAN, YELLOW or WAX:		
Raw, whole (USDA)	1 lb. (weighed untrimmed)	28
Boiled, drained (USDA) 1″ pieces	½ cup (2.9 oz.)	2
Canned, regular pack:		
(USDA):		
Solids & liq.	½ cup (4.2 oz.)	283
Drained, solids	½ cup (2.2 oz.)	146
Drained, liquid only	4 oz.	26
(Comstock) solids & liq.	½ cup	370
(Del Monte) solids & liq.	½ cup (4 oz.)	355
(Festal):		
Cut, solids & liq.	½ cup	332
French style, solids & liq.	½ cup (4 oz.)	383
(Larsen) *Freshlike*, cut, solids & liq.	½ cup (4.2 oz.)	320
Canned, dietetic or low calorie:		
(USDA):		

Food and Description	Measure or Quantity	Sodium (milligrams)
Solids & liq.	4-oz. serving	2
Drained solids	4-oz. serving	2
(Blue Boy) solids & liq.	4-oz. serving	2
(Featherweight) cut, solids & liq.	½ cup	<10
(Larsen) *Fresh-Lite*, solids & liq.	½ cup	6
Frozen:		
(USDA) cut, unthawed	4-oz. serving	1
(Frosty Acres)	3 oz.	5
(Larsen) cut	3 oz.	5
(McKenzie) cut	3 oz.	1
BEAR CLAWS (Dolly Madison):		
Cherry	2¾-oz. piece	250
Cinnamon	2¾-oz. piece	300
BEEF. Values for beef cuts are given below for "lean and fat" and for "lean only." Beef purchased by the consumer at the retail store usually is trimmed to about one-half inch layer of fat. This is the meat described as "lean and fat." If all the fat that can be cut off with a knife is removed, the remainder is the "lean only." These cuts still contain flecks of fat known as "marbling" distributed through the meat. Cooked meats are medium done. Choice grade cuts (USDA):		
Brisket:		
Raw	1 lb. (weighed with bone)	248
Braised, lean only	4 oz.	68
Chuck:		
Raw	1 lb. (weighed with bone)	248
Braised or pot-roasted, lean only	4 oz.	68

Food and Description	Measure or Quantity	Sodium (milligrams)
Dried (See **BEEF, CHIPPED**)		
Filet mignon. There are no data available on its composition. For dietary estimates, the data for sirloin, lean only, afford the closest approximation.		
Flank:		
Raw	1 lb.	295
Braised	4 oz.	68
Foreshank:		
Raw	1 lb. (weighed with bone)	165
Simmered:		
Lean & fat	4 oz.	68
Lean only	4 oz.	68
Ground:		
Lean:		
Raw	1 lb.	236
Raw	1 cup (8 oz.)	118
Broiled	4 oz.	54
Regular:		
Raw	1 lb.	295
Raw	1 cup (8 oz.)	147
Broiled	4 oz.	53
Heel of round:		
Raw	1 lb.	295
Roasted:		
Lean & fat	4 oz.	68
Lean only	4 oz.	68
Hindshank:		
Raw	1 lb. (weighed with bone)	136
Simmered:		
Lean & fat	4 oz.	68
Lean only	4 oz.	68
Neck:		
Raw	1 lb. (weighed with bone)	236
Pot-roasted:		
Lean & fat	4 oz.	51

Food and Description	Measure or Quantity	Sodium (milligrams)
Lean only	4 oz.	68
Plate:		
Raw	1 lb. (weighed with bone)	263
Simmered, lean & fat	4 oz.	68
Rib roast:		
Raw	1 lb. (weighed with bone)	271
Roasted, lean & fat	4 oz.	68
Round:		
Raw:		
Lean & fat	1 lb. (weighed with bone)	286
Lean & fat	1 lb. (weighed without bone)	295
Roasted:	1 lb. (weighed with bone)	286
Broiled:		
Lean & fat	4 oz.	68
Lean only	4 oz.	68
Steak, club:		
Raw	1 lb. (weighed without bone)	295
Broiled:		
Lean & fat	4 oz.	68
Lean only	4 oz.	68
Steak, porterhouse:		
Raw	1 lb. (weighed with bone)	268
Broiled:		
Lean & fat	4 oz.	68
Lean only	4 oz.	68
Steak, ribeye, broiled:		
One 10-oz. steak (weighed before cooking without bone) will give you lean & fat	7.3 oz	147
Steak, sirloin, double-bone:		
Raw	1 lb. (weighed with bone)	242

Food and Description	Measure or Quantity	Sodium (milligrams)
Broiled:		
Lean & fat	4 oz.	68
Lean only	4 oz.	68
One 16-oz. steak (weighed before cooking with bone) will give you:		
Lean & fat	4 oz.	167
Lean only	4 oz.	94
BEEF, CHIPPED:		
Home recipe (USDA) creamed	½ cup (4.3 oz.)	877
Frozen, creamed:		
(Banquet)	4-oz. pkg.	818
(Stouffer's)	11-oz. entree	1800
(Swanson)	10½-oz. entree	1545
BEEF, CORNED (See **CORNED BEEF**)		
BEEFAMATO COCKTAIL, canned (Mott's)	6 fl. oz.	240
BEEF BOUILLON, cubes or powder:		
(Borden) *Lite-Line*, instant, low sodium	1 tsp.	5
(Featherweight) cube or instant, low sodium	1 cube or 1 tsp.	10
(Herb-Ox):		
Cube	1 cube (3.7 g.)	500
Powder	1 packet (4.5 g.)	1040
*(Knorr)	8 fl. oz.	1220
(Wyler's) cube or instant	1 cube or 1 tsp.	930
BEEF DINNER or ENTREE:		
*Canned (Hunt's) *Entree Maker*, oriental	7.6-oz. serving	1122
Frozen:		
(Armour):		
Classics Lite, Steak Diane	10-oz. meal	440
Dining Lite, teriyaki	9-oz. meal	850
Dinner Classics:		
Sirloin roast	10.4-oz. meal	970
Sirloin tips	10½-oz. meal	820

Food and Description	Measure or Quantity	Sodium (milligrams)
(Banquet):		
Dinner:		
Chopped	11-oz. dinner	600
Extra Helping	16-oz. dinner	810
Platter	10-oz. meal	630
(Chun King) Szechuan	13-oz. entree	1810
(Healthy Choice) sirloin tips	11¾-oz. meal	350
(La Choy) *Fresh & Light*,		
broccoli	11-oz. meal	1299
(Morton) sliced	10-oz. dinner	950
(Stouffer's):		
Lean Cuisine:		
Oriental, with vegetables		
& rice	8⅝-oz. meal	900
Szechuan, with noodles		
& vegetables	9¼-oz. meal	680
Right Course:		
Dijon, with pasta &		
vegetables	9½-oz. meal	580
Fiesta, with corn pasta	8⅞-oz. meal	590
Ragout, with rice pilaf	10-oz. meal	550
(Swanson) *Hungry Man:*		
Chopped	17¼-oz. dinner	1640
Sliced, dinner	16-oz. dinner	1150
Sliced, entree	12¼-oz. entree	1040
(Weight Watchers):		
London broil in mushroom		
sauce	7.4-oz. meal	510
Sirloin tips & mushrooms		
in wine sauce	7½-oz. meal	940
BEEF, DRIED, packaged		
(Hormel) sliced	1 oz.	822
BEEF, GROUND, SEASONING		
MIX:		
*(Durkee) regular or with onion	1 cup	1099
(French's) with onion	1⅛-oz. pkg.	1760
BEEF HASH, ROAST, canned,		
Mary Kitchen (Hormel):		
Regular	7½-oz. serving	1142

Food and Description	Measure or Quantity	Sodium (milligrams)
Short Orders	7½-oz. can	1156
BEEF, PACKAGED:		
(Carl Buddig) smoked	1 oz.	430
(Hormel)	1 oz.	382
BEEF PEPPER ORIENTAL:		
Canned (La Choy)	¾ cup	1060
Frozen:		
(Chun King)	13-oz. meal	1300
(La Choy)	12-oz. dinner	1985
BEEF PIE:		
Home recipe (USDA) baked	4¼″ pie (8 oz. before baking)	645
Frozen:		
(Banquet)	7-oz. pie	870
(Morton)	7-oz. pie	740
(Stouffer's)	10-oz. pie	1300
(Swanson):		
Regular	8-oz. pie	900
Chunky	10-oz. pie	900
Hungry Man	16-oz. pie	1750
Hungry Man, steak burger	16-oz. pie	1520
BEEF SHORT RIBS, frozen:		
(Armour) Dinner Classics, boneless	9¾-oz.meal	790
(Stouffer's) boneless, with vegetable gravy	9-oz. meal	900
BEEF SOUP (See **SOUP**, Beef)		
BEEF SPREAD, ROAST, canned (Underwood)	½ of 4¾-oz. can	515
BEEF STEW:		
Home recipe (USDA)	1 cup	91
Canned, regular pack:		
(USDA)	1 cup (8.6 oz.)	1007
Dinty Moore (Hormel):		
Regular	⅓ of 24-oz. can	980
Short Orders	7½-oz. can	939
Canned, dietetic or low calorie:		
(Estee)	7½-oz. can	110
(Featherweight)	7½-oz. can	96

Food and Description	Measure or Quantity	Sodium (milligrams)
Frozen (Stouffer's)	10 oz.	1675
BEEF STEW SEASONING MIX:		
*(Durkee)	1 cup	975
(French's)	1⅞-oz. pkg.	4620
BEEF STOCK BASE (French's)	1 tsp. (4 g.)	500
BEEF STROGANOFF, frozen:		
(Armour) *Dinner Classics*	11¼-oz. meal	1090
(Stouffer's) with parsley, noodles	9¾-oz. meal	1090
(Weight Watchers)	9-oz. meal	900
***BEEF STROGANOFF SEASONING MIX** (Durkee)	1 cup	870
BEER, canned:		
Regular:		
Anheuser	12 fl. oz.	12
Blatz	12 fl. oz.	7
Budweiser	12 fl. oz.	12
Carlsberg	12 fl. oz.	12
C. Schmidt's	12 fl. oz.	17
King Cobra	12 fl. oz.	12
Old Style	12 fl. oz.	15
Ranier	12 fl. oz.	16
Schmidt	12 fl. oz.	7
Light:		
Budweiser Light	12 fl. oz.	5–15
Gablinger's	12 fl. oz.	21
Michelob Light	12 fl. oz.	5–15
Natural Light	12 fl. oz.	5–15
BEER, NEAR, *Kingsbury* (Heileman)	12 fl. oz.	28
BEET:		
Raw (USDA):		
Whole	1 lb. (weighed with skins, without tops)	190
Diced	½ cup (2.4 oz.)	40
Boiled (USDA) drained:		
Whole	2 beets (2″ dia., 3.5 oz.)	43

Food and Description	Measure or Quantity	Sodium (milligrams)
Diced	½ cup (3 oz.)	18
Sliced	½ cup (3.6 oz.)	44
Canned, regular pack, solids & liq.:		
(Blue Boy) harvard	½ cup	350
(Comstock):		
Regular	½ cup	100
Pickled	½ cup	500
(Del Monte):		
Pickled, sliced	½ cup (4 oz.)	375
Sliced, solids & liq.	½ cup (4. oz.)	290
(Larsen) *Freshlike*:		
Pickled	½ cup (4.3 oz.)	650
Sliced or whole	½ cup (4.7 oz.)	260
(Stokely-Van Camp):		
Cut	½ cup	253
Diced	½ cup	260
Harvard	½ cup (4½ oz.)	123
Pickled	½ cup (4.3 oz.)	290
Whole	½ cup (4.3 oz.)	223
Canned, dietetic pack, solids & liq.:		
(USDA)	½ cup (4.4 oz.)	57
(Comstock) water pack	½ cup	100
(Del Monte) no salt added	½ cup	100
(Featherweight) sliced	½ cup	55
(Larsen) *Fresh-Lite*, no salt added	½ cup	49
(S&W) *Nutradiet*, sliced	½ cup	40
BEET GREENS (USDA):		
Raw, whole	1 lb. (weighed untrimmed)	330
Boiled, leaves & stems, drained	½ cup (2.6 oz.)	55
BEET PUREE, canned, dietetic pack (Larsen)	1 cup	120
BERRY BEARS, *Fruit Corners* (General Mills)	.9-oz. pouch	20

Food and Description	Measure or Quantity	Sodium (milligrams)
BERRY CITRUS DRINK,		
chilled or frozen (Five Alive)	6 fl. oz.	20
BERRY DRINK:		
Canned, *Ssips* (Johanna Farms)	8.45-fl. oz. container	15
*Mix, dietetic, *Crystal Light*	8 fl. oz.	<1
Bigg Mixx, cereal (Kellogg's)		
plain or with raisins	½ cup	190
BIG MAC (See **McDONALD'S**)		
BISCUIT, home recipe (USDA)		
baking powder	1-oz. biscuit (2″ dia.)	175
BISCUIT DOUGH, refrigerated (Pillsbury):		
Baking powder, *1869 Brand*	1 biscuit	310
Ballard Oven Ready	1 biscuit	180
Butter	1 biscuit	180
Buttermilk:		
Regular	1 biscuit	180
Ballard Oven Ready	1 biscuit	180
Big Country	1 biscuit	320
1869 Brand	1 biscuit	310
Heat 'N Eat	1 biscuit	310
Hungry Jacks:		
Extra rich	1 biscuit	180
Flaky	1 biscuit	300
Fluffy	1 biscuit	280
Tender layer	1 biscuit	170
Big Country	1 biscuit	320
1869 Brand	1 biscuit	300
Country style	1 biscuit	180
Flaky, *Hungry Jack*:		
Regular	1 biscuit	300
Butter Tastin'	1 biscuit	280
Honey	1 biscuit	290
Heat 'N Eat	1 biscuit	305
Southern style, *Big Country*	1 biscut	320
***BISCUIT MIX** (USDA) baked		
from mix, with added milk	1-oz. biscuit	276

Food and Description	Measure or Quantity	Sodium (milligrams)
BITTERS (Angostura)	1 tsp. (4.6 g.)	Tr.
BLACKBERRY:		
Fresh (USDA) includes boysenberry, dewberry, youngsberry:		
With hulls	1 lb. (weighed untrimmed)	4
Hulled	½ cup (2.6 oz.)	Tr.
Canned, regular pack (USDA) solids & liq.:		
Juice pack	4-oz. serving	1
Light syrup	4-oz. serving	1
Heavy syrup	½ cup (4.6 oz.)	1
Extra heavy syrup	4-oz. serving	1
Frozen (USDA):		
Sweetened, unthawed	4-oz. serving	1
Unsweetened, unthawed	4-oz. serving	1
BLACKBERRY JELLY:		
Sweetened:		
(Home Brands)	1 T.	15
(Smucker's)	1 T.	<10
Dietetic (See **BLACKBERRY SPREAD**)		
BLACKBERRY JUICE, canned		
(USDA) unsweetened	½ cup	1
BLACKBERRY PRESERVE or JAM:		
Sweetened (Smucker's)	1 T. (.7 oz.)	0
Dietetic or low calorie:		
(Dia-Mel)	1 T.	<3
(Diet Delight)	1 T.	19
(Louis Sherry)	1 T.	<3
BLACKBERRY SPREAD, low sugar:		
(Diet Delight)	1 T.	45
(Smucker's)	1 T.	<10
BLACK-EYED PEA (See also **COWPEA**):		
Canned:		
(Allen's) regular	½ cup	370
(Goya)	½ cup	486

Food and Description	Measure or Quantity	Sodium (milligrams)
(Green Giant)	½ cup	300
(Trappey's):		
With bacon, in sauce	½ cup	410
With jalapeño pepper & bacon, in sauce	½ cup	480
Frozen:		
(USDA) boiled, drained	½ cup (3 oz.)	33
(Frosty Acres)	3.3 oz.	5
(Larsen)	3.3 oz.	5
(McKenzie)	3.3 oz.	19
(Southland)	⅕ of 16-oz. pkg.	5
BLANCMANGE (See PUDDING or PIE FILLING, Vanilla)		
BLINTZ, frozen:		
(Empire Kosher):		
Apple	2½-oz. piece	115
Blueberry	2½-oz. piece	116
Cheese	2½-oz. piece	126
Cherry	2½-oz. piece	105
Potato	2½-oz. piece	224
(King Kold) cheese	2½-oz. piece	250
BLOODY MARY MIX:		
(Holland House) *Smooth 'N Spicy*	6 fl. oz.	1974
(Libby's)	6 fl. oz.	1120
Tabasco	6 fl. oz.	788
BLUEBERRY:		
Fresh (USDA):		
Whole	1 lb. (weighed untrimmed)	4
Trimmed	½ cup (2.6 oz.)	<1
Canned solids & liq.:		
(USDA):		
Syrup pack, extra heavy	½ cup (4.4 oz.)	1
Water pack	½ cup (4.3 oz.)	1
(Thank You Brand):		
Heavy syrup	½ cup (4.3 oz.)	6
Water pack	½ cup (4.2 oz.)	<1
Frozen (USDA):		
Sweetened, solids & liq.	½ cup (4 oz.)	1

Food and Description	Measure or Quantity	Sodium (milligrams)
Unsweetened, solids & liq.	½ cup (2.9 oz.)	<1
BLUEBERRY PIE (See **PIE,** Blueberry)		
BLUEBERRY PRESERVE or JAM, sweetened (Smucker's)	1 T.	0
BLUEBERRY SQUARES, cereal (Kellogg's)	½ cup (1 oz.)	5
BLUEFISH (USDA):		
Raw:		
Whole	1 lb. (weighed whole)	171
Meat only	4 oz.	84
Baked or broiled, with butter or margarine	4.4-oz. piece (3½″ × 3″ × ½″)	130
Fried, prepared with egg, milk or water & bread crumbs	5.3-oz. piece (3½″ × 3″ × ½″)	219
BODY BUDDIES, cereal (General Mills) natural fruit flavor	1 cup (1 oz.)	280
BOLOGNA:		
(Ekrich):		
Beef:		
Regular	1 slice (8-oz. pkg.)	280
Smorgas Pac	¾-oz. slice	230
Thick sliced	1.5-oz. slice	400
Thick sliced	1.8-oz. slice	510
Garlic	1-oz. slice	290
German brand:		
Chub	1 oz.	360
Sliced	1-oz. slice	350
Lunch, chub	1 oz.	290
Meat:		
Regular	1-oz. slice	290
Smorgas Pac	¾-oz. slice	230
Smorgas Pac	1-oz. slice	310
Thick sliced	1.7-oz. slice	490
Thin sliced	1 slice	160
Ring:		

Food and Description	Measure or Quantity	Sodium (milligrams)
Regular	1 oz.	280
Pickled	1 oz.	290
Sandwich	1-oz. slice	310
(Hormel):		
Beef:		
Regular	1 slice	296
Ring, coarse ground	1 oz.	288
Coarse ground, ring	1 oz.	289
Fine ground, ring	1 oz.	298
Meat, regular	1 slice	300
(Ohse):		
Beef	1 oz.	310
15% chicken	1 oz.	320
Chicken, beef & pork	1 oz.	280
(Oscar Mayer):		
Beef:		
Regular	.5-oz. slice	152
Regular	1-oz. slice	304
Beef Lebanon	.8-oz. slice	302
Garlic beef	1-oz. slice	300
Meat:		
Regular	.5-oz. slice	156
Regular	1-oz. slice	312
With cheese	.8-oz. slice	232
BOO*BERRY, cereal		
(General Mills)	1 cup (1 oz.)	210
BORSCHT, canned:		
Regular:		
(Gold's)	8-oz. serving	1280
(Manischewitz) with beets	8-oz. serving	660
Dietetic or low calorie:		
(Gold's)	8-oz. serving	1160
(Manischewitz)	8-oz. serving	725
(Rokeach) unsalted	8-oz. serving	50
BOURBON WHISKEY, un-flavored (See **DISTILLED LIQUOR**)		
BOYSENBERRY:		
Fresh (See **BLACKBERRY**)		

Food and Description	Measure or Quantity	Sodium (milligrams)
Frozen (USDA) sweetened	10-oz. pkg.	3
BOYSENBERRY JELLY,		
sweetened (Smucker's)	1 T. (.7 oz.)	<10
BOYSENBERRY JUICE, canned		
(Smucker's)	8 fl. oz.	10
BOYSENBERRY PRESERVE		
or JAM:		
Sweetened:		
(Home Brands)	1 T.	15
(Smucker's)	1 T.	0
Dietetic or low calorie		
(Slenderella)	1 T. (.6 oz.)	16
BRAINS, all animals, raw (USDA)	1 oz.	35
BRAN:		
Crude (USDA)	1 oz.	3
Miller's (Elam's)	1 oz.	5
BRAN BREAKFAST CEREAL:		
(Kellogg's):		
All-Bran:		
Regular	⅓ cup (1 oz.)	260
With extra fiber	½ cup (1 oz.)	140
Bran Buds	⅓ cup (1 oz.)	170
Bran flakes	⅔ cup (1 oz.)	220
Fruitful Bran	⅔ cup (1.3 oz.)	230
Oat bran:		
Common Sense:		
Plain	½ cup (1 oz.)	270
With raisins	½ cup (1.3 oz.)	250
Cracklin' Oat Bran	½ cup (1 oz.)	150
Raisin	¾ cup (1.4 oz.)	230
(Loma Linda)	1 oz.	115
(Malt-O-Meal:		
40% bran	⅔ cup (1 oz.)	205
Raisin	¾ cup (1.4 oz.)	199
(Post):		
40% bran flakes	⅔ cup (1 oz.)	205
With raisins	⅔ cup (1 oz.)	198
(Ralston Purina):		
Bran News, apple or		

Food and Description	Measure or Quantity	Sodium (milligrams)
cinnamon	¾ cup (1 oz.)	160
Chex	⅔ cup (1 oz.)	200
Oat	1 cup (1.45 oz.)	150
BRANDY, unflavored (See **DISTILLED LIQUOR**		
BRAUNSCHWEIGER:		
(Eckrich) chub	1 oz.	400
(Hormel)	1 oz.	322
(Oscar Mayer):		
German brand	1-oz. serving	345
Sliced	1-oz. slice	327
Tube	1-oz. serving	321
BRAZIL NUT:		
Whole, in shell (USDA)	1 cup (4.3 oz.)	Tr.
Shelled (USDA)	½ cup (2½ oz.)	<1
Shelled (USDA)	4 nuts (.6 oz.)	<1
Roasted (Fisher)	¼ cup (1 oz.)	57
BREAD (listed by type or brand name):		
Apple cinnamon (Pritikin)	1-oz. slice	100
Autumn grain, *Merita* (Interstate Brands	1-oz. slice	150
Barbecue, *Millbrook* (Interstate Brands	1.23-oz. slice	220
Boston brown (USDA)	1.7-oz. slice (3″ × ¾″)	120
Bran (Roman Meal):		
5-Bran	1-oz. slice	136
Oat, light	.8-oz. slice	108
Rice	1-oz. slice	130
Bran'nola (Arnold)	1.3-oz. slice	135
Buttermaid, *Mrs. Karl's* (Interstate Brands)	1-oz. slice	170
Buttermilk, *Eddy's* (Interstate Brands)	1-oz. slice	160
Buttertop, *Eddy's* (Interstate Brands)	1-oz. slice	160
Cinnamon (Pepperidge Farm)	.9-oz. slice	100
Cracked wheat:		
(USDA) 18 slices to 1 lb.	.8-oz. slice	122

Food and Description	Measure or Quantity	Sodium (milligrams)
(Pepperidge Farm) thin	.9-oz. slice	145
(Roman Meal)	1-oz. slice	139
Crisp bread, *Wasa:*		
Mora	3¼-oz. slice	514
Rye:		
Golden	.4-oz. slice	43
Lite	.3-oz. slice	20
Sesame	.5-oz. slice	35
Sport	.4-oz. slice	66
Flatbread, *Ideal:*		
Bran	.2-oz. slice	47
Extra thin	.1-oz. slice	25
Whole grain	.2-oz. slice	47
French:		
(USDA)	.8-oz. slice	133
(Arnold) *Francisco,* regular	¹⁄₁₆ of loaf	110
Eddy's (Interstate Brands):		
Regular	1-oz. slice	180
Sour	1-oz. slice	170
Garlic (Arnold)	1-oz. slice	120
Hi-fibre (Monks')	1-oz. slice	110
Hillbilly		
Holsum (Interstate Brands)	1-oz. slice	160
Honey bran (Pepperidge Farm)	1.2-oz. slice	175
Honey wheatberry:		
(Arnold)	1.1-oz. slice	140
(Pepperidge Farm)	.9-oz. slice	163
Hunters grain, *Country Farms*		
(Interstate Brands)	1.5-oz. slice	210
Italian:		
(USDA)	1-oz. slice	166
(Arnold) *Francisco*	1 slice	110
Butternut (Interstate Brands)	1-oz. slice	180
(Pepperidge Farm)	2-oz. serving	320
Low sodium *Eddy's* (Interstate Brands)	1-oz. slice	20
Multi-grain:		
(Arnold) *Milk & Honey*	1-oz. slice	150
(Pepperidge Farm) thin	.5-oz. slice	75
(Pritikin)	1-oz. slice	80

Food and Description	Measure or Quantity	Sodium (milligrams)
(Weight Watchers)	.74-oz. slice	101
Oat (Arnold):		
Bran'nola	1.3-oz. slice	170
Milk & Honey	1-oz. slice	150
Oatmeal (Pepperidge Farm)	.9-oz. slice	185
Onion dill (Pritikin)	1-oz. slice	100
Potato, *Sweetheart* (Interstate Brands)	1-oz. slice	170
Protein (Thomas')	.7-oz. slice	94
Pumpernickel:		
(USDA) regular size	1.1-oz. slice (5″ × 4″ × ⅜″)	178
(USDA) snack size	7 g. (2½″ × 2″ × ¼″)	40
(Arnold)	1.1-oz. slice	200
(Levy's)	1.1-oz. slice	200
(Pepperidge Farm):		
Regular	1.1-oz. slice	305
Party	.2-oz. slice	55
Raisin:		
(USDA)	.9-oz. slice	91
(Arnold) tea	.9-oz. slice	85
Butternut (Interstate Brands)	1-oz. slice	130
(Monks') & cinnamon	1-oz. slice	85
(Pepperidge Farm) cinnamon	.9-oz. slice	95
(Pritikin)	1-oz. slice	110
(Weight Watchers)	.8-oz. slice	120
Rye:		
(USDA) light:		
Regular size	.9 oz. (4¾″ × 3¾″ × 7/16″ slice)	142
Snack size	7 g. (2½″ × 2″ × ¼″ slice)	39
(Arnold):		
Dill, with seeds	1.1-oz. slice	190
Jewish, with or without seeds	1.1-oz. slice	170
Melba thin	.7-oz. slice	110
(Levy's)	1.1-oz. slice	170

Food and Description	Measure or Quantity	Sodium (milligrams)
(Pepperidge Farm):		
Family	1.1-oz. slice	245
Party, fresh or frozen	.2-oz. slice	104
(Pritikin)	1-oz. slice	75
(Weight Watchers)	.74-oz. slice	102
Sahara (Thomas'):		
White:		
Regular	2-oz. piece	300
Mini	1-oz. piece	150
Large	3-oz. piece	440
Whole wheat:		
Regular	2-oz. piece	320
Mini	1-oz. piece	150
Salt rising (USDA)	.9-oz. slice	66
Sandwich (Roman Meal)	.8-oz. slice	114
7 Grain (Roman Meal):		
Regular	1-oz. slice	140
Light	.8-oz. slice	108
Sunflower & bran (Monks')	1-oz. slice	80
Sun grain (Roman Meal)	1-oz. slice	140
Texas toast, *Holsum* (Interstate Brands)	1.4-oz. slice	200
Toaster cake (See **TOASTER CAKE or PASTRY**)		
Vienna (USDA)	.8-oz. slice	133
Wheat (See also Cracked wheat, Honey wheatberry and Whole wheat):		
America's Own (Arnold):	1-oz. slice	155
Bran'nola:		
Dark	1.3-oz. slice	170
Hearty	1.3-oz. slice	200
Brick Oven	.8-oz. slice	100
Country	1.3-oz. slice	150
Less or Liteway	.8-oz. slice	120
Milk & Honey	1-oz. slice	160

Food and Description	Measure or Quantity	Sodium (milligrams)
Very thin	.5-oz. slice	65
(Pepperidge Farm):		
Family	.9-oz. slice	195
Sandwich	.8-oz. slice	115
(Roman Meal) light	.8-oz. slice	108
(Weight Watchers)	.74-oz. slice	101
Wheatberry (Roman Meal)		
light	.8-oz. slice	108
White:		
(USDA):		
Prepared with 1–4%		
non-fat dry milk	.8-oz. slice	117
Prepared with 5–6%		
non-fat dry milk	.8-oz. slice	114
America's Own, cottage	1-oz. slice	180
(Arnold):		
Brick Oven:		
.8-oz. slice	.8-oz. slice	130
2-lb. loaf	1.1-oz. slice	160
Country	1.3-oz. slice	200
Less	.8-oz. slice	120
Liteway	.8-oz. slice	130
Milk & Honey	1-oz. slice	160
Very thin	.5-oz. slice	85
(Monks')	1-oz. slice	95
(Pepperidge Farm):		
Regular	1.2-oz. slice	135
Toasting	1.1-oz. slice	230
Very thin slice	.6-oz. slice	85
(Roman Meal) light	.8-oz. slice	109
Regular	1-oz. slice	153
With buttermilk	1-oz. slice	170
Whole grain (Roman Meal)		
harvest recipe	1-oz. slice	139
Whole wheat:		
(USDA):		
Prepared with 2% non-fat		
dry milk	.8-oz. slice	121
Prepared with 2% non-fat		

Food and Description	Measure or Quantity	Sodium (milligrams)
dry milk	.9-oz. slice	132
Prepared with water	.9-oz. slice	132
(Arnold) stone ground	.8-oz. slice	100
(Monks')	1-oz. slice	110
(Pepperidge Farm):		
Thin sliced	.9-oz. slice	125
Very thin sliced	.6-oz. slice	80
(Roman Meal)	1-oz. slice	139
BREAD, CANNED, BROWN:		
(B&M) plain or raisin	½" slice (1.6 oz.)	220
(Friend's) plain or raisin	½" slice (1.6 oz.)	220
BREAD CRUMBS:		
(USDA) dry, grated, white bread	½ cup (1¾ oz.)	366
(4C):		
Plain:		
Regular	1 T.	77
Salt free	1 T.	0
Seasoned:		
Regular	1 T.	189
Salt free	1 T.	0
(Pepperidge Farm):		
Regular	1 oz.	255
Herb seasoned	1 oz.	260
(Progresso):		
Plain	1 T.	55
Italian style	1 T.	120
Onion	1 T.	160
*BREAD DOUGH:		
Frozen:		
(Pepperidge Farm):		
Country rye	⅒ of loaf (1 oz.)	185
Stone ground wheat	⅒ of loaf (1 oz.)	127
White	⅒ of loaf (1 oz.)	165
(Rich's)		
French	¹⁄₂₀ of loaf	138
Italian	¹⁄₂₀ of loaf	300
Raisin	¹⁄₂₀ of loaf	107
Wheat	.5-oz. slice	375

Food and Description	Measure or Quantity	Sodium (milligrams)
White	.8-oz. slice	96
Refrigerated (Pillsbury):		
French	1″ slice	120
Wheat or white	1″ slice	170
*BREAD MIX:		
Home Pride:		
French	⅜″ slice	160
Rye	⅜″ slice	180
White	⅜″ slice	130
(Pillsbury):		
Banana, blueberry nut or date	1/12 of loaf	150
Cranberry	1/12 of loaf	160
Nut	1/12 of loaf	190
BREAD PUDDING, with raisins, home recipe (USDA)	1 cup (9.3 oz.)	556
BREADFRUIT, fresh (USDA):		
Whole	1 lb. (weighed untrimmed)	17
Peeled & trimmed	4 oz.	17
BREAD STICK, dietetic (Stella D'Oro)	1 piece	<10
BREAD STICK DOUGH, refrigerated (Pillsbury) soft	1 piece	230
BREAKFAST WITH BARBIE, cereal (Ralston-Purina)	1 cup (1 oz.)	70
BREAKFAST DRINK, instant (Pillsbury):		
Chocolate or chocolate malt	1 pouch	190
Strawberry	1 pouch	180
Vanilla	1 pouch	210
BRITOS, frozen (Patio):		
Beef & bean	½ of 7¼-oz. pkg.	340
Chicken, spicy	½ of 7¼-oz. pkg.	330
Chili:		
Green	½ of 7¼-oz. pkg.	420
Red	½ of 7¼-oz. pkg.	370
Nacho beef	½ of 7¼-oz. pkg.	420
Nacho cheese	½ of 7¼-oz. pkg.	330

Food and Description	Measure or Quantity	Sodium (milligrams)
BROCCOLI:		
Raw (USDA):		
Whole	1 lb. (weighed untrimmed)	42
Large leaves removed	1 lb. (weighed partially trimmed)	53
Boiled (USDA) without salt:		
½″ pieces, drained	½ cup (2.8 oz.)	8
Whole, drained	1 med. stalk (6.3 oz.)	18
Frozen:		
(USDA) boiled, drained	10-oz. pkg.	34
(Birds Eye):		
With almonds & selected seasonings	⅓ of 10-oz. pkg.	216
Chopped	⅓ of 10-oz. pkg.	16
Cuts or deluxe florets	⅓ of 10-oz. pkg.	22
Spears:		
Regular	3.3 oz.	22
Deluxe, baby	⅓ of 10-oz. pkg.	13
(Frosty Acres)	3.3 oz.	20
(Green Giant):		
Cuts:		
In cream sauce:		
Regular	⅓ of 10-oz. pkg.	442
One serving	5-oz. pkg.	660
Harvest Fresh	⅓ of 9-oz. pkg.	150
Polybag	½ cup	15
Spears:		
In butter sauce:		
Regular	⅓ of 10-oz. pkg.	350
One serving	4½-oz. pkg.	420
Harvest Fresh	⅓ of 9-oz. pkg.	176
Polybag, individually frozen	2-oz. serving	15
(Larsen)	3.3 oz.	30
(McKenzie):		
Chopped	3.3 oz.	23

Food and Description	Measure or Quantity	Sodium (milligrams)
Spears	3.3 oz.	28
BROWNIE (See **COOKIE**)		
BRUSSELS SPROUTS:		
Raw (USDA)	1 lb.	54
Boiled (USDA) drained, 1¼"-1½" dia.	1 cup (7–8 sprouts, 5.5 oz.)	16
Frozen:		
(Birds Eye):		
Regular	⅓ of 10-oz. pkg.	15
With cheese sauce, baby	4½ oz.	495
(Frosty Acres)	3.3 oz.	12
(Green Giant):		
In butter sauce	⅓ of 10-oz. pkg.	280
Polybag	½ cup	10
(Larsen)	3.3 oz.	20
(McKenzie)	3.3 oz.	19
BULGUR (from hard red winter wheat) (USDA) canned:		
Unseasoned	4-oz. serving	679
Seasoned	4-oz. serving	522
BUN (See **ROLL or BUN**)		
BURGER KING:		
Apple pie	1 serving	412
Breakfast Croissan'wich:		
Bacon	1 sandwich	762
Ham	1 sandwich	987
Sausage	1 sandwich	1042
Cheeseburger:		
Regular	1 burger	439
Double:		
Plain	1 burger	615
Bacon	1 burger	728
Condiments:		
Ketchup	1 serving	121
Mustard	1 serving	31
Pickles	1 serving	60
Chicken specialty sandwich:		
Plain	1 sandwich	1280

Food and Description	Measure or Quantity	Sodium (milligrams)
Condiments:		
Lettuce	1 serving on sandwich	1
Mayonnaise	1 serving on sandwich	142
Chicken tenders	1 piece	106
Coffee, regular	1 serving	2
Danish, great	1 piece	288
Egg platter, scrambled:		
Bacon	1 serving	167
Croissant	1 serving	298
Eggs	1 serving	317
Hash browns	1 serving	193
Sausage	1 serving	405
French fries	1 regular order	160
French toast sticks	1 serving	498
Hamburger:		
Plain	1 burger	297
Condiments:		
Ketchup	1 serving on burger	121
Mustard	1 serving on burger	31
Pickles	1 serving on burger	60
Ham & cheese specialty sandwich:		
Plain	1 sandwich	1461
Condiments:		
Lettuce	1 serving on sandwich	1
Mayonnaise	1 serving on sandwich	71
Tomato	1 serving on sandwich	1
Milk:		
2% lowfat	1 serving	122
Whole	1 serving	119
Onion rings	1 order	665

Food and Description	Measure or Quantity	Sodium (milligrams)
Orange juice	1 serving	2
Salad dressing:		
Regular:		
Bleu cheese	1 serving	309
House	1 serving	269
1000 Island	1 serving	228
Dietetic, Italian	1 serving	426
Shakes, regular:		
Chocolate	1 serving	202
Strawberry	1 serving	213
Vanilla	1 serving	205
Whaler, fish sandwich:		
Plain	1 sandwich	389
Condiments:		
Lettuce	1 serving on sandwich	1
Tartar sauce	1 serving on sandwich	202
Whopper:		
Regular:		
Plain	1 burger	467
With cheese	1 burger	751
Condiments:		
Ketchup	1 serving on burger	183
Lettuce	1 serving on burger	2
Mayonnaise	1 serving on burger	107
Onion	1 serving on burger	1
Pickles	1 serving on burger	119
Tomato	1 serving on burger	1
Jr.:		
Plain	1 burger	297
With cheese	1 burger	439

Food and Description	Measure or Quantity	Sodium (milligrams)
Condiments:		
Ketchup	1 serving on burger	91
Lettuce	1 serving on burger	1
Mayonnaise	1 serving on burger	36
Pickles	1 serving on burger	60
Tomato	1 serving on burger	1
BURGUNDY WINE:		
(Gold Seal) 12% alcohol	3 fl. oz.	3
(Great Western) 12% alcohol	3 fl. oz.	36
BURGUNDY WINE, SPARKLING:		
(Barton & Guestier)	3 fl. oz.	2
(Gold Seal)	3 fl. oz.	3
BURRITO:		
*Canned (Old El Paso)	1 burrito	430
Frozen:		
(Hormel):		
Beef	1 burrito	780
Cheese	1 burrito	792
Chicken & rice	1 burrito (4 oz.)	594
Grande	5½-oz. serving	877
Hot chili	1 burrito	619
Little Juan (Fred's Frozen Foods):		
Bean & cheese	5-oz. serving	741
Beef & bean, spicy	10-oz. serving	1476
Beef & potato	5-oz. serving	736
Chili:		
Green	10-oz. serving	1973
Red	10-oz. serving	2197
Chili dog	5-oz. serving	772
Red hot	5-oz. serving	1109
(Old El Paso):		
Regular:		

Food and Description	Measure or Quantity	Sodium (milligrams)
Bean & cheese	1 piece	770
Beef & bean:		
Hot	1 piece	950
Medium	1 piece	730
Mild	1 piece	660
Dinner, festive,		
beef & bean	11-oz. dinner	1180
(Patio):		
Beef & bean:		
Regular	5-oz. serving	830
Green chili	5-oz. serving	710
Red chili	5-oz. serving	810
Red hot	5-oz. serving	800
(Swanson) bean & beef	15¼-oz. dinner	1630
(Van de Kamp's):		
Regular, crispy fried, with		
guacamole sauce	6 oz.	823
Sirloin, grande	11 oz.	1120
(Weight Watchers) beefsteak		
or chicken	7.6-oz. serving	790
BURRITO SEASONING MIX		
(Lawry's)	1½-oz. pkg.	2516
BUTTER:		
Salted:		
Solid:		
(USDA)	1 pat (1″ × ⅓″)	49
(USDA)	1 T. (.5 oz.)	138
(USDA)	½ cup (4 oz.)	1119
(Breakstone)	1 T. (.5 oz.)	95
(Land O'Lakes)	1 T.	100
(Sealtest)	1 T. (.5 oz.)	117
Whipped:		
(USDA)	1 T. (.3 oz.)	89
(Breakstone)	1 T. (.3 oz.)	64
(Land O'Lakes) lightly		
salted	1 T.	75
Unsalted:		
Solid:		
(USDA)	1 stick (4 oz.)	11

Food and Description	Measure or Quantity	Sodium (milligrams)
(USDA)	1 T. (.5 oz.)	1
(USDA)	1 pat (1″ × ⅓″)	<1
(Breakstone)	1 T.	<1
(Land O'Lakes)	1 T.	<1
Whipped (USDA)	1 T.	<1
BUTTER, SUBSTITUTE (See also **MARGARINE**), *Butter Buds:*		
Dry	⅛ oz.	170
Liquid	1 oz.	170
Sprinkles	1 tsp.	66
BUTTER BEAN (See **BEAN, LIMA**)		
BUTTERMILK (See **MILK**)		
BUTTERSCOTCH MORSELS		
(Nestlé) artificial	1 oz.	15

C

CABBAGE:
White (USDA):
Raw:

Whole	1 lb. (weighed untrimmed)	72
Finely shredded or chopped	1 cup (3.2 oz.)	18
Coarsely shredded or sliced	1 cup (2.5 oz.)	14
Wedge	3½″ × 4½″ (3½ oz.)	20

Boiled, without salt:

Shredded, in small amount of water, short time, drained	½ cup (2.6 oz.)	10
Wedges, in large amount of water, long time, drained	½ cup (3.2 o.z)	12

Food and Description	Measure or Quantity	Sodium (*milligrams*)
Dehydrated	1 oz.	54
Red:		
Raw (USDA) whole	1 lb. (weighed untrimmed)	93
Canned, solids & liq.:		
(Comstock)	½ cup	480
(Greenwood)	½ cup	475
Savory (USDA) raw:		
Whole	1 lb. (weighed untrimmed)	79
Coarsely shredded	1 cup (2.5 oz.)	15
CABBAGE, CHINESE or **CELERY,** raw (USDA):		
Whole	1 lb. (weighed untrimmed)	101
1″ pieces, leaves with stalk	½ cup (1.3 oz.)	9
CAKE (See also **CAKE MIX**):		
Not frozen:		
Plain:		
Home recipe, with butter & boiled white icing	⅑ of 9″ square	299
Home recipe, with butter & chocolate icing	⅑ of 9″ square	280
Angel food:		
Home recipe	1/12 of 8″ cake	113
(Dolly Madison)	⅙ of 10½-oz. cake	150
Apple (Dolly Madison) dutch *Buttercrumb*	1½-oz. piece	160
Apple spice (Entenmann's) fat & cholesterol free	1-oz. slice	80
Banana crunch (Entenmann's) fat & cholesterol free	1-oz. slice	90
Blueberry crunch (Entenmann's) fat & cholesterol free	1-oz. slice	85
Butter streusel (Dolly Madison) *Buttercrumb*	1½-oz. piece	170
Caramel, home recipe:		

Food and Description	Measure or Quantity	Sodium (*milligrams*)
Without icing	⅑ of 9″ square	262
With caramel icing	⅑ of 9¼″ square	214
Carrot (Dolly Madison)		
Lunch Cake	3¼-oz. serving	645
Chocolate:		
Home recipe with chocolate icing, 2-layer	1/12 of 9″ cake	234
(Dolly Madison) *Lunch Cake*	3¼-oz. pkg.	330
(Entenmann's) loaf, fat & cholesterol free	1-oz. slice	130
Coffee (Entenmann's) fat & cholesterol free:		
Cherry	1.3-oz. piece	70
Cinnamon apple	1.3-oz. piece	90
Crumb (See also **ROLL or BUN**) (Hostess)	1¼-oz. piece	98
Devil's food, home recipe:		
Without icing	3″ × 2″ × 1½″ piece	162
With chocolate icing, 2-layer	1/16 of 9″ cake	176
Fruit, home recipe:		
Dark	1/30 of 8¼″ loaf	24
Light, made with butter	1/30 of 8″ loaf	29
Golden (Entenmann's) fat & cholesterol free	1-oz. slice	90
Hawaiian spice (Dolly Madison) *Lunch Cake*	3¼-oz. pkg.	390
Honey 'n spice (Dolly Madison) *Lunch Cake*	3¼-oz. pkg.	370
Pineapple crunch (Entenmann's) fat & cholesterol free	1-oz. slice	85
Pound, home recipe:		
Equal weights flour, sugar, butter and eggs	3½″ × 3½″ slice (1.1 oz.)	33
Traditional, made with butter	3½″ × 3½″ slice (1.1 oz.)	53

Food and Description	Measure or Quantity	Sodium (milligrams)
Sponge, home recipe	1/12 of 10″ cake	110
White, home recipe:		
Made with butter, without icing, 2-layer	1/9 of 9″ wide, 3″ high cake	303
Made with butter, with coconut icing, 2-layer	1/12 of 9″ wide, 3″ high cake	270
White coconut (Dolly Madison) layer	1/12 of 30-oz. cake	240
Yellow, home recipe, made with butter, without icing, 2-layer	1/19 of cake	249
Frozen:		
Black forest (Weight Watchers)	3-oz. serving	280
Boston Cream:		
(Pepperidge Farm)	1/4 of 11¾-oz. cake	190
(Weight Watchers)	3-oz. serving	280
Butterscotch pecan (Pepperidge Farm) layer	1/10 of 17-oz. cake	110
Carrot:		
(Pepperidge Farm) with cream cheese icing	1/8 of 11¾-oz. cake	150
(Weight Watchers)	3-oz. serving	310
Cheese (Weight Watchers):		
Regular	3-oz. serving	280
Strawberry	3.9-oz. serving	230
Chocolate:		
(Pepperidge Farm):		
Layer:		
Fudge or mint	1/10 of 17-oz. cake	140
German	1/10 of 17-oz. cake	170
Supreme:		
Regular	1/8 of 11½-oz. cake	140
Dutch	1¾-oz. serving	115

Food and Description	Measure or Quantity	Sodium (milligrams)
(Weight Watchers):		
Regular	2½-oz. serving	250
German	2½-oz. serving	350
Coconut (Pepperidge Farm) layer	⅒ of 17-oz. cake	120
Devil's food (Pepperidge Farm) layer	⅒ of 17-oz. cake	135
Golden (Pepperidge Farm) layer	⅒ of 17-oz. cake	115
Grand Marnier (Pepperidge Farm) Supreme	1½ oz.	85
Lemon coconut (Pepperidge Farm) Supreme	¼ of 12¼-oz. cake	220
Pineapple cream (Pepperidge Farm) Supreme	⅟₁₂ of 24-oz. cake	130
Pound (Pepperidge Farm) butter	⅒ of 10¾-oz. cake	150
CAKE or COOKIE ICING		
(Pillsbury) all flavors	1 T.	0
CAKE ICING:		
Amaretto almond (Betty Crocker) *Creamy Deluxe*	⅟₁₂ of can	50
Butter pecan (Betty Crocker) *Creamy Deluxe*	⅟₁₂ of can	50
Caramel, home recipe (USDA)	4-oz. serving	94
Caramel pecan (Pillsbury) *Frosting Supreme*	⅟₁₂ of can	70
Cherry (Betty Crocker) *Creamy Deluxe*	⅟₁₂ of can	50
Chocolate:		
Home recipe (USDA)	4-oz. serving	168
(Betty Crocker) *Creamy Deluxe:*		
Regular	⅟₁₂ of can	60
Candy coated chips	⅟₁₂ of can	60
Chip	⅟₁₂ of can	30
Dinosaurs	⅟₁₂ of can	60

Food and Description	Measure or Quantity	Sodium (milligrams)
Fudge, dark dutch	1/12 of can	70
Milk	1/12 of can	55
Sour cream	1/12 of can	110
(Duncan Hines):		
Regular	1/12 of can	83
Fudge, dark dutch	1/12 of can	87
Milk	1/12 of can	79
(Pillsbury) *Frosting Supreme:*		
Chip	1/12 of can	70
Fudge	1/12 of can	80
Milk	1/12 of can	60
Mint	1/12 of can	80
Coconut, home recipe (USDA)	4-oz. serving	196
Coconut almond (Pillsbury) *Frosting Supreme*	1/12 of can	60
Coconut pecan (Pillsbury) *Frosting Supreme*	1/12 of can	60
Cream cheese:		
(Betty Crocker) *Creamy Deluxe*	1/12 of can	75
(Duncan Hines)	1/12 of can	111
(Pillsbury) *Frosting Supreme*	1/12 of can	115
Double dutch (Pillsbury) *Frosting Supreme*	1/12 of can	45
Lemon:		
(Betty Crocker) *Creamy Deluxe*	1/12 of can	70
(Pillsbury) *Frosting Supreme*	1/12 of can	80
Polka dot (Duncan Hines):		
Milk chocolate	1/12 of can	92
Pink vanilla	1/12 of can	72
Rainbow chip (Betty Crocker) *Creamy Deluxe*	1/12 of can	30
Rock road (Betty Crocker) *Creamy Deluxe*	1/12 of can	50
Strawberry (Pillsbury) *Frosting Supreme*	1/12 of can	75
Vanilla:		
(Betty Crocker) *Creamy Deluxe*	1/12 of can	30

Food and Description	Measure or Quantity	Sodium (milligrams)
(Duncan Hines)	$\frac{1}{12}$ of can	76
(Pillsbury) *Frosting Supreme:*		
Regular	$\frac{1}{12}$ of can	75
Sour cream	$\frac{1}{12}$ of can	80
White:		
Home recipe (USDA):		
Boiled	4-oz. serving	162
Uncooked	4-oz. serving	56
(Betty Crocker) *Creamy*		
Deluxe, sour cream	$\frac{1}{12}$ of can	50
*CAKE ICING MIX:		
Regular:		
Chocolate:		
(Betty Crocker):		
Fudge, creamy	$\frac{1}{12}$ of pkg.	70
Milk, creamy	$\frac{1}{12}$ of pkg.	40
(Pillsbury) *Frost It Hot*	$\frac{1}{8}$ of pkg.	50
Coconut almond (Pillsbury)	$\frac{1}{12}$ of pkg.	85
Coconut pecan:		
(Betty Crocker) creamy	$\frac{1}{12}$ of pkg.	50
(Pillsbury)	$\frac{1}{12}$ of pkg.	105
Lemon (Betty Crocker)		
creamy	$\frac{1}{12}$ of pkg.	100
White:		
(Betty Crocker):		
Fluffy	$\frac{1}{12}$ of pkg.	40
Sour cream, creamy	$\frac{1}{12}$ of pkg.	100
(Pillsbury) fluffy	$\frac{1}{12}$ of pkg.	50
Dietetic or low calorie		
(Estee)	$1\frac{1}{2}$ tsp.	0
CAKE MIX:		
Regular:		
Angel food:		
*(USDA)	$\frac{1}{12}$ of 10″ cake	
	(1.9 oz.)	77
(Betty Crocker):		
Confetti	$\frac{1}{12}$ of pkg.	300
Lemon custard	$\frac{1}{12}$ of pkg.	300
Traditional	$\frac{1}{12}$ of pkg.	170
White	$\frac{1}{12}$ of pkg.	300

Food and Description	Measure or Quantity	Sodium (milligrams)
(Duncan Hines)	$\frac{1}{12}$ of pkg.	119
*Apple cinnamon (Betty Crocker) *Supermoist*	$\frac{1}{12}$ of cake	280
*Apple streusel (Betty Crocker) *MicroRave*:		
Regular	$\frac{1}{6}$ of cake	190
No cholesterol recipe	$\frac{1}{6}$ of cake	200
*Banana (Pillsbury), *Pillsbury Plus*	$\frac{1}{12}$ of cake	290
*Black forest cherry (Pillsbury) *Bundt*	$\frac{1}{16}$ of cake	310
*Boston cream (Pillsbury) *Bundt*	$\frac{1}{16}$ of cake	310
*Butter (Pillsbury), *Pillsbury Plus*	$\frac{1}{12}$ of cake	370
Butter Brickle (Betty Crocker) *Supermoist*	$\frac{1}{12}$ of cake	280
*Butter pecan (Betty Crocker) layer, *Supermoist*	$\frac{1}{12}$ of cake	320
*Carrot (Betty Crocker) *Supermoist*	$\frac{1}{12}$ of cake	310
*Carrot'n spice, *Pillsbury Plus*	$\frac{1}{12}$ of cake	330
*Cheesecake:		
(Jello-O)	$\frac{1}{8}$ of 8″ cake	350
(Royal) No Bake:		
Lite	$\frac{1}{8}$ of cake	380
Real	$\frac{1}{8}$ of cake	370
*Cherry chip (Betty Crocker) layer, *Supermoist*	$\frac{1}{12}$ of cake	270
Chocolate:		
(Betty Crocker):		
MicroRave:		
Fudge, with vanilla frosting	$\frac{1}{6}$ of cake	300
German, with coconut pecan frosting	$\frac{1}{6}$ of cake	250
*Pudding recipe	$\frac{1}{6}$ of cake	250

Food and Description	Measure or Quantity	Sodium (milligrams)
Supermoist:		
Butter recipe	¹⁄₁₂ of cake	450
Chip	¹⁄₁₂ of cake	320
Chocolate chip	¹⁄₁₂ of cake	400
Fudge	¹⁄₁₂ of cake	470
German	¹⁄₁₂ of cake	420
Milk	¹⁄₁₂ of cake	340
Sour cream	¹⁄₁₂ of cake	430
(Duncan Hines) fudge, butter recipe	¹⁄₁₂ of pkg.	242
*(Pillsbury):		
Bundt:		
Fudge, Tunnel of	¹⁄₁₆ of cake	310
Macaroon	¹⁄₁₆ of cake	300
Microwave:		
Regular	⅛ of cake	260
Bundt, Tunnel of	⅛ of cake	320
With chocolate frosting	⅛ of cake	310
Double, supreme	⅛ of cake	340
With vanilla frosting	⅛ of cake	300
Pillsbury Plus:		
Chip	¹⁄₁₂ of cake	290
Dark	¹⁄₁₂ of cake	380
Fudge marble	¹⁄₁₂ of cake	300
German	¹⁄₁₂ of cake	340
*Cinnamon (Pillsbury) *Streusel Swirl*, microwave	⅛ of cake	180
*Cinnamon pecan streusel (Betty Crocker) *MicroRave*:		
Regular	⅙ of cake	210
No cholesterol recipe	⅙ of cake	220
*Coffee cake (Pillsbury), apple cinnamon	⅛ of cake	150
Devil's food:		
*(Betty Crocker):		
MicroRave, with chocolate frosting	⅙ of cake	250
Supermoist, layer	¹⁄₁₂ of cake	450

Food and Description	Measure or Quantity	Sodium (milligrams)
(Duncan Hines) deluxe	¹⁄₁₂ of pkg.	363
*(Pillsbury) *Pillsbury Plus*	¹⁄₁₂ of cake	370
Lemon:		
*(Betty Crocker):		
MicroRave, with lemon frosting	¹⁄₆ of cake	250
Pudding recipe	¹⁄₆ of cake	270
Supermoist	¹⁄₁₂ of cake	280
*(Pillsbury):		
Bundt, Tunnel of	¹⁄₁₆ of cake	300
Microwave:		
Plain	¹⁄₈ of cake	180
With lemon frosting	¹⁄₈ of cake	220
Supreme, deluxe	¹⁄₈ of cake	210
Pillsbury Plus	¹⁄₁₂ of cake	290
Streusel Swirl	¹⁄₁₆ of cake	340
*Marble (Betty Crocker) layer, *Supermoist*	¹⁄₁₂ of cake	290
*Pineapple cream (Pillsbury) *Bundt*	¹⁄₁₆ of cake	300
*Pound:		
(Betty Crocker) golden	¹⁄₁₂ of cake	155
(Dromedary)	½″ slice	340
*Rainbow chip (Betty Crocker), *Supermoist*	¹⁄₁₂ of cake	320
*Spice (Betty Crocker) *Supermoist*	¹⁄₁₂ of cake	320
*Strawberry, *Pillsbury Plus*	¹⁄₁₂ of cake	300
*Upside down (Betty Crocker) pineapple	¹⁄₉ of cake	210
*Vanilla (Betty Crocker) golden:		
MicroRave, with rainbow chip frosting	¹⁄₆ of cake	230
Supermoist	¹⁄₁₂ of cake	270
White:		
*(Betty Crocker) *Supermoist*:		

Food and Description	Measure or Quantity	Sodium (milligrams)
Regular	1/12 of cake	250
Sour cream	1/12 of cake	300
(Duncan Hines) deluxe	1/12 of pkg.	251
Pillsbury Plus	1/12 of cake	290
Yellow:		
*(Betty Crocker):		
MicroRave, with		
chocolate icing	1/6 of cake	210
Supermoist:		
Regular	1/12 of cake	300
Butter recipe	1/12 of cake	350
(Duncan Hines) deluxe	1/12 of pkg.	271
*(Pillsbury):		
Microwave:		
Plain	1/8 of cake	170
With chocolate		
frosting	1/8 of cake	220
*Dietetic or low calorie		
(Estee):		
Chocolate	1/10 of cake	100
Lemon pound or spice	1/10 of cake	65–70
CANADIAN WHISKY (See **DISTILLED LIQUOR**)		

CANDY. The following values of candies from the U.S. Department of Agriculture are representative of the types sold commercially. These values may be useful when individual brands or sizes are not known:

Almond:		
Chocolate-coated	1 cup (6.3 oz.)	106
Chocolate-coated	1 oz.	17
Sugar-coated or Jordan	1 oz.	6
Butterscotch	1 oz.	19
Candy corn	1 oz.	60
Caramel:		
Plain	1 oz.	64

Food and Description	Measure or Quantity	Sodium (milligrams)
Plain with nuts	1 oz.	58
Chocolate	1 oz.	64
Chocolate with nuts	1 oz.	58
Chocolate-flavored roll	1 oz.	56
Chocolate:		
Bittersweet	1 oz.	<1
Milk:		
Plain	1 oz.	27
With almonds	1 oz.	23
With peanuts	1 oz.	19
Semisweet	1 oz.	<1
Sweet	1 oz.	9
Chocolate discs, sugar-coated	1 oz.	20
Coconut center, chocolate-coated	1 oz.	56
Fondant, plain	1 oz.	60
Fondant, chocolate-covered	1 oz.	52
Fudge:		
Chocolate fudge	1 oz.	54
Chocolate fudge, chocolate-coated	1 oz.	65
Chocolate fudge with nuts	1 oz.	48
Chocolate fudge with nuts, chocolate-coated	1 oz.	58
Vanilla fudge	1 oz.	59
Vanilla fudge with nuts	1 oz.	53
With peanuts & caramel, chocolate-coated	1 oz.	36
Gum drops	1 oz.	10
Hard	1 oz.	9
Honeycombed hard candy, with peanut butter, chocolate-covered	1 oz.	46
Jelly beans	1 oz.	3
Marshmallows	1 oz.	11
Mints, uncoated	1 oz.	60
Nougat & caramel, chocolate-covered	1 oz.	49
Peanut bar	1 oz.	3

Food and Description	Measure or Quantity	Sodium (milligrams)
Peanut brittle	1 oz.	9
Peanuts, chocolate-covered	1 oz.	17
Raisins, chocolate-covered	1 oz.	18
Vanilla creams, chocolate-covered	1 oz.	52
CANDY, COMMERCIAL:		
Regular:		
Almond Joy (Hershey's)	1.76-oz. bar	70
Baby Ruth	2 oz.	120
Bar None (Hershey's)	1½ oz.	50
Bit-O-Honey (Nestlé)	1.7-oz.	130
Bonkers (Nabisco)	1 piece	0
Bridge mix (Nabisco)	1 piece (2 grams)	1
Butterfinger	2 oz.	100
Butternut (Hollywood Brands)	2¼-oz. bar	120
Canadamint (Necco)	.1-oz. piece	Tr.
Caramel Nip (Pearson's)	1 piece	17
Caramello (Hershey's)	1.6-oz. bar	60
Charleston Chew	2-oz. piece	80
Cherry, chocolate covered (Welch's) dark or milk	1 piece (.7 oz.)	10
Chocolate bar:		
Alpine white (Nestlé)	1 oz.	20
Brazil nut, *Cadbury's* (Peter Paul Cadbury)	2 oz.	82
Caramello, *Cadbury's* (Peter Paul Cadbury)	2 oz.	108
Crunch (Nestlé)	1¹⁄₁₆-oz. bar	50
Fruit & nut, *Cadbury's* (Peter Paul Cadbury)	2 oz.	77
Hazelnut, *Cadbury's* (Peter Paul Cadbury)	2 oz.	88
Milk:		
Cadbury's (Peter Paul Cadbury)	2 oz.	94
(Hershey's)	1.5-oz. bar	40
(Hershey's)	4-oz. bar	109
(Nestlé)	.35-oz. miniature	7
(Nestlé)	1¹⁄₁₆-oz. bar	21

Food and Description	Measure or Quantity	Sodium (milligrams)
Special Dark (Hershey's)	1.45-oz. bar	5
Special Dark (Hershey's)	4-oz. bar	14
Chocolate bar with almonds:		
Cadbury's (Peter Paul Cadbury)	2 oz.	82
(Hershey's) milk	1.55-oz. bar	60
(Nestlé)	1 oz.	15
Chocolate Parfait (Pearson's)	1 piece (.2 oz.)	17
Chocolate, petite (Andes)	1 piece (.15 oz.)	4
Chuckles, any flavor	1 oz.	10
Chunky (Nestlé)	1 oz.	15
Coffee Nips (Pearson's)	1 piece (.2 oz.)	17
Coffioca (Pearson's)	1 piece (6.5 g.)	17
Creme De Menthe (Andes)	1 piece (.2 oz.)	3
Eggs (Nabisco) *Chuckles*	½ oz.	5
5th Avenue Bar (Hershey's)	2.1-oz. serving	140
Fruit bears (Flavor Tree)	½ of 2.1-oz. pkg.	12
Fruit circus (Flavor Tree)	½ of 2.1-oz. pkg.	12
Fruit roll (Flavor Tree):		
Apple or apricot	¾-oz. piece	17
Cherry	¾-oz. piece	18
Fruit punch or grape	¾-oz. piece	12
Raspberry	¾-oz. piece	20
Strawberry	¾-oz. piece	11
Fudge (Nabisco) bar	1 piece (.7 oz.)	20
Fun fruit (Sunkist)	.9-oz. piece	10
Goobers (Nestlé)	1-oz. serving	10
Good Stuff (Nab)	1.8-oz. piece	90
Halvah (Sahadi)	1 oz.	45
Hard (Jolly Rancher):		
Apple; fire; grape; lemon; lemonade, pink; fruit punch; raspberry & watermelon	1 piece	5
Butterscotch	1 piece	37
Cherry; peppermint; strawberry	1 piece	3
Orange	1 piece	4

Food and Description	Measure or Quantity	Sodium (milligrams)
Holidays (M&M/Mars):		
Plain	1 oz.	40
Peanut	1 oz.	35
Jelly, *Chuckles*:		
Bar	1 oz.	10
Bean	½ oz.	15
Rings	1 oz.	10
Ju-Jubes (Nabisco) *Chuckles*	½ oz.	7
Kisses (Hershey's) milk chocolate	1 piece (5 g.)	4
Kit Kat (Hershey's)	1.62-oz. bar	60
Krackel Bar (Hershey's)	1.55-oz. bar	80
Licorice Nip (Pearson's)	1 piece (6.5 g.)	17
Lollipop (Life Savers)	1 piece	10
Mars Bar (M&M/Mars)	1.7-oz. serving	85
Marshmallow eggs (Nabisco) *Chuckles*	1 oz.	0
Mary Jane	.25-oz. piece	4
Mary Jane	1½-oz. piece	23
Milky Way (M&M/Mars)	2.24-oz. bar	150
Mint parfait (Andes)	.2-oz. piece	3
Mint pattie (Nabisco):		
Junior pattie	.1-oz. piece	<1
Peppermint	.5-oz. piece	5
M&M's (M&M/Mars):		
Peanut	1.83-oz. serving	60
Plain	1.69-oz. serving	65
Mounds (Hershey's)	1.95-oz. bar	85
Mr. Goodbar (Hershey's)	1.75-oz. serving	20
Munch bar (M&M/Mars)	1.43-oz. bar	110
My Buddy (Tom's)	1.8-oz. serving	60
Naturally Nut & Fruit Bar (Planters):		
Almond/apricot	1 oz.	75
Almond/pineapple	1 oz.	80
Peanut/raisin	1 oz.	70
Walnut/apple	1 oz.	90
Necco Wafers, assorted	2.02-oz. roll	5

Food and Description	Measure or Quantity	Sodium (milligrams)
Nougat center (Nabisco) *Chuckles*	1 oz.	10
Oh Henry! (Nestlé)	1-oz.	45
$100,000 Bar (Nestlé)	1¼-oz. bar	75
Orange slice (Nabisco) *Chuckles*	1 oz.	10
Park Avenue (Tom's)	1.8-oz. serving	120
Peanut bar (Planters)	1.6-oz. piece	110
Peanut butter cup (Reese's)	1 cup	90
Peanut Butter Pals (Tom's)	1.3-oz. serving	100
Peanut butter parfait (Pearson)	1 piece	17
Peanut, chocolate-covered (Nabisco)	1 piece	1
Peanut crunch (Saladi)	¾-oz. bar	10
Peanut parfait (Andes)	1 piece	11
Peanut Plank (Tom's)	1.7-oz. serving	30
Peanut roll (Tom's)	1¾-oz. serving	120
Pom Poms (Nabisco)	1 oz.	70
Powerhouse (Peter Paul Cadbury)	2 oz.	193
Raisin, chocolate-covered (Nabisco)	1 piece	<1
Reese's Pieces (Hershey's)	1.8-oz. pkg.	90
Rolo (Hershey's)	1 piece (6 g.)	14
Rolo (Hershey's)	1¾-oz. roll	109
Royals (M&M/Mars)	1½-oz. serving	34
Sesame crunch bar (Sahadi)	¾-oz. bar	55
Sesame Tahini (Sahadi)	1 oz.	75
Skittles (M&M/Mars)	1 oz.	13
Skor (Hershey's) toffee bar	1.4-oz. bar	125
Sky Bar (Necco)	1.5-oz. bar	57
Snickers (M&M/Mars)	2.16-oz. bar	170
Solitaires (Hershey's)	½ of 3.2-oz. bag	25
Spearmint leaves (Nabisco) *Chuckles*	1 oz.	15
Spice flavored sticks & drops (Nabisco) *Chuckles*	1 oz.	10

Food and Description	Measure or Quantity	Sodium (milligrams)
Spice flavored strings		
(Nabisco) *Chuckles*	1 oz.	10
Starburst (M&M/Mars)	1-oz. serving	15
Stars, chocolate (Nabisco)	1 piece	3
Sugar Babies (Nabisco)	1⅝-oz. pkg.	85
Sugar Daddy (Nabisco)	1⅜-oz. pop	85
Sugar Mama (Nabisco)	¾-oz. piece	30
3 *Musketeers Bar* (M&M/		
Mars)	2.13-oz. serving	120
Symphony (Hershey's):		
Almond butterscotch	1.4-oz.	40
Milk	1.4-oz.	35
Ting-A-Ling (Andes)	.2-oz. bar	7
Tootsie Roll:		
Regular:		
Chocolate	.23-oz. midgee	1
Chocolate	.63-oz. bar	4
Chocolate	¾-oz. bar	5
Chocolate	1-oz. bar	6
Chocolate	1¼-oz. bar	8
Flavored	.16-oz. square	1
Flavored	.23-oz. midgee	2
Pop:		
Caramel	.49-oz. pop	4
Chocolate	.49-oz. pop	4
Flavored	.49-oz. pop	Tr.
Pop drop:		
Caramel	.17-oz. piece	1
Chocolate	.17-oz. piece	Tr.
Flavored	.17-oz. piece	Tr.
Twix, cookie bar (M&M/		
Mars)	.85-oz. serving	48
Twix, cookie bar, peanut		
butter (M&M/Mars)	.8-oz. serving	69
Whatchamacallit (Hershey's)	1.8-oz. bar	130
Wispa (Peter Paul Cadbury)	1 oz.	47
Y&S Bites (Hershey's)	1 oz.	85
Dietetic or low calorie:		
Caramel (Estee)	1 piece	15

Food and Description	Measure or Quantity	Sodium (milligrams)
Carob bar, *Joan's Natural:*		
Coconut	1 section of 3-oz. bar (¼ oz.)	10
Coconut	3-oz. bar	117
Fruit & nut	1 section of 3-oz. bar (¼ oz.)	10
Fruit & nut	3-oz. bar	115
Honey bran	1 section of 3-oz. bar (¼ oz.)	9
Honey bran	3-oz. bar	114
Peanut	1 section of 3-oz. bar (¼ oz.)	9
Peanut	3-oz. bar	109
Chocolate or chocolate-flavored bar:		
Coconut (Estee)	1 section of 2½-oz. bar	5
Coconut (Estee)	2½-oz. bar	61
Crunch (Estee)	1 section of 2½-oz. bar	5
Crunch (Estee)	2½-oz. bar	65
Fruit & nut (Estee)	1 section of 2½-oz. bar	5
Fruit & nut (Estee)	2½-oz. bar	59
Milk (Estee)	1 section of 2½-oz. bar	6
Milk (Estee)	2½-oz. bar	68
Estee-Ets, peanut	1.4-g. piece	2
Gum drops (Estee) fruit and licorice	1 piece (2 g.)	0
Hard (Louis Sherry)	1 piece	2
Lollipop (Estee)	1 pop	5
Peanut brittle (Estee)	¼ oz.	30
Peanut butter cup (Estee)	1 piece (.3 oz.)	20
Raisin, chocolate-covered (Estee)	1 piece (1 g.)	2
CANDY APPLE COOLER DRINK, canned (Hi-C)	6 fl. oz.	17

Food and Description	Measure or Quantity	Sodium (milligrams)
CANNELONI, frozen:		
(Armour) *Dining Lite*,		
cheese	9-oz. meal	650
(Celentano) florentine	12-oz. pkg.	620
(Stouffer's) *Lean Cuisine*:		
Beef & pork with mornay		
sauce	9⅝-oz. meal	950
Cheese, with tomato sauce	9⅛-oz. meal	910
CANTALOUPE, fresh (USDA):		
Whole, medium	1 lb. (weighed with skin & cavity contents)	27
Cubed	½ cup (2.9 oz.)	10
CAP'N CRUNCH, cereal (Quaker):		
Regular	¾ cup (1 oz.)	185
Crunchberries	¾ cup (1 oz.)	166
Peanut butter	¾ cup (1 oz.)	210
CARAMBOLA, raw (USDA):		
Whole	1 lb. (weighed whole)	9
Flesh only	4 oz.	2
CARAWAY SEED (French's)	1 tsp.	Tr.
CARDAMOM SEED (French's)	1 tsp.	Tr.
CARL'S JR. RESTAURANT:		
Bacon	2 strips	200
Cake, chocolate	3.2-oz. piece	335
California roast beef 'n Swiss		
sandwich	1 sandwich	1070
Cheese:		
American	.6-oz. piece	290
Swiss	.6-oz. piece	221
Chicken sandwich:		
Charbroiler BBQ	6.3-oz. sandwich	955
Charbroiler Club	8.2-oz. sandwich	1165
Danish	3.5-oz. piece	550
Egg, scrambled	2.4-oz. serving	105
Fish filet sandwich	7.9-oz. sandwich	945
French toast dips, without		
syrup	4.7-oz. serving	576

Food and Description	Measure or Quantity	Sodium (milligrams)
Hamburger:		
Plain:		
Famous Star	8.1-oz. burger	890
Happy Star	3-oz. burger	445
Old Time Star	5.9-oz. burger	760
Super Star	10.6-oz. burger	990
Cheeseburger, *Western Bacon:*		
Regular	7.5-oz. burger	1415
Double	10.4-oz. burger	1620
Hot cakes, with margarine, excluding syrup	1 serving	1190
Milk, 2% lowfat	10 fl. oz.	550
Muffins:		
Blueberry	3½-oz. muffin	360
Bran	4-oz. muffin	300
English, with margarine	2-oz. serving	275
Onion rings	3.2-oz. serving	105
Orange juice	1 small serving	2
Potato:		
Baked:		
Bacon & cheese	1 potato	1820
Broccoli & cheese	1 potato	690
Cheese	1 potato	785
Fiesta	1 potato	1230
Lite	1 potato	35
Sour cream & chive	1 potato	140
French fries	1 regular order	626
Hash brown nuggets	3-oz. serving	350
Salad dressing:		
Regular:		
Bleu cheese	2-oz. serving	278
House	2-oz. serving	329
1000 Island	2-oz. serving	435
Dietetic, Italian	2-oz. serving	360
Sausage	1.5-oz. patty	275
Shake	1 regular size	255
Soft drink:		
Regular	1 regular drink	37
Dietetic	1 regular drink	13

Food and Description	Measure or Quantity	Sodium (milligrams)
Soup:		
Broccoli, cream of	6 fl. oz.	845
Chicken & noodle	6 fl. oz.	605
Chowder, Boston clam	6 fl. oz.	861
Vegetable	6 fl. oz.	807
Steak sandwich, country fried	7.2-oz. sandwich	1290
Sunrise Sandwich:		
Bacon	4.5-oz. sandwich	750
Sausage	6.1-oz. sandwich	990
Tea, iced	1 regular drink	0
Zucchini	4.3-oz. serving	480
CARP, raw (USDA):		
Whole	1 lb. (weighed whole)	68
Meat only	4 oz.	57
CARROT:		
Raw (USDA):		
Whole	1 lb. (weighed with full tops)	126
Partially trimmed	1 lb. (weighed without tops, with skins)	175
Trimmed	5½″ × 1″ carrot (1.8 oz.)	24
Trimmed	25 thin strips (1.8 oz.)	24
Chunks	½ cup (2.4 oz.)	32
Diced	½ cup (1½ oz.)	34
Grated or shredded	½ cup (1.9 oz.)	26
Slices	½ cup (2.2. oz.)	30
Strips	½ cup (2 oz.)	27
Boiled without salt, drained (USDA):		
Chunks	½ cup (2.9 oz.)	27
Diced	½ cup (2½ oz.)	23
Slices	½ cup (2.7 oz.)	25
Canned, regular pack, solids & liq.:		
(Comstock)	½ cup	320

Food and Description	Measure or Quantity	Sodium (milligrams)
(Del Monte), diced	½ cup (4 oz.)	265
(Stokely-Van Camp):		
Diced, solids & liq.	½ cup (4.3 oz.)	290
Sliced, solids & liq.	½ cup (4.3 oz.)	263
Canned, dietetic or low calorie, solids & liq.:		
(Blue Boy) sliced	½ of 8¼-oz. can	43
(Featherweight) sliced	½ cup	30
(Larsen) *Fresh-Lite*	½ cup (4.4 oz.)	40
(S&W) *Nutradiet*, sliced	½ cup	50
Dehydrated (USDA)	1 oz.	76
Frozen:		
(Birds Eye) baby, whole deluxe	⅓ of 10-oz. pkg.	45
(Frosty Acres):		
Crinkle cut	3.3 oz.	130
Whole, baby	3.3 oz.	45
(Green Giant) crinkle cuts in butter sauce	½ cup	315
(Larsen)	3.3 oz.	40
(McKenzie)	3.3-oz.	56
CASABA MELON, fresh (USDA):		
Whole	1 lb. (weighed whole)	27
Flesh	4 oz.	14
CASHEW NUT:		
(USDA) salted	1 oz.	57
(USDA) salted	½ cup (2.5 oz.)	140
(USDA) salted	5 large or 8 med.	21
(Beer Nuts)	1 oz.	65
(Eagle Snacks) *Honey Roast*	1 oz.	170
(Fisher) salted:		
Dry	1 oz.	140
Honey roasted	1 oz.	70
Oil:		
Whole or pieces	1 oz.	110
Halves	1 oz.	160
Lightly salted	1 oz.	40

Food and Description	Measure or Quantity	Sodium (milligrams)
(Guy's) whole, salted	1 oz.	140
(Planters):		
Dry:		
Salted	1 oz.	230
Unsalted	1 oz.	0
Honey roasted, with or		
without peanuts	1 oz.	170
Oil, salted, halves or		
fancy	1 oz.	135
(Tom's)	1 oz.	122
CASHEW BUTTER (Hain)	1 T.	2
CATAWBA WINE (Great		
Western) pink, 12% alcohol	3 fl. oz.	36
CATFISH:		
Raw, fillet (USDA)	4 oz.	68
Frozen (Mrs. Paul's) breaded &		
fried:		
Fillet	3.6-oz. fillet	243
Finger	½ of 8-oz. pkg.	260
CATSUP:		
Regular pack:		
(USDA)	1 T. (.6 oz.)	188
(USDA)	½ cup (4.8 oz.)	735
(Hunt's)	1 T. (.5 oz.)	160
(Smucker's)	1 T. (.6 oz.)	135
Dietetic or low calorie:		
(Del Monte) no salt added	1 T.	6
(Estee)	1 T.	20
(Hunt's)	1 T.	0
(Weight Watchers)	1 T.	165
CAULIFLOWER:		
Raw (USDA):		
Whole	1 lb. (weighed untrimmed)	23
Flowerbuds	½ cup (1.8 oz.)	6
Slices	½ cup (1.5 oz.)	5
Boiled (USDA) flowerbuds,		
without salt, drained	½ cup (2.2 oz.)	5
Frozen:		
(Birds Eye):		

Food and Description	Measure or Quantity	Sodium (milligrams)
Regular	⅓ of 10-oz. pkg.	18
With cheese sauce	5 oz.	558
(Frosty Acres)	3.3 oz.	15
(Green Giant):		
In cheese sauce	½ cup (3.3 oz.)	417
Polybag, cuts	½ cup	25
(Larsen)	3.3 oz.	45
(McKenzie)	3.3 oz.	28
CAVATELLI, frozen		
(Celentano)	⅕ of 16-oz. pkg.	5
CAVIAR, STURGEON (USDA)		
whole eggs	1 T. (.6 oz.)	352
CELERIAC ROOT, raw (USDA):		
Whole	1 lb. (weighed unpared)	390
Pared	4 oz.	113
CELERY, all varieties (USDA):		
Fresh:		
Whole	1 lb. (weighed untrimmed)	429
1 large outer stalk	8″ × 1½″ at root end (1.4 oz.)	50
Diced, chopped or cut in chunks	½ cup (2.1 oz.)	67
Slices	½ cup (1.9 oz.)	63
Boiled, drained solids:		
Diced or cut in chunks	½ cup (2.7 oz.)	67
Slices	½ cup (3 oz.)	74
Frozen (Larsen)	3½ oz.	90
CELERY CABBAGE (See **CABBAGE, CHINESE**)		
CELERY SALT (French's)	1 tsp. (4.6 g.)	1505
CELERY SEED (French's)	1 tsp. (2.4 g.)	4
CEREAL (See kind of cereal, such as **CORN FLAKES** or brand names such as *KIX, CHEX,* etc.)		
CEREAL BAR (Kellogg's)		
Smart Start:		
Common Sense, oat bran		

Food and Description	Measure or Quantity	Sodium (milligrams)
with raspberry filling or corn flakes with mixed berry filling	1½-oz. bar	160
Nutri-Grain or raisin bran	1½-oz. bar	170
Rice Krispies, with almonds	1-oz. bar	65
CERVELAT (Hormel) Viking, chub	1 oz.	325
CHABLIS WINE:		
(Great Western) 12% alcohol	3 fl. oz.	31
(Great Western) Diamond, 12% alcohol	3 fl. oz.	<1
CHAMPAGNE (Great Western)	3 fl. oz.	31
CHARD, Swiss (USDA):		
Raw, whole	1 lb. (weighed untrimmed)	613
Raw, trimmed	4 oz.	167
Boiled, without salt, drained solids	½ cup (3.4 oz.)	83
CHARLOTTE RUSSE, with ladyfingers, whipped cream filling, home recipe (USDA)	4 oz.	49
CHAYOTE, raw (USDA):		
Whole	1 lb. (weighed unpared)	19
Pared	4 oz.	6
CHEERIOS, cereal (General Mills):		
Regular	1¼ cups (1 oz.)	290
Honey-nut	¾ cup (1 oz.)	250
CHERRIOS-TO-GO (General Mills):		
Plain	¾-oz. pouch	220
Apple cinnamon	1-oz. pouch	180
Honey nut	1-oz. pouch	250
CHEESE:		
American or cheddar: (USDA):		
Natural	1″ cube (.6 oz.)	119

Food and Description	Measure or Quantity	Sodium (milligrams)
Natural, diced	1 cup (4.6 oz.)	917
Natural, grated or shredded	1 cup (3.9 oz.)	777
Natural, grated or shredded	1 T. (.7 g.)	48
Process	1″ cube (.6 oz.)	204
Churny Lite:		
Mild	1 oz.	210
Sharp	1 oz.	180
(Dorman's)	1 oz.	140
(Kraft):		
Regular:		
American singles	1 oz.	310
Cheddar	1 oz.	180
Old English, cheddar, sharp	1 oz.	440
(Land O'Lakes):		
American, process:		
Regular	1 oz.	450
Sharp	1 oz.	360
& Swiss	1 oz.	400
Cheddar, natural:		
Regular or *Chederella*	1 oz.	180
& bacon	1 oz.	350
Extra sharp	1 oz.	370
(Laughing Cow)	1 oz.	227
(Polly-O) cheddar, shredded	1 oz.	180
Bleu or blue:		
(Frigo)	1 oz.	511
(Sargento) cold pack or crumbled	1 oz.	396
Bonbino (Laughing Cow)	1 oz.	227
Brick (Land O'Lakes)	1 oz.	160
Brie (Sargento) *Danish Danko*	1 oz.	282
Burgercheese (Sargento)	1 oz.	406
Camembert (Sargento) *Danish Danko*	1 oz.	233
Cheddar (See American)		
Colby:		
Churny Lite	1 oz.	180
(Dorman's) *Lo-Chol*	1 oz.	140

Food and Description	Measure or Quantity	Sodium (milligrams)
(Kraft)	1 oz.	180
(Land O'Lakes)	1 oz.	170
Cottage:		
Unflavored:		
(USDA)	1 oz.	65
(USDA)	1 T.	34
(Borden):		
Regular, 4% milkfat:		
Salted	½ cup	400
Unsalted	½ cup	40
Dry curd, 0.5% milkfat	½ cup	20
Lite-Line, 1.5% milkfat	½ cup	400
(Breakstone's):		
Low fat	4 oz.	470
Smooth & creamy	4 oz.	370
Tangy	4 oz.	420
(Friendship):		
California-style	1 oz.	95
Low fat, no salt added	1 oz.	7
Low fat, pot style	1 oz.	101
Lactose reduced	1 oz.	87
(Johanna):		
Large or small curd	½ cup	450
Low fat	½ cup	430
No salt	½ cup	70
(Land O'Lakes)	1 oz.	120
(Sealtest) large or small curd	4 oz.	460
(Weight Watchers)	½ cup	420
Cream cheese:		
Plain, unwhipped:		
(USDA)	1 oz.	71
(Kraft) *Philadelphia Brand:*		
Regular	1 oz.	85
Lite	1 oz.	160
Flavored, unwhipped (Kraft) *Philadelphia Brand:*		

Food and Description	Measure or Quantity	Sodium (milligrams)
With chives & onion	1 oz.	100
With olives & pimiento	1 oz.	150
Edam:		
(House of Gold)	1 oz.	204
(Kaukauna)	1 oz.	275
(Land O'Lakes)	1 oz.	270
(Churny) *May-Bud*	1 oz.	275
(Sargento)	1 oz.	274
Farmer:		
(Friendship) no salt added	1 oz.	2
(Sargento)	1 oz.	132
Feta (Churny)	1 oz.	316
Gjetost (Sargento) Norwegian	1 oz.	170
Gouda:		
(Kaukauna) any flavor	1 oz.	230
(Land O'Lakes)	1 oz.	230
(Laughing Cow)	1 oz.	227
Wispride	1 oz.	298
Grated:		
(Kraft) Italian blend	1 oz.	435
(Polly-O)	1 oz.	530
Gruyère, *Swiss Knight*	1 oz.	362
Havarti (Sargento) creamy	1 oz.	198
Hoop (Friendship) no salt added	1 oz.	2
Jalapeño jack (Land O' Lakes)	1 oz.	430
Jarlsberg (Sargento) Norwegian, sliced	1 oz.	130
Kettle Moraine (Sargento) sliced	1 oz.	17
Limburger (Sargento) natural	1 oz.	227
Monterey Jack:		
(Churny) *Lite*	1 oz.	220
(Churny) *May-Bud*	1 oz.	150
(Kaukauna) natural	1 oz.	150
(Kraft)	1 oz.	190
(Land O'Lakes) regular or hot pepper	1 oz.	150
Mozzarella:		
(Dorman's) Light or *Lo-chol*	1 oz.	140

Food and Description	Measure or Quantity	Sodium (milligrams)
(Kraft) 100% natural	1 oz.	190
(Land O'Lakes)	1 oz.	150
(Polly-O):		
Fior di Latte	1 oz.	20
Lite	1 oz.	120
Part skim milk, regular or		
shredded	1 oz.	280
Smoked	1 oz.	240
Whole milk:		
Regular	1 oz.	280
Old fashioned:		
Regular	1 oz.	200
Shredded	1 oz.	220
Shredded or slices	1 oz.	220
Muenster:		
(Dorman's):		
Light or *Lo-chol*	1 oz.	140
Low sodium	1 oz.	95
(Kaukauna) natural	1 oz.	180
(Land O'Lakes)	1 oz.	180
Wispride	1 oz.	129
Parmesan:		
(Frigo):		
Regular	1 oz.	341
Grated	1 T. (6 g.)	88
(Polly-O) grated	1 oz.	530
(Progresso) grated	1 T.	95
(Sargento):		
Grated, non-dairy	1 T. (7 g.)	105
Wedge	1 oz.	454
Pizza (Sargento) shredded or		
sliced, non-dairy	1 oz.	306
Provolone:		
(Dorman's) Light	1 oz.	140
(Land O'Lakes)	1 oz.	250
Ricotta (Polly-O):		
Lite	1 oz.	32
Old fashioned	1 oz.	25

Food and Description	Measure or Quantity	Sodium (milligrams)
Part skim milk:		
Regular	1 oz.	22
No salt	1 oz.	10
Whole milk:		
Regular	1 oz.	22
No salt	1 oz.	10
Romano (Progresso) grated	1 T.	70
Roquefort, natural (USDA)	1 oz.	465
Samsoe (Sargento) Danish	1 oz.	198
Semi-soft:		
Bel Paese	1 oz.	196
Laughing Cow:		
Babybel	1 oz.	227
Bombel	1 oz.	227
Slim Jack (Dorman's)	1 oz.	140
String (Sargento)	1 oz.	150
Swiss:		
(Churny) *Lite*	1 oz.	45
(Dorman's):		
Light	1 oz.	60
Lo-chol	1 oz.	140
Low sodium	1 oz.	8
(Sargento) sliced:		
Domestic	1 oz.	74
Imported, Finland	1 oz.	74
Taco (Sargento) shredded	1 oz.	47
CHEESE DIP (See **DIP**)		
CHEESE FONDUE:		
Home recipe (USDA)	4 oz.	615
Swiss Knight	1-oz. serving	186
CHEESE FOOD, process:		
American or cheddar:		
(Borden) *Lite-Line:*		
American	1 oz.	410
Cheddar, sharp	1 oz.	440
Heart Beat (GFA):		
American	⅔-oz. piece	180
Sharp	⅔-oz. piece	210
(Land O'Lakes)	¾-oz. slice	260

Food and Description	Measure or Quantity	Sodium (milligrams)
(Shedd's) *Country Crock*	1 oz.	190
Wispride, cheddar:		
Regular	1 oz.	180
& port wine	1 oz.	190
Cheez-ola (Fisher) process	1 oz.	454
Colby (Pauly) low sodium	1 oz.	5
Cracker snack (Sargento)	1 oz.	406
Garlic & herb, *Wispride*	1 oz.	180
Italian herb (Land O'Lakes)	1 oz.	430
Jalapeño (Borden) *Lite-Line*	1 oz.	430
Low sodium:		
(Borden) *Lite-Line*	1 oz.	200
Heart Beat (GFA)	.7-oz. slice	90
Monterey Jack (Borden) *Lite-Line*	1 oz.	450
Muenster (Borden) *Lite-Line*	1 oz.	450
Mun-chee (Pauly) chunk	1 oz.	485
Neufchatel (Shedd's)		
Country Crock:		
Fresh garden vegetable or fresh herb & garlic	1 oz.	190
Fresh french onion	1 oz.	150
Onion (Land O'Lakes)	1 oz.	410
Pepperoni (Land O'Lakes)	1 oz.	430
Salami (Land O'Lakes)	1 oz.	410
Swiss:		
(Borden) *Lite-Line*	1 oz.	330
(Kraft) reduced fat, light natural	1 oz.	55
CHEESE SPREAD:		
American, process:		
(USDA)	1 T. (.5 oz.)	228
(Nabisco) *Easy Cheese*	1 tsp. (6 g.)	70
Wispride	1 oz.	304
Blue (Laughing Cow)	1 oz.	312
Cheddar:		
(Laughing Cow)	1 oz.	312
(Nabisco) *Easy Cheese:*		
Regular	1 tsp.	74

Food and Description	Measure or Quantity	Sodium (milligrams)
Chive	1 tsp.	68
Sharp	1 tsp.	64
Wispride, sharp	1 oz.	304
Cheese & bacon (Nabisco)		
Easy Cheese	1 tsp. (6 g.)	70
Count Down (Fisher)	1 oz.	435
Golden velvet (Land O'Lakes)	1 oz.	370
Gruyère (Laughing Cow) *La*		
Vache Qui Rit	1 oz.	312
Imitation (Fisher) *Chef's*		
Delight	1 oz.	380
Nacho (Nabisco) *Easy*		
Cheese	1 tsp.	68
Pimiento:		
(Pauly)	¾-oz. serving	386
(Price's)	1 oz.	335
Provolone (Laughing Cow)	1 oz.	312
Sharp (Pauly)	.8-oz. serving	437
Swiss (Pauly) process	.8-oz. serving	391
Velveeta (Kraft):		
Regular	1 oz.	430
Mexican, with jalapeño pepper	1 oz.	440
CHEESE STRAW (USDA)	5″ × ⅜″	
	piece (6 g.)	43
CHELOIS WINE (Great Western)		
12% alcohol	3 fl. oz.	37
CHERRY:		
Sour (USDA):		
Fresh:		
Whole	1 lb. (weighed with stems)	7
Whole	1 lb. (weighed without stems)	8
Pitted	½ cup (2.7 oz.)	2
Canned, syrup pack, pitted:		
Light syrup	4 oz. (with liq.)	1
Heavy syrup	½ cup (with liq.)	1
Extra heavy syrup	4 oz. (with liq.)	1
Canned, water pack, pitted,		
solids & liq.	½ cup (4.3 oz.)	2

Food and Description	Measure or Quantity	Sodium (milligrams)
Frozen, pitted:		
Sweetened	½ cup (4.6 oz.)	3
Unsweetened	4 oz.	2
Sweet:		
Fresh (USDA):		
Whole	1 lb. (weighed with stems)	8
Whole, with stems	½ cup (2.3 oz.)	1
Pitted	½ cup (2.9 oz.)	2
Canned, syrup pack:		
(USDA):		
Light syrup, pitted	4 oz. (with liq.)	1
Heavy syrup, pitted	½ cup (with liq., 4.2 oz.)	1
Extra heavy syrup, pitted	4 oz. (with liq.)	1
(Del Monte) solids & liq.:		
Dark	½ cup (4.3 oz.)	<10
Light	½ cup (4.3 oz.)	<10
(Stokely-Van Camp) pitted,		
solids & liq.	½ cup (4.2 oz.)	18
Canned, dietetic or water pack, solids & liq.:		
(Diet Delight)	½ cup (4.4 oz.)	5
(Featherweight):		
Dark	½ cup	<10
Light	½ cup	<10
CHERRY DRINK:		
Canned:		
(Hi-C)	6 fl. oz.	17
(Smucker's) black	8 fl. oz.	10
Squeezit (General Mills)	6¾-fl.-oz. container	30
Ssips (Johanna Farms)	8.45-fl.-oz. container	20
*Mix (Funny Face)	6 fl. oz.	0
CHERRY JELLY:		
Sweetened:		
(Home Brands)	1 T.	15
(Smucker's)	1 T.	<10

Food and Description	Measure or Quantity	Sodium (milligrams)
Dietetic or low calorie (Smucker's)	1 T.	<10
CHERRY PIE (See **PIE,** Cherry)		
CHERRY PIE FILLING (See **PIE FILLING,** Cherry)		
CHERRY PRESERVE or JAM:		
Sweetened (Home Brands)	1 T. (.7 oz.)	15
Dietetic (Louis Sherry)	1 T.	<3
CHERVIL (Spice Island)	1 tsp.	Tr.
CHESTNUT (USDA):		
Fresh:		
In shell	1 lb. (weighed in shell)	22
Shelled	4 oz.	7
Dried:		
In shell	1 lb. (weighed in shell)	45
Shelled	4 oz.	14
CHEWING GUM, sweetened or unsweetened:		
Beechies	1 tablet	0
Beech-Nut	1 stick	Tr.
Beemans	1 stick	
Big Red	1 stick	Tr.
Doublemint (Wrigley's)	1 stick	Tr.
Freedent (Wrigley's)	1 stick	Tr.
Juicy Fruit (Wrigley's)	1 stick	Tr.
Orbit, regular or bubble	1 stick	Tr.
Spearmint (Wrigley's)	1 stick	Tr.
CHEX, cereal (Ralston Purina):		
Bran (See **BRAN BREAKFAST CEREAL**)		
Corn	1 cup (1 oz.)	310
Double	⅔ cup (1 oz.)	190
Honey graham	⅔ cup (1 oz.)	180
Oat, honey nut	½ cup (1 oz.)	240
Rice	1⅛ cups (1 oz.)	280
Wheat	⅔ cup (1 oz.)	230

Food and Description	Measure or Quantity	Sodium (milligrams)
CHICKEN (See also **CHICKEN, CANNED**): (USDA):		
Broiler, cooked, meat only	4 oz.	75
Fryer, raw, ready-to-cook	1 lb. (weighed ready-to-cook)	0
Hen and cock:		
Stewed:		
Meat only	4 oz.	62
Chopped	½ cup (2.5 oz.)	40
Diced	½ cup (2.4 oz.)	37
Ground	½ cup (2 oz.)	31
Roaster:		
Roasted:		
Dark meat without skin	4 oz.	100
Light meat without skin	4 oz.	75
CHICKEN À LA KING:		
Home recipe (USDA)	1 cup (8.6 oz.)	760
Canned (Swanson)	½ of 10½-oz. can	690
Frozen		
(Armour):		
Classics Lite	11¼-oz. meal	630
Dining Lite, with rice	9-oz. meal	780
(Stouffer's) with rice	9½-oz. meal	900
(Weight Watchers)	9-oz. pkg.	940
CHICKEN BOUILLON/ BROTH, cube or powder (See also **SOUP**, Chicken):		
(Borden) *Lite-Line*	1 tsp.	5
(Herb-Ox):		
Cube	4-g. cube	950
Powder	5-g. packet	960
*(Knorr)	8 fl. oz.	1200
(Maggi)	1 cube	746
MBT	1 packet (.2 oz.)	575
(Wyler's):		
Cube	1 cube	900
Instant	1 tsp.	900
CHICKEN, CANNED, boned:		
(Featherweight) low sodium	5 oz.	99

Food and Description	Measure or Quantity	Sodium (milligrams)
(Hormel):		
Breast	6¾-oz. can	855
Dark	6¾-oz. can	933
White & dark:		
Regular	6¾-oz. can	857
Low sodium	6¾-oz. can	75
(Swanson):		
Regular	½ of 5-oz. can	240
Mixin' style	½ of 5-oz. can	225
White	½ of 5-oz. can	230
CHICKEN CHUNKS, frozen		
(Country Pride):		
Regular	¼ of 12-oz. pkg.	560
Southern fried	¼ of 12-oz. pkg.	690
CHICKEN DINNER or ENTREE:		
Canned:		
(Hunt's) *Minute Gourmet Microwave Entree Maker:*		
Barbecued:		
Without chicken	3.1 oz.	1040
With chicken	6.8 oz.	1110
Cacciatore:		
Without chicken	4.6 oz.	780
With chicken	8.3 oz.	840
Sweet & sour:		
Without chicken	4.1 oz.	360
With chicken	7.8 oz.	420
(Swanson) & dumplings	7½ oz.	960
Frozen:		
(Armour):		
Classics Lite:		
Breast medallions		
marsala	11-oz. meal	930
Burgundy	10-oz. meal	780
Oriental	10-oz. meal	660
Sweet & sour	11-oz. meal	820
Dining Lite, glazed	9-oz. meal	680

Food and Description	Measure or Quantity	Sodium (milligrams)
Dinner Classics:		
Glazed	10¾-oz. meal	960
Mesquite	9½-oz. meal	660
Parmigiana	11½-oz. meal	1060
With wine & mushroom sauce	10¾-oz. meal	900
(Banquet):		
Dinner:		
Regular:		
& dumplings	10-oz. meal	940
Fried	10-oz. meal	1100
Extra Helping:		
Fried	16-oz. meal	1470
Nuggets, with barbecue sauce	10-oz. meal	1390
Platter, boneless:		
Drumsnacker	7-oz. meal	690
Nuggets	6.4-oz. meal	630
Pattie	7½-oz. meal	760
(Celentano):		
Parmigiana, cutlets	9-oz. pkg.	490
Primavera	11½-oz. pkg.	620
(Chun King) entrees:		
Imperial	13-oz. entree	1540
Walnut, crunchy	13-oz. entree	1700
(Healthy Choice):		
A L'Orange	9½-oz. meal	90
Glazed	8½-oz. meal	340
Herb roasted	11-oz. meal	300
Mesquite	10½-oz. meal	270
Oriental	11¼-oz. meal	460
Parmigiana	11½-oz. meal	310
& pasta divan	11½-oz. meal	510
Sweet & sour	11½-oz. meal	260
(Kid Cuisine):		
Fried	7¼-oz. meal	1050
Nuggets	6¼-oz. meal	610
(La Choy) *Fresh and Lite*:		
Almond, with rice & vegetables	9¾-oz. meal	1092

Food and Description	Measure or Quantity	Sodium (milligrams)
Imperial	11-oz. meal	1269
Oriental, spicy	9¾-oz. meal	560
Sweet & sour	10-oz. meal	601
(Stouffer's):		
Regular:		
Cashew in sauce with rice	9½-oz. meal	1140
Creamed	6½-oz. meal	670
Divan	8½-oz. meal	780
Escalloped, & noodles	10-oz. meal	1230
Lean Cuisine:		
A l'orange, with almond rice	8-oz. meal	430
Breast:		
In herb cream sauce	9½-oz. meal	850
Marsala, with vegetables	8⅛-oz. meal	850
Parmesan	10-oz. meal	870
Cacciatore, with vermicelli	10⅞-oz. meal	250
Fiesta	8½-oz. meal	250
Glazed, with rice	8½-oz. meal	810
Oriental	9⅜-oz. meal	790
& vegetables, with vermicelli	11¾-oz. meal	980
Right Course:		
Italiano	9⅝-oz. meal	560
Sesame	10-oz. meal	590
Tenderloins:		
In barbecue sauce	8¾-oz. meal	590
In peanut sauce	9¼-oz. meal	570
(Swanson):		
Regular:		
& dumplings	7½-oz. meal	965
Fried, 4-compartment:		
Barbecue flavor	9¼-oz. meal	960
Breast portion	10¾-oz. meal	1580
Dark meat	10¼-oz. meal	1390
Hungry Man:		
Boneless	17½-oz. dinner	1640

Food and Description	Measure or Quantity	Sodium (milligrams)
Fried:		
Breast	14-oz. dinner	2120
Dark portion	14-oz. dinner	1680
Parmigiana	20-oz. dinner	2080
(Tyson):		
A l'orange	9½-oz. meal	670
Dijon	8½-oz. meal	840
Français	9½-oz. meal	1130
Kiev	9¼-oz. meal	1200
Marsala	10½-oz. meal	900
Mesquite	9½-oz. meal	700
Oriental	10¼-oz. meal	1140
Parmigiano	11¼-oz. meal	1100
Peking	10-oz. meal	860
Piccata	9-oz. meal	680
Sweet & sour	11-oz. meal	850
(Weight Watchers):		
Cordon bleu, breaded	8-oz. meal	880
Fettucini	8¼-oz. meal	550
Imperial	9¼-oz. meal	910
Nuggets	5.9-oz. meal	540
Patty, southern fried	6½-oz. meal	800
Sweet & sour tenders	10.2-oz. meal	600
CHICKEN & DUMPLINGS (See **CHICKEN DINNER or ENTREE**)		
CHICKEN FRICASSEE, home recipe (USDA)	1 cup (8½ oz.)	370
CHICKEN, FRIED, frozen:		
(Banquet):		
Assorted or hot & spicy	32-oz. pkg.	6005
Breast portion	11½-oz. pkg.	1420
Thigh & drumstick	12½-oz. pkg.	1580
(Swanson) Plump & Juicy:		
Assorted, regular	3¼ oz. serving	600
Breast portion	4½-oz. serving	830
Cutlet	3½-oz. serving	440
Dipsters	3-oz. serving	400
Drumlets	3-oz. serving	390
Nibbles (wings)	3¼-oz. serving	640

Food and Description	Measure or Quantity	Sodium (milligrams)
Take-out style	3¼-oz. serving	660
Thighs & drumsticks	3¼-oz. serving	550
CHICKEN GIZZARD (USDA):		
Raw	2-oz. serving	37
Simmered	2-oz. serving	32
*CHICKEN HELPER (General Mills):		
& biscuits, crispy	⅕ of pkg.	1240
& dumplings	⅕ of pkg.	1320
& mushroom	⅕ of pkg.	900
Potato & gravy	⅕ of pkg.	1000
& seasoned rice	⅕ of pkg.	1490
Stuffing	⅕ of pkg.	1600
Teriyaki	⅕ of pkg.	1010
Tetrazzini	⅕ of pkg.	870
CHICKEN LIVER (See **LIVER**)		
CHICKEN & NOODLES (See also **NOODLE & CHICKEN**):		
Home recipe (USDA)	1 cup (8½ oz.)	600
Frozen:		
(Armour):		
Dining Lite	9-oz. meal	570
Dinner Classics	11-oz. meal	660
(Stouffer's) home style	10-oz. meal	1090
CHICKEN NUGGETS, frozen		
(Country Pride)	¼ of 12-oz. pkg.	460
CHICKEN, PACKAGED:		
(Carl Buddig) smoked	1 oz.	340
(Eckrich) breast, sliced	1 slice	210
(Oscar Mayer) breast:		
Oven roasted	1-oz. slice	415
Smoked	1-oz. slice	398
(Weaver):		
Bologna	1 slice	185
Breast:		
Hickory smoked	1 slice	195
Oven roasted	1 slice	185
Roll	1 slice	153

Food and Description	Measure or Quantity	Sodium (milligrams)
CHICKEN PATTIE, frozen		
(Banquet) breaded & fried	12-oz. pkg.	2052
CHICKEN PIE:		
Home recipe (USDA) baked	8-oz. pie (4¼″ dia.)	581
Frozen:		
(Banquet)	7-oz. pie	860
(Morton)	7-oz. pie	740
(Stouffer's)	10-oz. pie	1260
(Swanson):		
Regular	8-oz. pie	840
Chunky	10-oz. pie	850
Hungry Man	16-oz. pie	1670
CHICKEN SALAD, canned		
(Carnation) *Spreadable*	¼ of 7½-oz. can	230
CHICKEN SOUP (See **SOUP,**		
Chicken)		
CHICKEN SPREAD, canned:	(Hormel):	
Lunche Loaf	1 oz.	304
Sandwich Makins	1 oz.	252
(Swanson)	1-oz. serving	140
(Underwood) chunky	½ of 4¾-oz. can	575
CHICKEN STEW:		
Canned, regular pack:		
(Libby's) with dumplings	⅓ of 24-oz. can	976
(Swanson)	7⅝-oz. serving	960
Canned, dietetic or low calorie		
(Featherweight)	7½-oz. can	53
CHICKEN STICKS, frozen		
(Country Pride)	12-oz. pkg.	1600
CHICKEN STOCK BASE		
(French's)	1 tsp. (3 g.)	475
CHICK-FIL-A:		
Brownie, fudge, with nuts	2.8-oz. serving	213
Chicken, without bun	3.6-oz. serving	801
Chicken nuggets:		
8-pack	4 oz.	1326
12-pack	6 oz.	1989
Chicken salad:		
Regular:		
Cup	3.4-oz. serving	543

Food and Description	Measure or Quantity	Sodium (milligrams)
Plate	11.8-oz. serving	1839
Chargrilled, golden	10.4-oz. serving	567
Sandwich:		
Regular, wheat bread	5.7-oz. sandwich	888
Chargrilled	5½-oz. sandwich	1121
Chicken sandwich:		
Regular	5¾-oz. sandwich	1174
Deluxe:		
Regular	7.45-oz. sandwich	1178
Chargrilled, with lettuce & tomato	7.15-oz. sandwich	1125
Cole slaw	3.7-oz. cup	158
Icedream	4½-oz.	51
Lemonade, regular	10-fl.-oz. serving	Tr.
Pie, lemon	4.1-oz. slice	300
Potato, *Waffle Potato Fries*	3-oz. serving	270
Potato salad	3.8-oz. cup	337
Salad, tossed:		
Plain	4½-oz. serving	19
With dressing:		
Honey french	6 oz.	519
Italian, lite	6 oz.	354
Ranch	6 oz.	206
1000 island	6 oz.	389
Soup, hearty breast of chicken, small	8½-fl.-oz. serving	530
CHICK PEAS or GARBANZOS:		
Dry (USDA)	1 cup (7.1 oz.)	52
Canned, regular pack, solids & liq:		
(Allen's)	½ cup	330
(Furman's)	⅓ cup (2.6 oz.)	275
(Goya)	½ cup (4 oz.)	480
(Progresso)	½ cup	390
CHICORY, WITLOOF, Belgian or French endive, raw, bleached head (USDA):		
Untrimmed	½ lb.	14

Food and Description	Measure or Quantity	Sodium (milligrams)
Trimmed, cut	½ cup (1.6 oz.)	1
CHILI or CHILI CON CARNE:		
Canned, beans only:		
(Comstock)	½ cup	540
(Hormel) in sauce	5 oz.	453
(Hunt's)	½ cup (3½ oz.)	490
Canned, regular pack, with beans:		
(USDA)	1 cup (8.8 oz.)	1328
(Gebhardt) hot	½ of 15-oz. can	1000
(Hormel):		
Regular:		
Hot	½ of 15-oz. can	1121
Mild	½ of 15-oz. can	1127
Short Orders:		
Hot	7½-oz. can	1086
Mild	7½-oz. can	1134
Just Rite:		
Regular	4 oz.	500
Hot	4 oz.	495
(Old El Paso)	½ cup	480
Canned, regular pack, without beans:		
(Gebhardt)	½ of 15-oz. can	1040
(Hormel):		
Regular:		
Hot	½ of 15-oz. can	985
Mild	½ of 15-oz. can	1012
Short Orders	7½-oz. can	961
Just Rite	4 oz.	515
(Old El Paso)	½ cup	510
Frozen, with beans (Stouffer's)	8¾-oz. meal	1265
*Mix, *Manwich, Chili Fixins*	8-oz. serving	980
CHILI MAC (Hormel) *Short Orders*	7½-oz. can	1418
CHILI SAUCE:		
Regular:		
(USDA)	1 T. (.5 oz.)	201
(El Molino) green, mild	1 T.	105

Food and Description	Measure or Quantity	Sodium (*milligrams*)
(La Victoria) green	1 T.	44
(Ortega) hot	1-oz. serving	181
Dietetic:		
(USDA) low sodium	1 T. (.5 oz.)	Tr.
(Featherweight)	1 T. (.5 oz.)	10
CHILI SEASONING MIX:		
*(Durkee)	1 cup	979
(French's) *Chili-O*, plain	1¾-oz. pkg.	3780
(Lawry's)	1.6-oz. pkg.	2291
CHIMICHANGA, frozen:		
Marquez (Fred's Frozen Foods):		
Beef, shredded	5 oz.	676
Chicken	5 oz.	630
(Old El Paso):		
Regular:		
Beef	1 piece	470
Chicken	1 piece	470
Dinner, festive:		
Beef	11-oz. dinner	1200
Beef & cheese	11-oz. dinner	1400
Entree:		
Bean & cheese	1 piece	700
Beef	1 piece	470
Beef & pork	1 piece	700
Chicken	1 piece	460
CHINESE DINNER, frozen (See individual listings such as **CHOP SUEY, CHOW MEIN,** etc.)		
CHIPS (See **CRACKERS, PUFFS and CHIPS; POTATO CHIPS**)		
CHOCOLATE, BAKING:		
(Baker's):		
Bitter or unsweetened	1-oz. square	1
Milk, chips	1 oz.	25
Semi-sweet:		
Regular	1-oz. square	<1
Chips	¼ cup (1½ oz.)	<9
Sweetened, *German's*	1-oz. square	<1

Food and Description	Measure or Quantity	Sodium (milligrams)
(Hershey's):		
Bitter or unsweetened	1-oz. square	5
Milk:		
Chips:		
Regular	1 oz.	55
Vanilla	1 oz.	43
Chunks	1 oz.	25
Semi-sweet, chips	1 oz.	3
(Nestlé):		
Bitter or unsweetened,		
Choco-Bake	1-oz. packet	5
Semi-sweet, morsels	1 oz.	0
Sweetened, milk, morsels	1 oz.	20
CHOCOLATE CAKE (See **CAKE,** Chocolate)		
CHOCOLATE CANDY (See **CANDY**)		
CHOCOLATE, HOT (See also **COCOA**)		
home recipe (USDA)	1 cup (8.8 oz.)	120
CHOCOLATE ICE CREAM (See **ICE CREAM,** Chocolate)		
CHOCOLATE PIE (See **PIE,** Chocolate)		
CHOCOLATE PUDDING or PIE FILLING (See **PUDDING or PIE FILLING,** Chocolate)		
CHOCOLATE SYRUP (See **SYRUP,** Chocolate)		
CHOP SUEY:		
Home recipe (USDA) with meat	1 cup (8.8 oz.)	1052
Canned (USDA) with meat	1 cup (8.8 oz.)	1378
Frozen (Stouffer's) beef, with rice	12-oz. pkg.	1590
*Mix (Durkee)	1¾ cups	5582
CHOW CHOW (USDA):		
Sour	1 oz.	379
Sweet	1 oz.	149

Food and Description	Measure or Quantity	Sodium (milligrams)
CHOW MEIN:		
Home recipe (USDA) chicken, without noodles	8-oz. serving	652
Canned, regular pack:		
(Chun King) chicken, *Divider-Pak*	¼ of pkg.	821
(La Choy):		
Beef	¾ cup	900
*Beef, bi-pack	¾ cup	840
Chicken	¾ cup	890
*Chicken, bi-pack	¾ cup	980
Meatless	¾ cup	820
*Pepper oriental, bi-pack	¾ cup	950
*Pork, bi-pack	¾ cup	970
Shrimp	¾ cup	820
*Shrimp, bi-pack	¾ cup	860
Frozen:		
(Armour) *Dining Lite*, chicken & rice	9-oz. meal	650
(Chun King) chicken	13-oz. entree	1560
(Healthy Choice) chicken	8½-oz. meal	440
(La Choy):		
Regular:		
Chicken:		
Dinner	12-oz. dinner	1740
Entree	⅔ cup	720
Shrimp:		
Dinner	12-oz. dinner	1740
Entree	⅔ cup	820
Fresh & Lite, imperial chicken	11-oz. entree	950
(Stouffer's):		
Regular, without noodles	8-oz. meal	1080
Lean Cuisine, with rice	11¼-oz. meal	980
(Van de Kamp's) Mandarin:		
Beef	11-oz. meal	1700
Chicken	11-oz. meal	1180
CHOW MEIN NOODLES (See **NOODLE, CHOW MEIN**)		

Food and Description	Measure or Quantity	Sodium (milligrams)
CHOW MEIN SEASONING MIX (Kikkoman)	1⅛-oz. pkg.	3
CHURCH'S FRIED CHICKEN:		
Chicken, fried:		
Breast	4.3-oz. serving	560
Leg	2.9-oz. serving	286
Thigh	4.2-oz. serving	448
Wing-breast	4.8-oz. serving	583
Corn, with butter oil	1 serving	20
French fries	1 regular order (3 oz.)	126
CIDER (See **APPLE CIDER**)		
CINNAMON, GROUND:		
(USDA)	1 tsp. (2.3 g.)	1
(French's)	1 tsp. (1.7 g.)	Tr.
CINNAMON SUGAR (French's)	1 tsp.	0
CINNAMON TOAST CRUNCH,		
cereal (General Mills)	¾ cup (1 oz.)	220
CITRON, CANDIED (USDA)	1 oz.	82
*****CITRUS BERRY BLEND,**		
mix, dietetic (Sunkist)	8 fl. oz.	20
CITRUS COOLER DRINK,		
canned (Hi-C)	6 fl. oz.	17
CLAM:		
Raw (USDA):		
Hard or round, meat only	1 cup (8 oz.)	465
Soft, meat only	1 cup (8 oz.)	82
Canned (Gorton's) minced,		
drained solids	1 can	1280
Frozen:		
(Gorton's) fried strips,		
crunchy	3½ oz.	430
(Mrs. Paul's) batter fried,		
light	½ of 5-oz. pkg.	385
CLAMATO COCKTAIL, canned		
(Mott's)	6 fl. oz.	815
CLOVE, GROUND (French's)	1 tsp. (1.7 g.)	4

Food and Description	Measure or Quantity	Sodium (milligrams)
CLUB SODA (See **SOFT DRINK**)		
CLUSTERS, cereal (General Mills)	½ cup (1 oz.)	140
COCOA:		
Dry:		
(USDA):		
Low fat	1 T. (5 g.)	<1
Medium-low fat	1 T. (5 g.)	<1
Medium-high fat	1 T. (5 g.)	<1
High fat	1 T.	<1
(Hershey's) unsweetened, American process	⅓ cup (1 oz.)	10
Home recipe (USDA)	1 cup (8.8 oz.)	128
Mix, regular pack:		
(Alba '66) instant, low fat, regular and chocolate with marshmallow flavor	6 fl. oz.	89
(Carnation) instant	1-oz. pkg.	120
(Hershey's) instant	3 T. (¾ oz.)	45
(Nestlé)	1.5-oz. pkg.	110
(Ovaltine) hot'n rich	1-oz. packet	183
Swiss Miss:		
Regular:		
Double rich	1 envelope	160
Milk chocolate	1 envelope	170
With mini marshmallows	1 envelope	150
European creme:		
Amaretto	1 envelope	120
Chocolate	1 envelope	180
Creme de menthe or mocha	1 envelope	120
Mix, dietetic or low calorie:		
(Carnation) *70 Calorie*	.73-oz. pkg.	125
(Ovaltine) reduced calorie	.45-oz. packet	88
Swiss Miss:		
Lite	1 envelope	160
Milk chocolate	1 envelope	190
with sugar-free marshmallows	1 envelope	130

Food and Description	Measure or Quantity	Sodium (milligrams)
(Weight Watchers)	1 envelope	160
COCOA KRISPIES, cereal (Kellogg's)	¾ cup (1 oz.)	190
COCOA PUFFS, cereal (General Mills)	1 cup (1 oz.)	170
COCONUT:		
Fresh (USDA):		
Whole	1 lb. (weighed in shell)	54
Meat only	4 oz.	26
Meat only	2″ × 2″ × ½″ piece (1.6 oz.)	10
Grated or shredded, loosely packed	½ cup (1.4 oz.)	15
Dried, canned or packaged: (Baker's):		
Angel Flake, bag	⅓ cup	73
Cookie	⅓ cup	109
Premium shred	⅓ cup	84
(Durkee) shredded	¼ cup	5
COCONUT, CREAM OF, canned:		
(Coco Lopez)	1 T.	5
(Holland House)	1 oz.	21
COCO WHEATS, cereal:	1 T. (.42 oz.)	3
Regular	1 T.	4
Instant	1¼ oz.	70
COD (USDA):		
Raw:		
Whole	1 lb.	98
Meat only	4 oz.	79
Broiled	4 oz.	124
Dehydrated, lightly salted	4 oz.	9185
Frozen:		
(Frionor) *Norway Gourmet*	4-oz. fillet	106
(Gorton's) *Fishmarket Fresh*	5 oz.	90
(National Sea Products):		
Plain, raw	5 oz.	95
*Breaded:		
Butter crumb	4 oz. cooked	150

Food and Description	Measure or Quantity	Sodium (milligrams)
Lemon pepper crumb (Van de Kamp's) *Today's*	4 oz. cooked	300
Catch	4 oz.	150
COD DINNER or ENTREE,		
frozen (Frionor) *Norway Gourmet:*		
With dill sauce	4.5-oz. fillet	169
With toasted bread crumbs	4.5-oz. fillet	359
COD LIVER OIL (Hain)	any quantity	0
COFFEE:		
Ground:		
(Chase & Sanborn) drip or electric perk; *Max-Pax;* (Maxwell House) regular or *Electra-Perk*; (Yuban) regular, drip or *Electra Matic*	6 fl. oz.	Tr.
Mellow Roast	6 fl. oz.	1
Decaffeinated:		
Brim, regular, drip or electric perk	6 fl. oz.	5
Decaf, Nescafé	6 fl. oz.	<10
Sanka	6 fl. oz.	1
Freeze-dried, *Taster's Choice*	6 fl. oz.	0
Instant:		
(Chase & Sanborn)	5 fl. oz.	1
(General Foods) *International Coffee:*		
Café Amaretto	6 fl. oz.	25
Café Francais	6 fl. oz.	24
Café Irish Crème	6 fl. oz.	19
Café Vienna	6 fl. oz.	93
Irish Mocha Mint	6 fl. oz.	24
Orange Cappuccino	6 fl. oz.	98
Suisse Mocha	6 fl. oz.	24
Mellow Roast	6 fl. oz.	2
Sunrise	6 fl. oz.	0
COFFEE SOUTHERN, liqueur	1 fl. oz.	Tr.
COGNAC (See **DISTILLED LIQUOR**)		

Food and Description	Measure or Quantity	Sodium (milligrams)
COLA SOFT DRINK (See **SOFT DRINK,** Cola)		
COLD DUCK WINE (Great Western) pink, 12% alcohol	3 fl. oz.	31
COLESLAW, solids & liq. (USDA):		
Prepared with commercial French dressing	4-oz. serving	304
Prepared with homemade French dressing	4-oz. serving	149
Prepared with mayonnaise	4-oz. serving	136
Prepared with mayonnaise type salad dressing	1 cup (4.2 oz.)	149
COLLARDS:		
Raw (USDA) leaves, including stems	1 lb.	195
Canned (Sunshine) chopped, solids & liq.	½ cup (4.1 oz.)	378
Frozen:		
(USDA):		
Not thawed	10-oz. pkg.	51
Boiled, chopped, drained	½ cup (3 oz.)	14
(Frosty Acres)	3.3 oz.	45
(McKenzie) chopped	3.3 oz.	56
(Southland) chopped	⅕ of 16-oz. pkg.	45
COLLINS MIXER (See **SOFT DRINK,** Tom Collins)		
COMPLETE, cereal (Elam's)	1-oz. serving	5
CONCORD WINE:		
(Gold Seal) 13-14% alcohol	3 fl. oz.	3
(Pleasant Valley) red, 12½% alcohol	3 fl. oz.	23
COOKIE (Listed below by type or brand name. See also **COOKIE, DIETETIC; COOKIE DOUGH; COOKIE, HOME RECIPE; COOKIE MIX**)		
Almond supreme (Pepperidge Farm)	1 piece	21

Food and Description	Measure or Quantity	Sodium (milligrams)
Animal:	1 piece (3 g.)	9
(USDA)	1 oz.	86
(FFV)	1 piece (.1 oz.)	13
(Gerber)	1 piece	10
(Nabisco) *Barnum's*	1 piece	11
(Ralston)	1 piece	7
(Sunshine)	1 piece	13
(Tom's)	1.7 oz.	200
Apple Newtons (Nabisco)	1 piece	30
Apple & raisin (Archway)	1 piece	169
Apricot-raspberry (Pepperidge Farm)	1 cookie	26
Assortment:		
(Nabisco) *Famous Assortment*:		
Baronet creme sandwich	1 piece	25
Biscos sugar wafer	1 piece	6
Butter flavored	1 piece	23
Cameo creme sandwich	1 piece	28
Kettle cookie	1 piece	29
Lorna Doone	1 piece	34
Oreo, chocolate	1 piece	57
(Pepperidge Farm):		
Butter	1 piece	27
Champagne, Original Pirouettes	1 piece	18
Seville	1 piece	25
Southport	1 piece	35
Blueberry (Pepperidge Farm)	1 piece	23
Blueberry Newtons (Nabisco)	1 piece	53
Bordeaux (Pepperidge Farm)	1 cookie	23
Brown edge wafer (Nabisco)	1 piece	16
Brownie:		
(Hostess):		
Large	2-oz. piece	122
Small	1¼-oz. piece	76
(Nabisco) *Almost Home*	1 piece	75
(Pepperidge Farm):		
Chocolate nut	1 piece (.4 oz.)	27

Food and Description	Measure or Quantity	Sodium (milligrams)
Nut, large	1 piece (.9 oz.)	65
Brussels (Pepperidge Farm):		
Regular	1 cookie	32
Mint	1 cookie	40
Butter flavored:		
(Nabisco)	1 piece	23
(Sunshine)	1 piece	37
Cappucino (Pepperidge Farm)	1 cookie	20
Capri (Pepperidge Farm)	1 cookie	45
Caramel Pattie (FFV)	1 piece	62
Cherry Newtons (Nabisco)	1 piece	53
Chessman (Pepperidge Farm)	1 cookie	26
Chocolate & chocolate covered:		
(USDA)	1 oz.	39
(Keebler) fudge stripes	1 piece	50
(Nabisco):		
Famous Wafer	1 cookie	40
Pinwheels, cake	1.1-oz. piece	35
Snaps	1 piece	20
(Sunshine) nugget	1 cookie	18
Chocolate chip:		
(USDA)	1 oz.	114
(Archway) & toffee	1 piece	160
(Keebler) *Rich 'n Chips*	1 piece	70
(Nabisco):		
Almost Home:		
Fudge	1 cookie	65
Real	1 cookie	50
Chips Ahoy!:		
Regular	1 cookie	32
Chewy	1 cookie	55
Chips 'n More:		
Coconut	1 cookie	47
Fudge	1 cookie	30
Original	1 cookie	35
Snaps	1 cookie	17
(Pepperidge Farm):		
Old fashioned	1 cookie	30
Chocolate	1 cookie	25

Food and Description	Measure or Quantity	Sodium (milligrams)
(Sunshine):		
Chip-A-Roos:		
Regular	1 cookie	50
Chocolate	1 cookie	80
Chippy Chews, any flavor	1 cookie	35
(Tom's)	1½ g.	110
Chocolate peanut bar (Nabisco)	1 cookie	65
Cinnamon raisin (Nabisco)		
Almost Home	1 cookie	47
Coconut fudge (FFV)	1 piece	32
Creme stick (Dutch Twin)	1 piece	3
Danish (Nabisco) imported	1 cookie	14
Date nut granola (Pepperidge		
Farm) Kitchen Hearth	1 cookie	32
Date pecan (Pepperidge Farm)	1 cookie	20
Devil's food cake (Nabisco)	1⅓-oz. piece	90
Dinosaurs (FFV)	1 oz.	110
Dutch cocoa (Archway)	1 piece	110
Fig bar:		
(FFV):		
Vanilla	1 piece	55
Whole wheat	1 piece	50
(Nabisco) *Fig Newtons*	1 piece (.6 oz.)	50
(Sunshine) Chewies	1 cookie	30
(Tom's)	1.8-oz. serving	130
Fruit stick (Nabisco) *Almost Home*:		
Apple	1 cookie	30
Blueberry	1 cookie	90
Cherry	1 cookie	100
Iced dutch apple	1 cookie	40
Geneva (Pepperidge Farm)	1 piece	21
Ginger Boys (FFV)	1 oz.	170
Gingerman (Pepperidge Farm)	1 piece	25
Gingersnap:		
(Archway)	1 cookie	20
(FFV)	1 oz.	140
(Nabisco) old fashioned	1 cookie	50
(Sunshine)	1 cookie	23

Food and Description	Measure or Quantity	Sodium (milligrams)
Golden fruit raisin (Sunshine)	1 piece (smallest portion after breaking on score line)	40
Hazelnut (Pepperidge Farm)	1 piece	37
Heyday (Nabisco)	1 cookie	45
Jelly tarts (FFV)	1 piece	55
Ladyfinger (USDA)	3¼″ × 1¾″ × 1⅛″	8
Lemon (Archway) frosty	1 piece	150
Lemon (Sunshine) cooler	1 cookie	22
Lemon nut crunch (Pepperidge Farm)	1 piece	25
Lido (Pepperidge Farm)	1 piece	42
Macaroon (Nabisco) soft	1 piece	65
Mallo Puffs (Sunshine)	1 cookie	60
Marshmallow (Nabisco):		
Mallomars	1 piece	17
Puffs, cocoa covered	1 piece	55
Sandwich	1 piece	20
Twirls	1 cookie	55
Milano (Pepperidge Farm)	1 piece	26
Mint fudge (FFV)	1 piece	25
Molasses:		
(Archway)	1 cookie	155
(Nabisco) *Pantry*	1 cookie	65
Molasses crisp (Pepperidge Farm)	1 piece	25
Nassau (Pepperidge Farm)	1 piece	45
Nilla wafer (Nabisco)	1 piece	14
Oatmeal:		
(Archway):		
Regular	1 cookie	90
Apple filled	1 cookie	115
Date filled	1 cookie	105
(FFV):		
Regular	1 piece	30
Bars:		
Apple	1 piece	55
Raisins	1 piece	40

Food and Description	Measure or Quantity	Sodium (milligrams)
Raspberry	1 piece	50
(Keebler) old fashioned:	1 piece	115
(Nabisco) *Bakers Bonus*	1 cookie	45
(Pepperidge Farm):		
Irish	1 piece	40
Raisin	1 piece	57
(Sunshine):		
Country style	1 cookie	60
Peanut sandwich	1 cookie	65
Orange Milano (Pepperidge Farm)	1 piece	35
Orbits (Sunshine):		
Butter flavored	1 cookie	19
Chocolate	1 cookie	21
Orleans (Pepperidge Farm)	1 piece	10
Peach apricot bar (FFV)	1 piece	50
Peanut or peanut butter:		
(Nabisco):		
Almost Home:		
Regular	1 cookie	47
Fudge	1 cookie	45
Creme pattie	1 piece	25
Nutter Butter, sandwich	1 piece	50
(Sunshine) wafer	1 cookie	17
Pecan Sandies (Keebler)	1 piece	52
Praline pecan (FFV)	1 piece	40
Raisin (Nabisco) *Almost Home*:		
Fudge chocolate chip	1 cookie	42
Iced applesauce	1 cookie	35
Iced oatmeal	1 cookie	40
Oatmeal	1 cookie	50
Raspberry filled (Archway)	1 piece	90
Rocky road (Archway)	1 piece	85
Royal Dainty (FFV)	1 piece	45
Royal kreem pilot bread (FFV)	1 piece	60
Sandwich:		
(FFV):		
Mint	1 piece	25
Peanut butter	1 piece	55

Food and Description	Measure or Quantity	Sodium (milligrams)
(Keebler):		
Fudge creme	1 cookie	30
Oatmeal creme	1 cookie	60
Pitter Patter	1 cookie	120
(Nabisco):		
Almost Home		
Baronet	1 cookie	25
Cameo	1 cookie	28
Gaity, fudge chocolate	1 cookie	
Giggles:		
Chocolate	1 cookie	35
Vanilla	1 cookie	25
I Screame	1 cookie	35
Mystic Mint	1 cookie	47
Oreo:		
Regular	1 cookie	57
Double Stuf	1 cookie	60
Mint	1 cookie	80
(Sunshine):		
Regular:		
Chocolate fudge	1 cookie	55
Cup custard	1 cookie	75
Hydrox	1 cookie	45
Vienna Fingers	1 cookie	60
Chips 'n Middles:		
Fudge	1 cookie	65
Peanut butter	1 cookie	70
Tru Blu	1 cookie	75
Shortbread:		
(FFV) regular or *Double*		
Pleasure	1 piece	45
(Nabisco):		
Lorna Doone	1 piece	33
Pecan	1 piece	40
Striped	1 piece	37
(Pepperidge Farm)	1 piece	43
Social Tea (Nabisco)	1 piece	18
Sprinkles (Sunshine)	1 piece	65
Strawberry (Pepperidge Farm)	1 piece	23

Food and Description	Measure or Quantity	Sodium (milligrams)
Strawberry filled (Archway)	1 piece	100
Sugar:		
(Nabisco) rings	1 piece	50
(Pepperidge Farm)	1 piece	38
Sugar wafer:		
(Keebler) *Krisp Kreem*	1 piece	14
(Nabisco) *Biscos*	1 piece	4
(Sunshine) wafer	1 piece	12
Sugar Heroes (Nabisco)	1 piece	11
Tahiti (Pepperidge Farm)	1 piece	25
Tango (FVV)	1 piece	25
Toy (Sunshine)	1 piece	18
Trolly Cakes (FFV)	1 piece	40
Vanilla wafer (FFV)	1 oz. serving	100
Waffle creme (Nabisco) *Biscos*	1 piece	10
COOKIE, DIETETIC:		
Chocolate chip		
(Estee)	1 piece	0
Coconut:		
(Estee)	1 piece	0
(Stella D'Oro)	1 piece	<10
Egg biscuit (Stella D'Oro)	1 piece	<10
Fruit & honey (Entenmann's)		
fat & cholesterol free	1 piece	55
Fudge (Estee)	1 piece	0
Kichel (Stella D'Oro)	1 piece	<10
Lemon (Estee) thin	1 piece	0
Oatmeal raisin:		
(Entenmann's) fat &		
cholesterol free	1 piece	60
(Estee)	1 piece	0
Peach apricot pastry (Stella D'Oro)	1 piece	<10
Prune pastry (Stella D'Oro)	1 piece	<10
Sandwich (Estee) original	1 piece	5
Sesame (Stella D'Oro)	1 piece	<10
Wafer (Estee):		
Chocolate covered	1 piece	10
Creme filled	1 piece	5

Food and Description	Measure or Quantity	Sodium (milligrams)
COOKIE CRISP, cereal (Ralston-Purina):		
Chocolate chip	1 cup (1 oz.)	190
Vanilla	1 cup (1 oz.)	220
COOKIE DOUGH:		
Refrigerated:		
(USDA):		
Unbaked, plain	1 oz.	141
Baked, plain	1 oz.	155
*(Pillsbury):		
Brownie, fudge:		
Regular	¹⁄₂₄ of pkg.	115
Microwave, with chocolate-flavored chips	¹⁄₉ of pkg.	110
Chocolate chip	1 piece	55
Chocolate chocolate chip	1 cookie	35
Oatmeal raisin	1 cookie	55
Peanut butter	1 piece	75
Sugar	1 piece	70
*Frozen (Rich's):		
Chocolate chip	1 piece	120
Oatmeal	1 piece	90
Oatmeal with raisin	1 piece	73
Oatmeal, super jumbo	1 piece	226
Peanut butter	1 piece	185
Ranger	1 piece	90
Sugar	1 piece	111
COOKIE, HOME RECIPE (USDA):		
Brownie with nuts	1¾″ × 1¾″ × ⅞″	50
Chocolate chip	1 oz.	99
Sugar, soft, thick	1 oz.	90
COOKIE MIX:		
Regular:		
Brownie:		
*(Betty Crocker):		
Regular:		
Caramel swirl	¹⁄₂₄ of pkg.	115

Food and Description	Measure or Quantity	Sodium (milligrams)
Chocolate chip	¹⁄₂₄ of pkg.	75
Frosted	¹⁄₂₄ of pkg.	120
Fudge:		
Regular	¹⁄₁₆ of pkg.	105
Family size	¹⁄₁₆ of pkg.	100
German chocolate	¹⁄₂₄ of pkg.	110
Supreme	¹⁄₂₄ of pkg.	85
Walnut	¹⁄₂₄ of pkg.	80
MicroRave:		
Frosted	1 brownie	120
Fudge	1 brownie	110
Walnut	1 brownie	95
(Duncan Hines):		
Chewey recipe	¹⁄₂₄ of pkg.	84
Fudge, original	¹⁄₂₄ of pkg.	99
Milk chocolate	¹⁄₂₄ of pkg.	91
Peanut butter	¹⁄₂₄ of pkg.	93
Truffle	¹⁄₂₄ of pkg.	130
Turtle	¹⁄₂₄ of pkg.	136
Gold Medal, fudge	¹⁄₁₆ of pkg.	85
*(Pillsbury) fudge:		
Deluxe:		
Plain	¹⁄₁₆ of pkg.	100
Family size	¹⁄₂₄ of pkg.	95
Walnut	¹⁄₁₆ of pkg.	90
Microwave	¹⁄₉ of pkg.	105
Ultimate:		
Caramel fudge chunk, chunky triple fudge or double fudge	¹⁄₁₆ of pkg.	105
Rocky road	¹⁄₁₆ of pkg.	95
Chocolate chip:		
*(Betty Crocker) *Big Batch*	1 cookie	50
(Duncan Hines)	¹⁄₃₆ of pkg.	41
Date bar (Betty Crocker)	¹⁄₃₂ of pkg.	35
Oatmeal (Duncan Hines) raisin	¹⁄₃₆ of pkg.	31
Peanut butter (Duncan Hines)	¹⁄₃₆ of pkg.	57

Food and Description	Measure or Quantity	Sodium (milligrams)
Sugar (Duncan Hines) golden	⅟₃₆ of pkg.	33
*Dietetic (Estee) brownie	2″ × 2″ piece	5
COOKING FATS (See **FAT, COOKING**)		
CORIANDER (HHS/FAO)		
Raw:		
Untrimmed	1 lb.	333
Leaves only	4 oz.	107
CORIANDER SEED (French's)	1 tsp. (1.4 grams)	Tr.
CORN:		
Fresh, white or yellow (USDA):		
Raw:		
Untrimmed, on the cob	1 lb. (weighed in husk)	Tr.
Trimmed, on cob	1 lb. (husk removed)	Tr.
Boiled:		
Kernels, cut from cob, drained	1 cup (5.8 oz.)	Tr.
Whole	4.9-oz. ear (5″ × 1¾″)	Tr.
Canned, regular pack:		
(USDA):		
Golden or yellow, whole kernel, solids & liq., vacuum pack	½ cup (3.7 oz.)	250
Golden or yellow, whole kernel, wet pack	½ cup (4.5 oz.)	302
Golden or yellow, whole kernel, drained solids, wet pack	½ cup (3 oz.)	203
White kernel, solids & liq.	½ cup (4.5 oz.)	302
White kernel, drained solids	½ cup (2.8 oz.)	189
White, whole kernel, drained liq., wet pack	4 oz.	268
Cream style	½ cup (4.4 oz.)	295
(Allen's) whole kernel, solids & liq.	½ cup (4.2 oz.)	300

Food and Description	Measure or Quantity	Sodium (milligrams)
(Comstock) solids & liq.:		
Cream style	½ cup	350
Whole kernel	½ cup	440
(Del Monte):		
Cream style, golden or white	½ cup	355
Whole kernel, solids & liq.	½ cup	355
(Green Giant) solids & liq.:		
Cream style, golden kernel	½ of 8½-oz. can	390
Whole kernel:		
Golden or yellow	¼ of 17-oz. can	280
Golden or yellow, vacuum pack	½ of 7-oz. can	280
Golden, *Mexicorn*	½ of 7-oz. can	330
White, vacuum pack	½ of 7½-oz. can	290
(Larsen) *Freshlike:*		
Cream style, golden	½ cup	290
Whole kernel:		
Regular, solids & liq.	½ cup	320
Vacuum pack:		
Plain	½ cup	260
With pepper	½ cup	300
(Le Sueur) golden, whole kernel, solids & liq.	¼ of 17-oz. can	376
(Libby's):		
Cream style	½ cup (4.3 oz.)	295
Whole kernel, solids & liq.	½ cup (4.4 oz.)	264
(Stokely-Van Camp):		
Cream style:		
Golden	½ cup (4½ oz.)	383
White	½ cup (4.6 oz.)	360
Whole kernel:		
Golden or yellow, solids & liq.	½ cup (4.5 oz.)	290
Golden, vacuum pack	½ cup (4.4 oz.)	418
White, solids & liq.	½ cup (4.5 oz.)	248
Canned, dietetic pack:		
(USDA):		
Whole kernel:		
Solids & liq.	4 oz.	2

Food and Description	Measure or Quantity	Sodium (milligrams)
Drained solids	4 oz.	2
Liquid only	4 oz.	2
Cream style	4 oz.	2
(Del Monte) no salt added, solids & liq.	½ cup	<10
(Diet Delight) whole kernel, solids & liq.	½ cup (4.4 oz.)	5
(Green Giant) no salt or sugar added	½ cup	0
(Larsen) *Fresh-Lite*, solids & liq.	½ cup	5
(S&W) *Nutradiet:*		
Cream style	½ cup	<10
Whole kernel, solids & liquid	½ cup	<10
Frozen:		
(USDA):		
On the cob, boiled, drained	5″ ear (4 oz.)	1
Whole kernel, boiled, drained	½ cup (3.2 oz.)	<1
(Birds Eye):		
On the cob:		
Regular	4.4 oz. serving	4
Big Ears	5.7-oz. serving	5
Little ears	4.6-oz. serving	4
Whole kernel:		
Cob corn, deluxe, baby	⅓ of 8-oz. pkg.	12
Deluxe, petite	⅓ of 8-oz. pkg.	2
Sweet:		
Regular	¼ of 12-oz. pkg.	3
In butter sauce	⅓ of 10-oz. pkg.	245
Deluxe, tender	⅓ of 10-oz. pkg.	3
(Frosty Acres):		
On the cob:		
Whole	1 ear	0
Piece	1 piece	0
Cut	3.3 oz.	0

Food and Description	Measure or Quantity	Sodium (milligrams)
(Green Giant):		
On the cob:		
Nibblers, regular or supersweet	1 ear	5
Niblets, regular or supersweet	1 ear	10
One Serving	1 half ear	5
Cream style	½ cup (4.4 oz.)	370
Whole kernel:		
Butter sauce:		
Golden	½ cup (4 oz.)	310
Niblets, One Serving	4½-oz. container	350
White, shoepeg	½ cup (4 oz.)	280
Harvest Fresh:		
Niblets	⅓ of 9-oz. pkg.	140
White, shoepeg	⅓ of 9-oz. pkg.	225
Polybag:		
Niblets:		
Regular	½ cup	120
Supersweet	½ cup	125
White	½ cup	5
(Larsen):		
On the cob	1 piece	5
Cut	3.3 oz.	5
(McKenzie):		
On the cob	5″ ear (4.4 oz.)	25
Whole kernel	3.3 oz.	19
(Ore-Ida) cob corn	5.3 oz. ear	35
CORNBREAD, home recipe (USDA):		
Corn pone, prepared with white, whole-ground cornmeal	4 oz.	449
Johnnycake, prepared with yellow, degermed cornmeal	4 oz.	782
Southern style, prepared with degermed cornmeal	2½″ × 2½″ × 1⅝″ piece (2.9 oz.)	491
Southern style, prepared with whole-ground cornmeal	4 oz.	712

Food and Description	Measure or Quantity	Sodium (milligrams)
Spoon bread, prepared with white, whole-ground cornmeal	4 oz.	547
CORNBREAD MIX:		
(USDA):		
Dry	1 oz.	328
*Prepared with egg and milk	2⅜″ muffin (1.4 oz.)	298
*(Aunt Jemima)	⅙ of pkg.	600
*_Gold Medal_ (General Mills):		
White	⅙ of mix	490
Yellow	⅙ of mix	500
*(Pillsbury) _Ballard_	⅛ of pkg.	570
***CORN DOG,** frozen		
(Hormel)	1 wiener	656
CORNED BEEF:		
Uncooked (USDA) boneless, medium fat	1 lb.	5897
Cooked (USDA) medium fat, boneless	4 oz.	1973
Canned:		
(Libby's)	⅓ of 7-oz. can	720
Dietetic (Featherweight) loaf	2½ oz.	53
Packaged:		
(Carl Buddig) smoked	1 oz.	380
(Eckrich)	1 oz.	340
(Hebrew National):		
1st cut	1 oz.	200
Full	1 oz.	210
(Oscar Mayer)	.6 oz.	202
CORNED BEEF HASH, canned:		
(USDA) with potato	1 cup (7.8 oz.)	1197
(Libby's)	1 cup (8 oz.)	1330
Mary Kitchen (Hormel):		
Regular	7½-oz. serving	1386
Short Orders	7½-oz. can	1368
CORNED BEEF SPREAD		
(Underwood)	½ of 4½-oz. can	605
CORN FLAKE CRUMBS		
(Kellogg's)	¼ cup (1 oz.)	290

Food and Description	Measure or Quantity	Sodium (milligrams)
CORN FLAKES, cereal:		
(USDA):		
Regular	1 cup (.9 oz.)	291
Crushed	1 cup (3 oz.)	704
Frosted	1 cup (1.4 oz.)	310
(General Mills) *Country*	1 cup (1 oz.)	280
(Kellogg's):		
Regular	1 cup (1 oz.)	290
Sugar frosted	¾ cup (1 oz.)	200
(Malt-O-Meal):		
Regular	1 cup (1 oz.)	268
Sugar frosted	¾ cup (1 oz.)	186
(Post) *Post Toasties*	1¼ cups (1 oz.)	310
(Ralston-Purina):		
Regular	1 cup (1 oz.)	267
Sugar frosted	¾ cup (1 oz.)	179
CORN FRITTER (See **FRITTER**)		
CORN GRITS (See **HOMINY GRITS**)		
CORNMEAL, white or yellow:		
Dry:		
Bolted:		
(USDA)	1 cup (4.3 oz.)	1
(Aunt Jemima/Quaker)	1 cup (4 oz.)	1
Degermed (USDA)	1 cup (4.9 oz.)	Tr.
Self-rising, degermed:		
(USDA)	1 cup (5 oz.)	1946
(Aunt Jemima)	1 cup (6 oz.)	2292
CORN POPS, cereal (Kellogg's)	1 cup (1 oz.)	95
CORN PUDDING, home recipe (USDA)	1 cup (8.6 oz.)	1068
CORN PUREE, canned (Larsen)	½ cup	6
CORNSTARCH:		
(USDA)	1 cup (4.5 oz.)	Tr.
(Argo; Duryea's or Kingsford's)	1 T. (9.5 g.)	Tr.
CORN STICK (See **CORNBREAD**)		

Food and Description	Measure or Quantity	Sodium (milligrams)
COTTAGE PUDDING, home recipe (USDA):		
Without sauce	2 oz.	170
With chocolate sauce	2 oz.	132
With strawberry sauce	2 oz.	132
COUGH DROP:		
(Beech-Nut)	1 drop (2 g.)	<1
(Pine Bros.)	1 drop (3 g.)	0
COUNT CHOCULA, cereal (General Mills)	1 cup (1 oz.)	205
COUNTRY CRISP, cereal (Post)	¾ cup (1 oz.)	197
COWPEA (USDA):		
Immature seeds:		
Raw, whole	1 lb. (weighed in pods)	5
Raw, shelled	½ cup (2.5 oz.)	1
Boiled, without salt, drained solids	½ cup (2.9 oz.)	<1
Canned, solids & liq.	4 oz.	268
Frozen (See **BLACK-EYED PEA**, frozen)		
Young pods, with seeds:		
Raw, whole	1 lb. (weighed untrimmed)	17
Boiled, drained solids	4 oz.	3
Mature seeds, dry:		
Raw	1 lb.	159
Raw	½ cup (3 oz.)	29
Boiled	½ cup (4.4 oz.)	10
CRAB, all species:		
Canned (USDA) drained solids	4 oz.	1134
Frozen (Wakefield's) Alaska King, thawed & drained	4 oz.	Tr.
CRAB, DEVILED:		
Home recipe (USDA)	1 cup (8.5 oz.)	2081
Frozen (Mrs. Paul's):		
Breaded & french-fried	3-oz. piece	385
Breaded & fried, miniatures	½ of 7-oz. pkg.	195

Food and Description	Measure or Quantity	Sodium (milligrams)
CRAB, IMITATION (See **SURIMI**)		
CRAB IMPERIAL:		
Home recipe (USDA)	1 cup (7.8 oz.)	1602
Frozen (Gorton's) *Light Recipe*, stuffed	1 pkg.	950
CRABAPPLE, fresh (USDA):		
Whole	1 lb. (weighed whole)	4
Flesh only	4 oz.	1
CRABAPPLE JELLY, sweetened:		
(Home Brands)	1 T.	15
(Smucker's)	1 T.	<10
CRACKED WHEAT CEREAL (See **WHEAT CEREAL, CRACKED**)		
CRACKERS, PUFFS and CHIPS (See also individual listings such as **POTATO CHIPS,** etc.):		
Arrowroot biscuit (Nabisco) *National*	1 piece (5 g.)	13
Bacon flavored thins (Nabisco)	1 piece (2 g.)	30
Bugles (General Mills):	15 pieces (1 oz.)	300
Regular	1 oz.	290
Nacho	1 oz.	250
Butter (Pepperidge Farm)	1 piece	33
Cafe (Sunshine)	1 piece (smallest portion after breaking on scoreline)	45
Cheese-flavored (See also individual brand names in this grouping):		
(USDA)	1 oz.	295
American Heritage (Sunshine):		
Cheddar	1 piece	30
Parmesan	1 piece	45
Better Blue Cheese (Nabisco)	1 piece	26
Better Cheddar (Nabisco)	1 piece	20

Food and Description	Measure or Quantity	Sodium (milligrams)
Better Nacho (Nabisco)	1 piece	24
Better Swiss (Nabisco)	1 piece	23
Cheddar Sticks (Flavor Tree)	1 oz.	445
Cheese Bites (Tom's)	1½ oz.	540
Chee•Tos:		
Crunchy:		
Regular	1 oz.	280
Light	1 oz.	360
Puffed balls	1 oz.	360
Puffs	1 oz.	330
Cheez Balls (Planters)	1 oz.	270
Cheez Curls (Planters)	1 oz.	290
Cheez-It (Sunshine)	1 piece	11
Corn cheese (Tom's):		
Crunchy	1⅝ oz.	270
Puffed, baked	1⅛ oz.	300
Dip In A Chip (Nabisco)	1 piece	16
(Dixie Bell)	1 piece	10
(Eagle)	1 oz.	330
Nachips (Old El Paso)	1 oz.	193
Nips (Nabisco)	1 piece	10
(Ralston)	1 piece	10
Tid-Bit (Nabisco)	1 piece (<1 g.)	12
Cheese & peanut butter sandwich (USDA)	1 oz.	281
Chicken in a Biskit (Nabisco)	1 piece (2 g.)	19
Club cracker (Keebler)	1 piece	39
Corn chips:		
Dipsy Doodle (Wise)	1 oz.	180
(Flavor Tree)	1 oz.	260
Fritos:		
Regular	1 oz.	230
Bar-B-Q	1 oz.	320
Chili cheese	1 oz.	310
Crisp 'N Thin or king size	1 oz.	210
Happy Heart (TKI Foods)	⅜ oz.	50
Heart Lovers (TKI Foods)	⅜ oz.	50
(Laura Scudder's)	1 oz.	125
(Planters)	1 oz.	224
Pringles	1 oz.	210

Food and Description	Measure or Quantity	Sodium (milligrams)
(Tom's):		
Regular	1 oz.	200
BBQ	1 oz.	220
Corn Snacker's (Weight Watchers):		
Lightly salted	.5-oz. pkg.	190
Nacho cheese	.5-oz. pkg.	240
Corn Stick (Flavor Tree)	1 oz.	220
Crown Pilot (Nabisco)	1 piece (.6 oz.)	70
English Water Biscuit (Pepperidge Farm)	1 piece	22
Escort (Nabisco)	1 piece	38
Goldfish (Pepperidge Farm), Tiny:		
Cheddar cheese, lightly salted, pizza or pretzel	1 piece	4
Parmesan	1 piece	6
Graham:		
(USDA)	2½″ sq. (7 g.)	47
(Dixie Belle) sugar-honey coated	1 piece	26
(Keebler) cinnamon crisp or honey	1 piece	21
(Ralston) sugar-honey coated	1 piece	26
(Sunshine):		
Cinnamon	1 piece (after breaking on scoreline)	24
Honey	1 piece (after breaking on scoreline)	22
Great Snackers (Weight Watchers:		
Barbecue or cheese	.5-oz. pkg.	170
Toasted onion	.5-oz. pkg.	120
Hi-Ho (Sunshine)	1 piece	31
Meal Mates (Nabisco)	1 piece	53
Nacho Rings (Tom's)	1 oz.	330
Oat thins (Nabisco)	1 piece	11

Food and Description	Measure or Quantity	Sodium (milligrams)
Ocean Crisp (FFV)	1 piece	120
Onion rings (Wise)	1 oz.	360
Oyster:		
(USDA)	10 pieces (.4 oz.)	110
(USDA)	1 cup (1 oz.)	312
(Dixie Belle)	1 piece	11
(Nabisco):		
Dandy	1 piece	11
Oysterettes	1 piece	8
(Ralston)	1 piece	11
(Sunshine)	1 piece	12
Party (Estee)	½ oz.	50
Party mix (Flavor Tree):		
Regular	1 oz.	400
No salt added	1 oz.	10
Peanut brittle & cheese (Eagle)	1.8-oz. serving	450
Pizza Crunchies (Planters)	1 oz.	160
Rich & Crisp (Dixie Belle)	1 piece	18
Ritz (Nabisco):		
Regular	1 piece	30
Low salt	1 piece	15
Ritz Bits (Nabisco):		
Regular	1 piece	5
Cheese	1 piece	6
Cheese sandwich	1 piece	22
Low salt	1 piece	3
Peanut butter	1 piece	13
Royal Lunch (Nabisco)	1 piece (1.7 g.)	80
Rye toast (Keebler)	1 piece	29
RyKrisp:		
Regular	1 triple cracker	37
Seasoned or sesame	1 triple cracker	52
Saltine:		
(Dixie Belle)		
Regular	1 piece	36
Unsalted top	1 piece	21
(Keebler) *Zesta*	1 piece	41

Food and Description	Measure or Quantity	Sodium (milligrams)
(Nabisco) *Premium*:		
Regular	1 piece	36
Bits	1 piece	10
Fat free or low salt	1 piece	23
Unsalted tops	1 piece	27
Whole wheat, *Premium Plus*	1 piece	26
(Ralston):		
Regular	1 piece	36
Unsalted Top	1 piece	21
(Sunshine) *Krispy*:		
Regular	1 piece	42
Unsalted	1 piece	24
Schooners (FFV):		
Regular	½ oz.	130
Whole wheat	½ oz.	160
Sesame (Estee)	½ oz.	120
Sesame crunch (Flavor Tree)	1 oz.	70
Sesame stick (Flavor Tree):		
Plain	1 oz.	405
With bran	1 oz.	370
No salt added	1 oz.	10
Sesame toast (Keebler)	1 piece	20
Snackers (Dixie Belle)	1 piece	23
Snackin' Crisp (Durkee) *O&C*	1 oz.	257
Snack sticks (Pepperidge Farm):		
Cheese	1 piece	43
Pumpernickel	1 piece	48
Sesame or cheese	1 piece	43
Sociables (Nabisco)	1 piece (2 g.)	22
Soda:		
(USDA)	1 oz.	312
(USDA)	2½" sq. (6 g.)	60
Sour cream & onion stick (Flavor Tree)	1 oz.	415
Spirals (Wise):		
Corn	1 oz.	125
Nacho cheese	1 oz.	190
Taco chip (Laura Scudder's) mini	1 oz.	200

Food and Description	Measure or Quantity	Sodium (milligrams)
Tortilla chip:		
Doritos:		
Regular	1 oz.	230
Cool Ranch:		
Regular	1 oz.	190
Light	1 oz.	240
Nacho cheese:		
Regular	1 oz.	240
Light	1 oz.	290
Salsa Rio	1 oz.	170
Taco flavored	1 oz.	220
(Eagle):		
Regular:		
Nacho	1 oz.	200
Ranch	1 oz.	150
Restaurant style	1 oz.	100
Strips	1 oz.	140
Del Mara	1 oz.	140
(La Famous):		
Regular	1 oz.	180
No salt added	1 oz.	5
(Laura Scudder's)	1 oz.	90
(Old El Paso):		
Crispy corn	1 oz.	105
Nachips	1 oz.	80
Santitas:		
Regular	1 oz.	75
Strips	1 oz.	65
(Tom's)	1 oz.	173
Tostitos:		
Jalapeño & cheese	1 oz.	160
Sharp nacho	1 oz.	200
Traditional	1 oz.	170
Tortilla strip (Laura Scudder's)	1 oz.	140
Town House (Keebler)	1 piece	29
Triscuit (Nabisco):		
Regular or wheat & bran	1 piece	25
Bits	1 piece	9
Low salt	1 piece	12
Tuc (Keebler)	1 piece	28

Food and Description	Measure or Quantity	Sodium (milligrams)
Twigs (Nabisco)	1 piece	28
Uneeda Biscuit (Nabisco)	1 piece	50
Unsalted (Estee)	1 piece	0
Vegetable thins (Nabisco)	1 piece	20
Waverly (Nabisco):		
Regular	1 piece	40
Low salt	1 piece	20
Wheat (Pepperidge Farm):		
Cracked	1 piece	50
Hearty	1 piece	45
Wheat nuts (Flavor Tree)	1 oz.	185
Wheat snack (Dixie Belle)	1 piece	12
Wheat Snax (Estee)	1 oz.	150
Wheat Thins (Nabisco):		
Regular	1 piece	15
Low salt	1 piece	7
Nutty	1 piece	24
Wheat toast (Keebler)	1 piece	30
Wheat wafer (Estee) *6 Calorie*	1 piece	0
CRACKER CRUMBS, GRAHAM:		
(USDA)	1 cup (3 oz.)	576
(Nabisco)	⅛ of 9″ pie shell or 2 T. (.5 oz.)	90
(Nabisco)	1 cup (3 oz.)	540
(Sunshine)	½ cup (2¼ oz.)	495
CRACKER MEAL:		
(USDA)	1 T. (.4 oz.)	110
(Nabisco) unsalted	½ cup (1.5 oz.)	0
CRANAPPLE juice drink (Ocean Spray) canned:		
Regular pack	6 fl. oz.	<3
Low calorie or dietetic	6 fl. oz.	<5
CRANBERRY:		
Fresh:		
(USDA)		
Untrimmed	1 lb. (weighed with stems)	9
Trimmed, stems removed	1 cup (4 oz.)	2
(Ocean Spray)	½ cup (2 oz.)	<1
Dehydrated (USDA)	1 oz.	5

Food and Description	Measure or Quantity	Sodium (milligrams)
CRANBERRY JUICE COCKTAIL:		
Canned:		
Regular pack:		
(Ardmore Farms)	6 fl. oz.	<1
(Ocean Spray)	6 fl. oz.	<2
Dietetic or low calorie		
(Ocean Spray)	6 fl. oz.	<13
*Frozen (Sunkist)	6 fl. oz.	8
CRANBERRY SAUCE:		
Home recipe (USDA) sweetened, unstrained	4 oz.	1
Canned:		
(USDA) sweetened, strained	½ cup (4.8 oz.)	1
(Ocean Spray):		
Jellied	2-oz. serving	5
Whole berry	2-oz. serving	6
CRAN-FRUIT (Ocean Spray):		
& apple	2 oz.	20
& orange, raspberry or strawberry	2 oz.	10
CRANICOT, drink (Ocean Spray)	6 fl. oz.	<5
CRAN-RASPBERRY JUICE DRINK (Ocean Spray)	6 fl. oz.	10
CRAZY COW, cereal (General Mills) chocolate	1 cup (1 oz.)	185
CREAM (See also **CREAM SUBSTITUTE**):		
Half & half:		
(USDA)	1 T.	7
(USDA)	½ cup (4.3 oz.)	56
(Johanna)	1 T. (.5 oz.)	6
(Land O'Lakes)	1 T.	5
Light, table or coffee:		
(USDA)	1 T. (.5 oz.)	6
(Johanna) 18% butterfat	1 T.	6
(Sealtest)	1 T. (.5 oz.)	6
Light whipping:		
(USDA)	1 cup (8.4 oz.)	86

Food and Description	Measure or Quantity	Sodium (milligrams)
(USDA)	1 T. (.5 oz.)	5
(Sealtest) 30% fat	1 T. (.5 oz.)	5
Heavy whipping (unwhipped):		
(USDA)	1 cup (8.4 oz.)	76
(Dean)	1 T. (.5 oz.)	5
(Johanna) 36% butterfat	1 T.	6
(Land O'Lakes) gourmet	1 T. (.5 oz.)	5
Sour:		
(USDA)	1 cup (8.1 oz.)	99
(Dean)	1 T. (.5 oz.)	6
(Friendship):		
Regular	1 T.	7
Light	1 T.	12
(Johanna)	1 T.	8
(Land O'Lakes):		
Regular	1 T.	10
Light:		
Plain	1 T.	15
With chives	1 T.	75
(Weight Watchers)	1 T.	20
Sour, imitation (Pet)	1 T. (.5 oz.)	25
CREAM PUFF:		
Home recipe (USDA) with custard filling	3½″ × 2″ piece (4.6 oz.)	108
Frozen (Rich's):		
Bavarian	1⅓-oz. piece	83
Chocolate	1⅓-oz. piece	83
CREAM SUBSTITUTE:		
(Carnation) *Coffee-mate*	1 tsp. (1.9 g.)	4
Coffee Rich, frozen, liquid	½ oz.	7
Cremora (Borden)	1 tsp.	5
Mocha Mix (Presto Food Products)	1 T.	5
N-Rich (Swiss Miss)	1 tsp. (2-g. packet)	2
CREME DE MENTHE LIQUEUR, green or white (Leroux)	1 fl. oz.	<1

Food and Description	Measure or Quantity	Sodium (milligrams)
CREPE, frozen (Mrs. Paul's):		
Crab	½ of 5½-oz. pkg.	578
Shrimp	½ of 5½-oz. pkg.	523
CRESS, garden (USDA):		
Raw, whole	1 lb. (weighed untrimmed)	45
Boiled, without salt, drained	1 cup (4.8 oz.)	14
CRISPIX, cereal (Kellogg's)	¾ cup (1 oz.)	220
CRISP RICE cereal:		
Regular (Ralston Purina)	1 cup (1 oz.)	208
Low Sodium (Van Brode)	1 cup (1 oz.)	2
CRISPY WHEAT 'N RAISINS cereal (General Mills)	¾ cup (1 oz.)	140
CROAKER (USDA):		
Atlantic:		
Raw, whole	1 lb. (weighed whole)	134
Raw, meat only	4 oz.	99
Baked	4 oz.	136
CROUTON (Kellogg's) *Croutettes*	⅔ cup (.7 oz.)	260
CRULLER (See **DOUGHNUT**)		
CUCUMBER, fresh (USDA):		
Eaten with skin	½ lb. (weighed whole)	13
Eaten without skin	½ lb. (weighed with skin)	10
Unpared, 10-oz. cucumber	7½″ × 2″ pared cucumber (7.3 oz.)	12
Pared	6 slices (2″ × ⅛″)	Tr.
Pared and diced	½ cup (2.5 oz.)	4
CUMIN SEED (French's)	1 tsp. (1.6 oz.)	3
CUPCAKE:		
Home recipe (USDA):		
Without icing	1.4-oz. cupcake	120
With chocolate icing	1.8-oz. cupcake	114
With boiled white icing	1.8-oz. cupcake	131
With uncooked white icing	1.8-oz. cupcake	114
Commercial type (Dolly Madison)	1.6-oz. cupcake	290

Food and Description	Measure or Quantity	Sodium (milligrams)
Chocolate	1¾-oz. cupcake	249
Orange	1½-oz. cupcake	170
CURRANT:		
Fresh (USDA):		
Black European:		
Whole	1 lb. (weighed with stems)	13
Stems removed	4 oz.	3
Red and white:		
Whole	1 lb. (weighed with stems)	9
Stems removed	1 cup (3.9 oz.)	2
Dried:		
(Del Monte) Zante	½ cup (2.4 oz.)	<10
(Sun-Maid) Zante	½ cup (2.5 oz.)	18
CURRANT JELLY, sweetened:		
(Home Brands)	1 T.	15
(Smucker's)	1 T. (.7 oz.)	<10
CUSTARD:		
Home recipe (USDA) baked	½ cup (4.7 oz.)	104
Canned (Thank You Brand) egg	½ cup (4.6 oz.)	195
C.W. POST, cereal, granola	¼ cup (1 oz.)	78

D

DAIQUIRI COCKTAIL MIX:		
Dry (Holland House)	.56-oz. pkg.	21
*Frozen (Bacardi)	4 fl. oz.	9
Liquid:		
*(Bar-Tender's)	3½ fl. oz.	50
(Holland House)	1 fl. oz.	4
DAIRY CRISP, cereal (Pet)		
high calcium	¼ cup (1 oz.)	140

Food and Description	Measure or Quantity	Sodium (milligrams)
DAIRY QUEEN/BRAZIER:		
Banana split	13.5-oz. serving	150
Brownie Delight, hot fudge	9.4-oz. serving	225
Buster Bar	5¼-oz. piece	175
Chicken sandwich	7.8-oz. sandwich	870
Cone:		
Plain, any flavor:		
Small	3-oz. cone	47
Regular	5-oz. cone	80
Large	7½-oz. cone	115
Dipped, chocolate:		
Small	3¼-oz. cone	55
Regular	5½-oz. cone	100
Large	8¼-oz. cone	145
Dilly Bar	3-oz. piece	50
Double Delight	9-oz. serving	150
DQ Sandwich	2.1-oz. sandwich	40
Fish sandwich:		
Plain	6-oz. sandwich	875
With cheese	6¼-oz. sandwich	1035
Float	14-oz. serving	85
Freeze, vanilla	14-oz. serving	180
French fries:		
Regular	2½-oz. serving	115
Large	4-oz. serving	185
Hamburger:		
Plain:		
Single	5.2-oz. burger	630
Double	7.5-oz. burger	660
Triple	9.6-oz. burger	690
With cheese:		
Single	5.7-oz. burger	790
Double	8.4-oz. burger	980
Triple	10.62-oz. burger	1010
Hot dog:		
Regular:		
Plain	3.5-oz. serving	830
With cheese	4-oz. serving	990
With chili	4½-oz. serving	985

Food and Description	Measure or Quantity	Sodium (milligrams)
Super:		
Plain	6.2-oz. serving	1365
With cheese	6.9-oz. serving	1605
With chili	7.7-oz. serving	1595
Lettuce	½ oz.	<10
Malt, chocolate:		
Small	10¼-oz. serving	180
Regular	14¾-oz. serving	260
Large	20¾-oz. serving	360
Mr. Misty:		
Plain:		
Small	8¼-oz. serving	<10
Regular	11.64-oz. serving	<10
Large	15½-oz. serving	<10
Kiss	3.14-oz. serving	<10
Float	14.5-oz. serving	95
Freeze	14.5-oz. serving	140
Onion rings	3-oz. serving	140
Parfait	10-oz. serving	140
Peanut Butter Parfait	10¾-oz. serving	250
Shake, chocolate:		
Small	10¼-oz. serving	180
Regular	14¾-oz. serving	260
Large	20¾-oz. serving	360
Strawberry shortcake	11-oz. serving	215
Sundae, chocolate:		
Small	3¾-oz. serving	75
Regular	6¼-oz. serving	120
Large	8¾-oz. serving	165
Tomato	½ oz.	<10
DANDELION GREENS		
(USDA):		
Raw, trimmed	1 lb.	345
Boiled, without salt, drained	½ cup (3.2 oz.)	40
DATE, dry:		
Domestic:		
(USDA):		
With pits	1 lb. (weighed with pits)	4
Without pits	4 oz.	1

Food and Description	Measure or Quantity	Sodium (milligrams)
Without pits, chopped	1 cup (6.1 oz.)	2
(Dole) California, pitted	½ cup	0
Imported (Bordo) Iraq	2 oz.	5
DENNY'S:		
BLT	1 serving	945
Chef salad	1 salad	14
Chicken:		
Sandwich, breast	1 sandwich	1512
Steak, fried	1 serving	620
Stir fry	1 serving	774
Club sandwich	1 sandwich	1689
Denny Burger	1 burger	428
Eggs, omelet, made with		
Egg Beaters	1 omelet	2673
Grand Slam	1 serving	2673
Halibut	1 serving	935
Patty melt	1 serving	1186
Super Bird	1 serving	1902
Turkey sandwich, sliced	1 serving	1263
DEWBERRY, fresh (See **BLACKBERRY,** fresh)		
DILL SEED (French's)	1 tsp. (2.1 g.)	Tr.
DINERSAURS, cereal (Ralston-Purina)	1 cup (1 oz.)	70
DIP:		
Acapulco (Ortega):		
Plain	1 oz.	1
With American cheese	1 oz.	172
With cheddar cheese	1 oz.	106
With Monterey Jack cheese	1 oz.	124
Bean (Eagle)	1 oz.	140
Bleu cheese (Dean) tang	1 oz.	14
Chili (La Victoria)	1 T.	90
Chili bean (Old El Paso)	1 T.	50
Guacamole (Calavo)	1 oz.	142
Hot bean (Hain)	1 T.	62
Jalapeño (Wise)	1 T.	50
Onion (Hain)	1 T.	67
Taco:		
(Hain)	1 T.	87

Food and Description	Measure or Quantity	Sodium (milligrams)
(Old El Paso)	1 T.	37
(Wise)	1 T.	57
DISTILLED LIQUOR. The values below would apply to unflavored bourbon whiskey, brandy, Canadian whiskey, gin, Irish whiskey, rum, rye whiskey, Scotch whiskey, tequila and vodka. The proof is twice the alcohol percent and the following values apply to all brands (USDA):		
80 proof	1 fl. oz.	<1
86 proof	1 fl. oz.	<1
90 proof	1 fl. oz.	<1
94 proof	1 fl. oz.	<1
100 proof	1 fl. oz.	<1
DOCK, including **SHEEP SORREL** (USDA):		
Raw, whole	1 lb. (weighed untrimmed)	16
Boiled, without salt, drained	4 oz.	3
DOUGHNUT:		
(USDA):		
Cake type	1.1-oz. piece	160
Yeast-leavened	.6-oz. piece	40
Commercial type (Dolly Madison):		
Regular:		
Plain, chocolate-coated or powdered sugar	1¼-oz. piece	240
Coconut crunch	1¼-oz. piece	350
Dunkin' Stix	1⅜-oz. piece	190
Gems:		
Chocolate coated	.5-oz. piece	90
Cinnamon sugar	.5-oz. piece	82
Coconut crunch	.5-oz. piece	62
Powdered sugar	.5-oz. piece	60
Jumbo:		
Plain or cinnamon sugar	1.6-oz. piece	220

Food and Description	Measure or Quantity	Sodium (milligrams)
Sugar	1.7-oz. piece	160
Old fashioned:		
Cinnamon chip	2.2-oz. piece	230
Chocolate glazed	2.2-oz. piece	250
Chocolate iced	2.2-oz. piece	190
Glazed	2.2-oz. piece	210
Orange crush	2.2-oz. piece	220
Powdered sugar	1.8-oz. piece	250
White iced	2.2-oz. piece	180
DRUM, raw (USDA):		
Freshwater:		
Whole	1 lb. (weighed whole)	83
Meat only	4 oz.	79
Red:		
Whole	1 lb. (weighed whole)	102
Meat only	4 oz.	62
DRUMSTICK, frozen, in a cone:		
Ice cream:		
Topped with peanuts	1 piece	82
Topped with peanuts & cone bisque	1 piece	72
Ice milk:		
Topped with peanuts	1 piece	87
Topped with peanuts & cone bisque	1 piece	77
DUCK, raw (USDA) domesticated meat only	4 oz.	84
DULCITO, frozen (Hormel):		
Apple	4 oz.	350
Cherry	4 oz.	345

Food and Description	Measure or Quantity	Sodium (milligrams)

E

ECLAIR:
  Home recipe (USDA) with
    custard filling & chocolate icing | 4-oz. piece | 93
  Frozen (Rich's) chocolate | 2.6-oz. piece | 194
ECTO COOLER DRINK,
  canned (Hi-C) | 6 fl. oz. | 17
EGG (USDA) (See also **EGG, SUBSTITUTE**):
  Chicken:
    Raw:

Food and Description	Measure or Quantity	Sodium (milligrams)
White only	1 large egg (1.2 oz.)	48
White only	1 cup (9 oz.)	372
Yolk only	1 large egg (.6 oz.)	9
Yolk only	1 cup (8.5 oz.)	125
Whole, small	1 egg (1.3 oz.)	45
Whole, medium	1 egg (1.5 oz.)	53
Whole, large	1 egg (1.8 oz.)	61
Whole	1 cup (8.8 oz.)	306
Whole, extra large	1 egg (2 oz.)	70
Whole, jumbo	1 egg (2.3 oz.)	79
Cooked:		
Boiled, without salt	1 large egg (1.8 oz.)	61
Fried in butter	1 large egg	155
Omelet, mixed with milk & cooked in fat	1 large egg	159
Poached	1 large egg	130
Scrambled, mixed with milk & cooked in fat	1 large egg	164

Food and Description	Measure or Quantity	Sodium (milligrams)
Scrambled, mixed with milk & cooked in fat	1 cup (7.8 oz.)	565
Dried:		
Whole	1 cup (3.8 oz.)	461
White, powder	1 oz.	313
Yolk	1 cup (3.4 oz.)	96
Duck, raw, whole	1 egg (2.8 oz.)	98
EGG, SUBSTITUTE:		
Egg Beaters (Fleischmann) plain	¼ cup (2.1 oz.)	80
Egg Magic (Featherweight)	½ envelope	123
*Scramblers (Morningstar Farms)	1 egg equivalent	75
Second Nature (Avoset)	3 T.	68
EGG DINNER or ENTREE, frozen (Swanson):		
Omelet:		
With cheese sauce & ham	7-oz. meal	1160
Spanish style	8-oz. meal	840
Scrambled with sausage & potatoes	6¼-oz. meal	790
*EGG FOO YOUNG, canned:		
(Chun King) stir fry	5-oz. serving	517
(La Choy)	1 patty plus ¼ cup sauce	760
EGG MIX (Durkee):		
*Omelet:		
With bacon	½ of pkg.	276
Puffy	½ of pkg.	333
Western	½ of pkg.	823
Scrambled:		
With bacon	1.3-oz. pkg.	476
Plain	.8-oz. pkg.	320
EGG NOG, dairy:		
(Borden)	½ cup	80
(Johanna)	½ cup	69
EGG NOG COCKTAIL (Mr. Boston)	3 fl. oz.	71

Food and Description	Measure or Quantity	Sodium (milligrams)
EGGPLANT:		
Raw (USDA) whole	1 lb. (weighed untrimmed)	7
Boiled (USDA) without salt, drained, diced	1 cup (7.1 oz.)	2
Frozen:		
(Buitoni) parmigiana	5-oz. serving	669
(Celentano):		
Parmigiana	½ of 16-oz. pkg.	400
Rollettes	11-oz. pkg.	210
(Mrs. Paul's):		
Parmigiana	½ of 11-oz. pkg.	905
Sticks, breaded and fried	½ of 7-oz. pkg.	610
(Weight Watchers) parmigiana, 1-compartment meal	13-oz. meal	1073
EGG ROLL, frozen:		
(Chun King):		
Regular:		
Chicken	3.6-oz. piece	600
Meat & shrimp	3.6-oz. piece	680
Shrimp	3.6-oz. piece	480
Restaurant style, pork	3-oz. piece	450
(La Choy):		
Chicken	.5-oz. piece	62
Lobster	.5-oz. piece	70
Lobster	3-oz. piece	485
Meat & shrimp	.24-oz. piece	42
Meat & shrimp	.5-oz. piece	73
Shrimp	.5-oz. piece	70
Shrimp	3-oz. piece	575
EGG ROLL DINNER or ENTREE, frozen:		
(La Choy) entrees:		
Almond chicken	2 egg rolls	1020
Beef & broccoli	2 egg rolls	1060
Spicy oriental chicken	2 egg rolls	690
Sweet & sour pork	2 egg rolls	720
(Van de Kamp's) Cantonese	10½-oz. meal	1100

Food and Description	Measure or Quantity	Sodium (milligrams)
ELDERBERRY JELLY, sweet-ened (Smucker's)	1 T.	<10
ELDERBERRY PRESERVE or JAM, sweetened (Smucker's)	1 T.	Tr.
EL POLLO LOCO, restaurant:		
Beans	3½-oz. serving	450
Chicken, 2-piece	4.8-oz. serving	460
Coleslaw	2.8-oz. serving	160
Combo	16-oz. serving	890
Corn	3.3-oz. serving	110
Dole Whip	4½-oz. serving	18
Potato salad	4.3-oz. serving	500
Rice	2½-oz. serving	250
Salsa	1.8-oz. serving	90
Tortilla:		
Corn	3.3-oz. serving	70
Flour	3.3-oz. serving	450
ENCHILADA:		
Canned (Old El Paso) beef	1 enchilada	325
Frozen:		
Beef:		
(Banquet):		
Dinner	12-oz. dinner	1810
Entree, family	2-lb. pkg.	5908
(Fred's Frozen Foods)		
Marquez	7½-oz. serving	915
(Hormel)	1 enchilada	573
(Old El Paso):		
Dinner	11-oz. dinner	1200
Entree	1 piece	720
(Swanson):		
Regular:		
Dinner	15-oz. dinner	1400
Entree	11¼-oz. entree	1190
Hungry Man	16-oz. entree	2010
(Van de Kamp's):		
Dinner, regular	12-oz. dinner	2177
Entree:		
Regular	7½-oz. entree	1201

Food and Description	Measure or Quantity	Sodium (milligrams)
Shredded	5½-oz. serving	930
(Weight Watchers) ranchero	9.1-oz. meal	930
Cheese:		
(Banquet) dinner	12-oz. dinner	2170
(Hormel)	1 enchilada	676
(Old El Paso):		
Dinner, festive	11-oz. dinner	1200
Entree	1 piece	830
(Patio)	12¼-oz. meal	2010
(Van de Kamp's):		
Dinner	12-oz. dinner	1664
Entree:		
Regular	7½-oz. meal	963
Ranchero	5½-oz. serving	540
(Weight Watchers)		
ranchero	8.87-oz. meal	900
Chicken:		
(Old El Paso):		
Dinner, festive	11-oz. meal	770
Entree:		
Regular	1 piece	740
With sour cream sauce	1 piece	520
(Weight Watchers) suiza	9.37-oz. meal	970
ENCHILADA SAUCE:		
Canned:		
(El Molino) hot	1 T.	50
(La Victoria)	1 T.	93
(Old El Paso):		
Green chili	¼ cup	400
Hot	¼ cup	248
Mild	¼ cup	250
(Rosarita)	1 oz.	143
*Mix (Durkee)	1 cup	96
ENCHILADA SEASONING		
MIX (Lawry's)	1.62-oz. pkg.	1723
ENDIVE, BELGIAN or		
FRENCH (See **CHICORY,**		
WITLOOF)		

Food and Description	Measure or Quantity	Sodium (milligrams)
ENDIVE, CURLY, raw (USDA):		
Untrimmed	1 lb.	56
Trimmed	½ lb.	32
Cut up or shredded	1 cup (2.5 oz.)	10

F

Food and Description	Measure or Quantity	Sodium (milligrams)
FAJITA, frozen:		
(Healthy Choice):		
Beef	7-oz. serving	250
Chicken	7-oz. serving	310
(Weight Watchers):		
Beef	6¾-oz. serving	730
Chicken	6¾-oz. serving	590
FAJITA SEASONING MIX		
(Lawry's)	1.27-oz. pkg.	2118
FARINA:		
Regular:		
Dry:		
(USDA)	1 cup (6 oz.)	3
(H-O) cream, enriched	1 cup (6.1 oz.)	Tr.
(H-O) cream, enriched	1 T.	<1
(3-Minute Brand)	2½ T.	<5
Cooked:		
*(USDA)	1 cup (8.4 oz.)	343
*(USDA)	4 oz.	163
*(Pillsbury) made with water and salt	⅔ cup	270
Quick-cooking:		
Dry (USDA)	1 oz.	71
Cooked (USDA)	1 cup (8.6 oz.)	466
Instant-cooking (USDA):		
Dry	1 oz.	2

Food and Description	Measure or Quantity	Sodium (milligrams)
Cooked	4 oz.	213
FAT, COOKING	Any quantity	0
FENNEL SEED (French's)	1 tsp. (2.1 grams)	2
FETTUCINI, frozen:		
(Armour Classics):		
Dining Lite, & broccoli	9-oz. meal	1020
Dinner Classics, chicken	11-oz. meal	660
(Green Giant) primavera	9½-oz. pkg.	610
(Healthy Choice):		
Alfredo	8-oz. meal	410
Chicken	8½-oz. meal	370
(Stouffer's) Alfredo	½ of 10-oz. pkg.	560
FIBER ONE, cereal (General Mills)	½ cup (1 oz.)	140
FIG:		
Fresh (USDA):		
Regular size	1 lb.	9
Small	1.3-oz. fig (1½″ dia.)	<1
Candied (Bama)	1 T. (.7 oz.)	<1
Canned, regular pack, solids & liq.:		
(USDA):		
Light syrup	4 oz.	2
Heavy syrup	3 figs & 2 T. syrup (4 oz.)	2
Heavy syrup	½ cup (4.4 oz.)	3
Extra heavy syrup	½ cup	<10
Canned, unsweetened or dietetic:		
(USDA) water pack, solids & liq.	4 oz.	2
(Diet Delight) Kadota, solids & liq.	½ cup (4.4 oz.)	4
(Featherweight) Kadota, water pack, solids & liq.	½ cup	<10
Dried (USDA):		
Chopped	1 cup (6 oz.)	58
Whole	.7-oz. fig (2″ × 1″)	7

Food and Description	Measure or Quantity	Sodium (milligrams)
FIG JUICE, canned (Sunsweet)	6 fl. oz.	24
FIGURINES (Pillsbury):		
Chocolate, chocolate peanut butter or vanilla	1 bar	45
Chocolate caramel	1 bar	55
FILBERT or HAZELNUT:		
(USDA):		
Whole	1 lb.	4
Shelled	1 oz.	<1
(Fisher) oil dipped, salted	½ cup (2 oz.)	114
FISH (See individual listings)		
***FISH BOUILLON** (Knorr)	8 fl. oz.	1130
FISH CAKE, frozen (Mrs. Paul's) thins, breaded and fried	½ of 10-oz. pkg.	1020
FISH & CHIPS, frozen:		
(Gorton's)	1 pkg.	1380
(Swanson):		
Dinner:		
Regular	10½-oz. dinner	970
Hungry Man	14¾-oz. dinner	1350
Entree	5½-oz. entree	585
(Van de Kamp's) batter dipped, french-fried	7-oz. pkg.	640
FISH DINNER, frozen:		
(Gorton's) fillet, almondine or in herb butter	1 pkg.	450
(Kid Cuisine) nuggets	7-oz. meal	750
(Morton)	9¾-oz. dinner	910
(Mrs. Paul's):		
Regular, parmesan	5 oz.	540
Light:		
Dijon	8½ oz.	650
Florentine	9 oz.	1025
Mornay	10 oz.	665
(Stouffer's) *Lean Cuisine:*		
Divan	12⅜-oz.	785
Florentine	9 oz.	815

Food and Description	Measure or Quantity	Sodium (milligrams)
(Van de Kamp's) fillet, regular	12-oz. dinner	1820
(Weight Watchers):		
Au gratin	9¼-oz. meal	700
Oven fried	7.1-oz. serving	500
FISH FILLET, frozen:		
(Frionor) *Norway Gourmet,* breaded	1.5-oz. piece	150
(Gorton's):		
Regular:		
Batter dipped, crispy	1 piece	290
Crunchy	1 piece	200
Microwave	1 piece	200
Potato crisp	1 piece	190
Light Recipe:		
Lightly breaded	1 piece	380
Tempura batter	1 piece	400
(Mrs. Paul's):		
Batter fried, light:		
Regular	3-oz. piece	415
Crunchy	2¼-oz. piece	417
Supreme	3.6-oz. piece	505
Breaded & fried:		
Crispy crunchy	2.1-oz. piece	325
Light & natural	6-oz. piece	770
Buttered	2½-oz. piece	390
FISH KABOBS, frozen		
(Van de Kamp's) batter dipped, french-fried	4-oz. serving	430
FISH NUGGET, frozen		
(Frionor) *Bunch O' Crunch,* breaded	.5-oz. piece	37
FISH SANDWICH, frozen		
(Frionor) *Bunch O' Crunch,* microwave	5-oz. sandwich	635
FISH STICK, frozen:		
(Frionor) *Bunch O'Crunch,* breaded	.7-oz. piece	70

Food and Description	Measure or Quantity	Sodium (milligrams)
(Gorton's):		
Batter dipped, crispy	1 piece	120
Crunchy:		
Regular	1 piece	70
Microwave	1 piece	70
Potato crisp	1 piece	97
Value pack	1 piece	105
(Mrs. Paul's):		
Batter fried, light & crunchy	1 stick (.8 oz.)	199
Breaded and fried	1 stick (¾ oz.)	114
(Van de Kamp's) batter dipped, French-fried:		
Regular	1-oz. piece	83
Light & crispy	.9-oz. piece	75
FLOUNDER:		
Raw (USDA):		
Whole	1 lb.	117
Meat only	4 oz.	88
Baked (USDA)	4 oz.	269
Frozen:		
(Frionor) *Norway Gourmet*	4-oz. fillet	350
(Gorton's):		
Fishmarket Fresh	5 oz.	170
Light Recipe:		
Fillet, entree	1 piece	710
Stuffed	1 pkg.	880
Microwave entree, stuffed	1 pkg.	850
(Mrs. Paul's) fillets:		
Batter fried, crunchy, light	2¼-oz. piece	555
Breaded & fried:		
Crispy, crunchy	2-oz. piece	400
Light & natural	3-oz. piece	487
(Van de Kamp's) *Today's Catch*	4 oz.	130
FLOUR:		
(USDA):		
Chestnut	1 oz.	3
Corn	1 cup (3.9 oz.)	1

Food and Description	Measure or Quantity	Sodium (milligrams)
Fish, from whole fish	1 oz.	48
Potato	1 oz.	10
Rice, stirred, spooned	1 cup (5.6 oz.)	8
Rye:		
Light:		
Unsifted, spooned	1 cup (3.6 oz.)	1
Sifted, spooned	1 cup (3.1 oz.)	4
Medium:	1 oz.	<1
Dark, unstirred or stirred	1 cup (4.5 oz.)	1
Sunflower seed, partially defatted	1 oz.	16
Wheat:		
All-purpose:		
Unsifted, dipped	1 cup (5 oz.)	3
Unsifted, spooned	1 cup (4.4 oz.)	3
Sifted, spooned	1 cup (4.1 oz.)	2
Bread:		
Unsifted, dipped	1 cup (4.8 oz.)	3
Unsifted, spooned	1 cup (4.3 oz.)	2
Sifted, spooned	1 cup (4.1 oz.)	2
Cake:		
Unsifted, dipped	1 cup (4.2 oz.)	2
Unsifted, spooned	1 cup (3.9 oz.)	2
Sifted, spooned	1 cup (3.5 oz.)	2
Gluten:		
Unsifted, dipped	1 cup (5 oz.)	3
Unsifted, spooned	1 cup (4.8 oz.)	3
Sifted, spooned	1 cup (4.8 oz.)	3
Self-rising:		
Unsifted, dipped	1 cup (4.6 oz.)	1403
Unsifted, spooned	1 cup (4.5 oz.)	1370
Sifted, spooned	1 cup (3.7 oz.)	1144
(Aunt Jemima) self-rising	¼ cup (1 oz.)	368
Ballard:		
All-purpose	¼ cup	<2
Self-rising	¼ cup	323
Bisquick (Betty Crocker)	¼ cup	350
Drifted Snow	¼ cup	<2

Food and Description	Measure or Quantity	Sodium (milligrams)
(Elam's):		
Brown rice, stone ground, whole grain	¼ cup	2
Buckwheat, pure	¼ cup	2
Pastry	1 oz.	2
Rye, stone ground, whole grain	¼ cup	3
Soy	1 oz.	5
Whole wheat, stone ground, whole grain	1 oz.	5
Gold Medal (Betty Crocker):		
All-purpose or unbleached	¼ cup	<2
High protein	¼ cup	<2
Self-rising	¼ cup	380
La Pina	¼ cup	Tr.
(Pillsbury):		
All purpose	¼ cup	0
All purpose, unbleached	¼ cup	1
Bread	¼ cup	0
Rye, medium	¼ cup	1
Sauce & gravy	1 T.	<5
Self-rising	¼ cup	322
Whole wheat	¼ cup	3
Presto, self-rising	¼ cup (1 oz.)	322
Purasnow:		
Regular	¼ cup (1 oz.)	1
Self-rising	¼ cup (1 oz.)	380
Red Band:		
Regular or unbleached	¼ cup (1 oz.)	1
Self-rising	¼ cup (1 oz.)	380
Red Star, self-rising	¼ cup (1 oz.)	380
Softasilk	¼ cup (1 oz.)	<5
Swans Down, cake:		
Regular	¼ cup	0
Self-rising	¼ cup	188
White Deer	¼ cup (1 oz.)	1
Wondra	¼ cup (1 oz.)	<3
FRANKEN*BERRY, cereal (General Mills)	1 cup (1 oz.)	210

Food and Description	Measure or Quantity	Sodium (milligrams)
FRANKFURTER, raw or cooked:		
(USDA):		
Raw, all kinds	1 frankfurter (10 per lb.)	499
(Eckrich):		
Beef	1.2-oz. frankfurter	380
Beef	1.6-oz. frankfurter	480
Beef	2-oz. frankfurter	620
Cheese	2-oz. frankfurter	650
Meat	1.2-oz. frankfurter	360
Meat	1.6-oz. frankfurter	470
Meat	2-oz. frankfurter	630
(Empire Kosher):		
Chicken	2 oz.	634
Turkey	2 oz.	746
(Hebrew National):		
Beef:		
Regular	1.7-oz. frankfurter	410
Lite	1.7-oz. frankfurter	360
Collagen	2.3-oz. frankfurter	555
Natural casing	2-oz. frankfurter	482
(Hormel):		
Beef	1 frankfurter (12-oz. pkg.)	362
Beef	1 frankfurter (1-lb. pkg.)	463
Chili, *Frank 'N Stuff*	1 frankfurter (00 oz.)	517
Meat	1 frankfurter (12-oz. pkg.)	378
Meat	1 frankfurter (1-lb. pkg.)	486
Wrangler's, smoked:		
Beef	1 frankfurter (00 oz.)	619
Cheese	1 frankfurter (00 oz.)	546
Range Brand	1 frankfurter (00 oz.)	600

Food and Description	Measure or Quantity	Sodium (milligrams)
(Morrison & Schiff) skinless	1.7-oz. frankfurter	410
(Ohse):		
Beef	1 oz.	280
Wiener:		
Regular	1 oz.	300
Chicken, beef & pork	1 oz.	260
(Oscar Mayer):		
Bacon & cheddar	1.6-oz. frankfurter	502
Beef:		
Regular	1.6-oz. frankfurter	459
Regular	2-oz. frankfurter	574
Regular	4-oz. frankfurter	1147
Bun-Length	2-oz. frankfurter	570
With cheese	1.6-oz. frankfurter	503
Cheese	1.6-oz. frankfurter	483
Little Wieners	.32-oz. frankfurter	92
Wiener:		
Regular	1.6-oz. frankfurter	466
Regular	2-oz. frankfurter	582
Bun-Length	2-oz. frankfurter	574
FRANKS AND BEANS (See **BEAN & FRANKFURTER**)		
FRENCH TOAST, frozen (Aunt Jemima):		
Regular	1½-oz. slice	216
Cinnamon swirl	1½-oz. slice	179
FRENCH TOAST & SAUSAGE, frozen (Swanson) plain	6½-oz. meal	770
FRITTER:		
Home recipe, corn (USDA)	2″ × 1½″ fritter (1.2 oz.)	541
Frozen (Mrs. Paul's):		
Apple	2-oz. fritter	385
Corn	2-oz. fritter	363
FROOT LOOPS, cereal (Kellogg's)	1 cup (1 oz.)	135
FROSTED RICE, cereal (Ralston-Purina)	1 cup	151
FROSTEE (Borden):		
Chocolate	1 cup	160

Food and Description	Measure or Quantity	Sodium (milligrams)
Strawberry	1 cup	150
FROSTING (See **CAKE ICING**)		
FROZEN DESSERT (See also **TOFUTTI**):		
(Baskin-Robbins)		
Low, Lite 'n Luscious	½ cup (4 fl. oz.)	50
Eskimo bar, chocolate covered	2½-fl.-oz. bar	40
Mocha Mix (Presto Food Products):		
Bar, vanilla, with chocolate coating	4-fl.-oz. bar	76
Bulk:		
Dutch chocolate	½ cup	90
Heavenly hash	½ cup	113
Mocha almond fudge or toasted almond	½ cup	75
Neopolitan or vanilla	½ cup	80
Peach	½ cup	64
Strawberry swirl	½ cup	65
FRUIT N'APPLE JUICE,		
canned or *frozen (Tree Top)	6 fl. oz.	10
FRUIT N'BERRY JUICE,		
canned or *frozen (Tree Top)	6 fl. oz.	10
FRUIT BITS, dried (Sun-Maid)	1-oz. serving	24
FRUIT N'CHERRY JUICE,		
canned or *frozen (Tree Top)	6 fl. oz.	10
FRUIT N'CITRUS JUICE,		
canned (Tree Top)	6 fl. oz.	10
FRUIT COCKTAIL:		
Canned, regular pack, solids & liq.:		
(USDA):		
Light syrup	4 oz.	6
Heavy syrup	½ cup (4.5 oz.)	6
Extra heavy syrup	4 oz.	6
(Del Monte) heavy syrup, regular or chunky fruit	½ cup (4½ oz.)	5
(Hunt's)	4 oz.	7

Food and Description	Measure or Quantity	Sodium (milligrams)
Canned, dietetic or unsweetened, solids & liq.:		
(USDA) water pack	4 oz.	6
(Del Monte) *Lite*	½ cup (4¼ oz.)	5
(Diet Delight)	½ cup (4.4 oz.)	5
(Libby's) water pack	½ cup (4.3 oz.)	10
FRUIT COMPOTE, canned		
(Rokeach)	½ cup (4 oz.)	4
FRUIT & CREAM BAR		
(Dole):		
Blueberry, chocolate-banana, chocolate-strawberry, raspberry or strawberry	1 bar	20
Peach	1 bar	15
FRUIT & FIBER, cereal (Post)	⅔ cup (1¼-oz.)	167
FRUIT & JUICE BAR:		
(Dole):		
Regular:		
Cherry, dark, sweet	1 bar	6
Peach passion fruit	1 bar	<1
Pina Colada	1 bar	4
Pineapple or pineapple-orange-banana	1 bar	5
Raspberry	1 bar	13
Strawberry	1 bar	9
Fresh Lites:		
Cherry	1 bar	12
Lemon	1 bar	30
Pineapple-orange	1 bar	6
Raspberry	1 bar	11
Sun Tops	1 bar	5
(Weight Watchers)	1.7-oz. bar	10
FRUIT, MIXED:		
Canned, regular (Hunt's)		
Snack Pack	5-oz. container	5
Canned, dietetic or low calorie (Del Monte) *Lite,* solids & liq.	½ cup	5

Food and Description	Measure or Quantity	Sodium (milligrams)
Dried:		
(Del Monte)	2 oz.	10
(Sun-Maid/Sunsweet)	2 oz.	11
FRUIT & NUT MIX (Carnation)	.9-oz. pkg.	10
FRUIT PUNCH:		
Canned:		
Bama (Borden)	8.45-fl.-oz. container	15
Capri Sun	6¾ oz.	1
(Hi-C)	6 fl. oz.	17
(Lincoln) party	6 fl. oz.	30
(Minute Maid):		
Regular	8.45-fl.-oz. container	24
On The Go	10-fl.-oz. bottle	29
Ssips (Johanna Farms)	8.45-fl. oz. container	<10
Chilled:		
Five Alive (Snow Crop)	6 fl. oz.	1
(Minute Maid)	6 fl. oz.	17
(Sunkist)	8.45 fl. oz.	0
*Mix:		
Regular (Funny Face)	6 fl. oz.	<10
Dietetic:		
Crystal Light	6 fl. oz.	<1
(Sunkist)	6 fl. oz.	15
FRUIT ROLL:		
Fruit Roll-Ups, Fruit Corners (General Mills):		
Cherry, fruit punch, grape or raspberry	.5-oz. roll	40
Strawberry	.5-oz. roll	45
Watermelon	.5-oz. roll	10
(Sunkist)	.5-oz. roll	10
FRUIT SALAD:		
Canned, regular pack, solids & liq.:		
(USDA):		
Light syrup	4 oz.	1

Food and Description	Measure or Quantity	Sodium (milligrams)
Heavy syrup	½ cup (4.3 oz.)	1
Extra heavy syrup	4 oz.	1
(Del Monte):		
Fruit for salad	½ cup (4.3 oz.)	<10
Tropical	½ cup (4.2 oz.)	<10
(Dole) tropical & passion		
fruit juice	½ cup (4 oz.)	10
(Libby's) heavy syrup	½ cup (4.4 oz.)	8
Canned, unsweetened or dietetic pack, solids & liq.:		
(USDA) water pack	4 oz.	1
(Diet Delight) juice pack	½ cup (4.4 oz.)	
FRUIT SLUSH (Wyler's) any flavor	4 fl. oz.	10
FRUIT WRINKLES, *Fruit Corners* (General Mills):		
Cherry or strawberry	1 pouch	115
Fruit punch	1 pouch	100
Grape	1 pouch	90
Watermelon	1 pouch	50
FRUITY YUMMY MUMMY, Cereal (General Mills)	1 cup (1 oz.)	160

G

GARFIELD AND FRIENDS		
(General Mills):		
Pouch:		
1-2 Punch	.9-oz. pouch	70
Very strawberry	.9-oz. pouch	60
Roll:		
Fruit party	.5-oz. roll	40
Wild blueberry	.5-oz. roll	20

Food and Description	Measure or Quantity	Sodium (milligrams)
GARLIC, raw (USDA):		
Whole	2 oz. (weighed with skin)	10
Peeled	1 oz.	5
GARLIC FLAKES (Gilroy)	1 tsp. (1.5 grams)	<1
GARLIC POWDER (Lawry's)	1 tsp.	5
GARLIC SALT (Lawry's)	1 tsp. (5.7 grams)	968
GAZPACHO SOUP, canned (Crosse & Blackwell)	½ of 13-oz. can	1653
GELATIN, unflavored, dry (Knox)	1 envelope	10
GELATIN DESSERT:		
Canned, dietetic (Dia-Mel; Louis Sherry)	4 oz.	5
Powder:		
*Regular:		
(Jello):		
Apricot, black cherry, mixed fruit, orange, peach, raspberry, strawberry or strawberry-banana	½ cup	55
Blackberry	½ cup	54
Cherry	½ cup	77
Grape, concord	½ cup	40
Lemon or wild strawberry	½ cup	81
Lime	½ cup	62
Orange-pineapple	½ cup	70
Raspberry, black	½ cup	39
(Royal) all fruit flavors	½ cup (4.9 oz.)	90–100
*Dietetic or low calorie:		
Carmel Kosher, all flavors	½ cup	<10
(Estee)	½ cup	10
(Featherweight) all flavors, artificially sweetened	½ cup	2
(Jell-O):		
Cherry	½ cup	80
Lime	½ cup	60

Food and Description	Measure or Quantity	Sodium (milligrams)
Orange	½ cup	56
Raspberry or strawberry	½ cup	56
(Louis Sherry) *Shimmer*	½ cup	10
(Royal)	½ cup	70
GELATIN, DRINKING (Knox)		
orange	1 envelope	20
GIN, unflavored (see **DISTILLED LIQUOR**)		
GINGERBREAD:		
Home recipe (USDA)	1.9-oz piece (2″ × 2″ × 2″)	130
*Mix:		
(USDA)	⅑ of 8″ sq. (2.2 oz.)	192
(Betty Crocker)	⅑ of pkg.	330
(Pillsbury)	3″ sq. (⅑ of pkg.)	310
GINGER ROOT, fresh (USDA):		
With skin	1 oz.	2
Without skin	1 oz.	2
GOLDEN GRAHAMS, cereal (General Mills)	¾ cup (1 oz.)	280
GOOBER GRAPE (Smucker's)	1 T.	60
GOOSE, domesticated (USDA) roasted, meat only	4 oz.	141
GOOSEBERRY (USDA):		
Fresh	1 lb.	5
Fresh	1 cup (5.3 oz.)	2
Canned, water pack, solids & liq.	4 oz.	1
GRAHAM CRACKER (See **CRACKERS, PUFFS AND CHIPS**)		
GRANOLA BAR:		
Nature Valley (General Mills):		
Cinnamon or peanut butter	.8-oz. bar	70
Oat-bran–honey graham	.8-oz. bar	90
Oats 'N Honey	.8-oz. bar	65
(Hershey's) chocolate covered:		
Chocolate chip, cocoa creme or cookies & creme	1.2-oz. piece	50

Food and Description	Measure or Quantity	Sodium (milligrams)
Peanut butter	1.2-oz. piece	65
GRANOLA CEREAL,		
Nature Valley:		
Cinnamon raisin or toasted oat	⅓ cup (1 oz.)	90
Coconut & honey	⅓ cup (1 oz.)	35
Fruit & nut	⅓ cup (1 oz.)	80
Sun Country (Kretschmer)	¼ cup (1 oz.)	10
GRAPE:		
Fresh:		
American type (slip skin), Concord, Delaware, Niagara, Catawba and Scuppernong:		
(USDA)	½ lb. (weighed with stem, skin & seeds)	4
(USDA)	½ cup (2.7 oz.)	1
(USDA)	3½″ × 3″ bunch (3.5 oz.)	2
European type (adherent skin), Malaga, Muscat, Thompson seedless, Emperor & Flame Tokay:		
(USDA)	½ lb. (weighed with stem & seeds)	6
(USDA) whole	20 grapes (¾″ dia.)	2
(USDA) whole	½ cup (.3 oz.)	3
Canned, solids & liq.:		
(USDA) Thompson, seedless, heavy syrup	4 oz.	5
(USDA) Thompson, seedless, water pack	4 oz.	5
(Featherweight) water pack, seedless	½ cup	<10
(Thank You Brand) in heavy syrup	½ cup (4.1 oz.)	6
GRAPEADE, chilled or frozen (Minute Maid)	6 fl. oz.	18

Food and Description	Measure or Quantity	Sodium (milligrams)
GRAPE APPLE DRINK,		
canned (Mott's)	10-fl.-oz.	
	container	<1
GRAPE DRINK:		
Canned:		
Bama (Borden)	8.45-fl.-oz.	
	container	25
(Capri Sun)	6¾ fl. oz.	19
(Hi-C)	6 fl. oz.	17
(Lincoln)	6 fl. oz.	30
Ssips (Johanna Farms)	8.45-fl.-oz.	
	container	20
(Sunkist)	8.45 fl. oz.	0
Chilled (Sunkist)	8.45 fl.-oz.	
	container	0
*Mix:		
Regular (Funny Face)	6 fl. oz.	0
Dietetic (Sunkist)	6 fl. oz.	19
GRAPE JAM, sweetened		
(Smucker's)	1 T.	5
GRAPE JELLY:		
Sweetened:		
(Bama)	1 T.	7
(Home Brands)	1 T.	15
Dietetic (See **GRAPE SPREAD)**		
GRAPE JUICE:		
Canned:		
(USDA)	½ cup (4.4 oz.)	3
(Ardmore Farms)	6 fl. oz.	2
(Minute Maid)	8.45-fl.-oz.	
	container	30
(Seneca Foods)	6 fl. oz.	4
Sippin' Pak (Borden)	8.45-fl.-oz.	
	container	25
(Tree Ripe)	8.45-fl.-oz.	
	container	7
*(Welch's):		
Regular	6 fl. oz.	5
Red or white	6 fl. oz.	15

Food and Description	Measure or Quantity	Sodium (milligrams)
Sparkling red or white	6 fl. oz.	30
Chilled (Minute Maid)	6 fl. oz.	21
*Frozen, sweetened:		
(USDA)	½ cup (4.4 oz.)	1
(Minute Maid)	6 fl. oz.	2
(Ocean Spray)	6 fl. oz.	10
GRAPE JUICE DRINK:		
Canned, *Squeezit* (General Mills)	6¾-fl.-oz. container	30
*Frozen:		
(Ocean Spray)	6 fl. oz.	10
(Sunkist)	6 fl. oz.	3
GRAPE NUTS, cereal		
(Post):		
Regular	¼ cup (1 oz.)	170
Flakes	⅞ cup (1 oz.)	110
Raisin	¼ cup (1 oz.)	141
GRAPE SPREAD, low sugar:		
(Diet Delight)	1 T. (.6 oz.)	15
(Estee)	1 T. (.6 oz.)	Tr.
(Featherweight)	1 T.	40–50
(Louis Sherry)	1 T.	<3
(Smucker's) regular	1 T.	34
GRAPEFRUIT:		
Fresh (USDA):		
White:		
Seeded type	1 lb. (weighed with seeds & skin)	2
Seedless type	1 lb. (weighed with skin)	2
Seeded type	½ med. grapefruit (3¾" dia., 8.5 oz.)	1
Pink and red:		
Seeded type	1 lb. (weighed with seeds & skin)	2
Seedless type	1 lb. (weighed with skin)	2

Food and Description	Measure or Quantity	Sodium (milligrams)
Seeded type	½ med. grapefruit (3¾″ dia., 8.5 oz.)	1
Canned, syrup pack (Del Monte) solids & liq.	½ cup	2
Canned, unsweetened or dietetic pack, solids & liq.:		
(USDA) water pack	½ cup (4.2 oz.)	5
Del Monte) sections	½ cup	2
(Diet Delight) sections, juice pack	½ cup (4.3 oz.)	5
(Featherweight) sections, juice pack	½ of 8-oz. can	<10
GRAPEFRUIT JUICE:		
Fresh (USDA) pink, red or white, all varieties	½ cup (4.3 oz.)	1
Canned:		
Sweetened:		
(USDA)	½ cup (4.4 oz.)	1
(Del Monte)	6 fl. oz.	2
(Johanna Farms)	6 fl. oz.	4
(Minute Maid) *On The Go*	10 fl. oz.	31
(Mott's)	9.5-fl.-oz. can	5
Unsweetened:		
(USDA)	½ cup (4.4 oz.)	1
(Del Monte)	6 fl. oz.	<10
(Libby's)	6 fl. oz.	0
(Ocean Spray)	6 fl. oz. (6.5 oz.)	10
(Texsun) pink	6 fl. oz.	2
(Tree Top)	6 fl.-oz.	0
Chilled:		
(Minute Maid)	6 fl. oz.	19
(Sunkist)	6 fl. oz.	2
*Frozen:		
Sweetened (USDA) diluted with 3 parts water	½ cup (4.4 oz.)	1
Unsweetened:		
(USDA) diluted with 3 parts water	½ cup (4.4 oz.)	1
(Minute Maid)	6 fl. oz.	19

Food and Description	Measure or Quantity	Sodium (milligrams)
(Sunkist)	6 fl. oz.	1
*Dehydrated crystals (USDA) reconstituted	½ cup (4.4 oz.)	1
GRAPEFRUIT JUICE COCKTAIL:		
Canned (Ocean Spray) pink	6 fl. oz.	15
Chilled (Minute Maid)	6 fl. oz.	18
*Frozen (Minute Maid)	6 fl. oz.	18
GRAVY:		
Canned:		
Au jus (Franco-American)	2-oz. serving	290
Beef (Franco-American)	2-oz. serving	310
Brown:		
(Franco-American) with onion	2-oz. serving	340
(La Choy)	1 oz.	73
Chicken (Franco-American) Regular or giblet	2-oz. serving	320
Mushroom (Franco-American)	2-oz. serving	320
Pork (Franco-American)	2-oz. serving	350
Turkey (Franco-American)	2-oz. serving	300
Mix, regular:		
Au jus:		
*French's) *Gravy Makins*	1 cup	1040
*(Lawry's)	1 cup	3454
*Brown:		
With onions	1 cup	1356
(French's) *Gravy Makins*	1 cup	1000
(Knorr) classic	1 cup	1200
(Lawry's)	1 cup	1500
(Pillsbury)	1 cup	1200
(Spatini)	1-oz. serving	205
Chicken:		
*(French's) *Gravy Makins*	1 cup	1080
*(Pillsbury)	1 cup	920
*Homestyle:		
(French's) *Gravy Makins*	1 cup	1000
(Pillsbury)	1 cup	1200

Food and Description	Measure or Quantity	Sodium (milligrams)
*Mushroom: (French's)		
Gravy Makins	1 cup	1000
*Onion: (French's)		
Gravy Makins	1 cup	1080
GRAVY MASTER	1 tsp. (.2 oz.)	127
GREAT BEGINNINGS (Hormel):		
With chunky beef	5 oz.	904
With chunky chicken or pork	5 oz.	567
With chunky turkey	5 oz.	585
GREENS, MIXED, canned:		
(Allen's)	½ cup	100
(Sunshine) solids & liq.	½ cup (4.1 oz.)	468
GREEN PEA (See **PEA, GREEN**)		
GRENADINE SYRUP (Rose's)	1 fl. oz.	27
GRITS (See **HOMINY GRITS**)		
GUACAMOLE SEASONING MIX		
(Lawry's)	.7-oz. pkg.	1495
GUAVA, COMMON, fresh (USDA):		
Whole	1 lb. (weighed untrimmed)	18
Whole	1 guava (2.8 oz.)	3
Flesh only	4 oz.	5
GUAVA, STRAWBERRY, fresh (USDA):		
Whole	1 lb. (weighed untrimmed)	18
Flesh only	4 oz.	<5
GUAVA FRUIT DRINK, canned		
Mauna La'i	6 fl. oz.	10
GUAVA JELLY (Smucker's)	1 T.	<10
GUAVA NECTAR, canned		
(Libby's)	6 fl. oz.	5
GUAVA-PASSION FRUIT DRINK, canned *Mauna La'l*	6 fl. oz.	10

Food and Description	Measure or Quantity	Sodium (milligrams)

H

HADDOCK:
  Raw (USDA):

Whole	1 lb.	133
Meat only	4 oz.	69
Fried, breaded (USDA)	4″ × 3″ × ½″ fillet (3.5 oz.)	176
Frozen:		
(Frionor) *Norway Gourmet*	4-oz. fillet	149
(Gorton's):		
Fishmarket Fresh	5 oz.	120
Microwave entree in lemon butter	1 pkg.	730
(Mrs. Paul's):		
Batter fried, crunchy & light	2 oz.	400
Breaded & fried:		
Crispy, crunchy	6 oz.	960
Light & natural	2¼ oz.	468
(Van de Kamp's) batter dipped, french-fried	2-oz. piece	215
HAKE, raw (USDA):		
Whole	1 lb.	144
Meat only	4 oz.	84
HALF & HALF (milk & cream) (see **CREAM**)		
HALIBUT:		
Atlantic & Pacific (USDA):		
Raw:		
Whole	1 lb. (weighed whole)	145

Food and Description	Measure or Quantity	Sodium (milligrams)
Meat only	4 oz.	61
Broiled	4.4 oz. (4″ × 3″ × ½″ steak)	168
Frozen (Van de Kamp's) batter dipped, French-fried	½ of 8-oz. pkg.	440
HAM (See also **PORK**):		
Canned:		
(Hormel):		
Black Label	4 oz. (1½-lb. ham)	1324
Black Label	4 oz. (5-lb. ham)	1245
Chopped	3 oz. (8-lb. ham)	1062
Chunk	6¾-oz. serving	2241
Curemaster	4 oz.	1361
EXL	4 oz.	1382
Patties	1 patty	456
(Oscar Mayer) *Jubilee,* extra lean, cooked	¹⁄₁₂ of 3-lb. ham (4 oz.)	1144
(Swift):		
Hostess	¼″ slice (3.5 oz.)	1231
Premium	1¾-oz. slice (5″ × 2″ × ¼″)	535
Canned, deviled:		
(Hormel)	1 T.	108
(Underwood)	1 T. (.5 oz.)	142
Packaged, cooked:		
(Carl Buddig) smoked	1 oz.	400
(Eckrich):		
Chopped:		
Regular	1-oz. slice	330
Smorgas pac	¾-oz. slice	250
Cooked	1.2-oz. slice	470
Danish	1.3-oz. slice	487
Loaf	1-oz. slice	330
Smoked, cured:		
Regular	¾-oz. slice	270
Slender-sliced	1 oz.	360
(Hormel) chopped	1 slice	347

Food and Description	Measure or Quantity	Sodium (milligrams)
(Ohse):		
Chopped or cooked	1 oz.	260
Smoked:		
Regular	1 oz.	320
95% fat free	1 oz.	310
Turkey ham	1 oz.	370
(Oscar Mayer):		
Baked, cooked	.7-oz. slice	235
Black pepper, cracked	.7-oz. slice	284
Boiled	.7-oz. slice	275
Breakfast	1½-oz. slice	582
Chopped	1-oz. slice	324
Honey	.7-oz. slice	268
Lower salt	.7-oz. slice	166
Slice, *Jubilee*	1-oz. serving	335
Steak, *Jubilee*	2-oz. serving	756
Smoked, cooked	¾-oz. slice	265
HAM & ASPARAGUS BAKE, frozen (Stouffer's)	9½-oz. meal	900
HAMBURGER (See **BEEF,** Ground; *McDONALD'S; BURGER KING;* etc.)		
*HAMBURGER MIX		
Hamburger Helper (General Mills):		
Beef noodle	⅕ of pkg.	1050
Beef Romanoff	⅕ of pkg.	1070
Cheeseburger macaroni	⅕ of pkg.	1030
Chili, with beans	¼ of pkg.	1740
Chili tomato	⅕ of pkg.	1410
Hash	⅕ of pkg.	1020
Lasagna	⅕ of pkg.	1050
Pizzabake	⅙ of pkg.	840
Pizza dish	⅕ of pkg.	1010
Potato stroganoff	⅕ of pkg.	950
Spaghetti	⅕ of pkg.	1110
HAM & CHEESE:		
Canned (Hormel):		
Loaf	3 oz.	1135

Food and Description	Measure or Quantity	Sodium (milligrams)
Patties	1 patty	468
Packaged:		
(Eckrich)	1-oz. slice	350
(Hormel) loaf	1 slice	334
HAM DINNER, frozen:		
(Armour) *Dinner Classics*,		
steak	10¾-oz. meal	1320
(Banquet)	10-oz. meal	1180
(Morton)	10-oz. meal	700
HAM SALAD SPREAD:		
(Carnation) spreadable	1½-oz. serving	264
(Oscar Mayer)	1-oz. serving	259
HARDEE'S:		
Apple turnover	3.2-oz. piece	250
Big Cookie	1.7-oz. serving	240
Big Country Breakfast:		
Bacon	7.65-oz. serving	1540
Country ham	8.96-oz. serving	2870
Ham	8.85-oz. serving	1780
Sausage	9.7-oz. serving	1980
Biscuit:		
Bacon	3.3-oz. serving	950
Bacon & egg	4.4-oz. serving	990
Bacon, egg & cheese	4.8-oz. serving	1220
Chicken	5.1-oz. serving	1330
Country ham:		
Plain	3.8-oz. serving	1550
& egg	4.9-oz. serving	1600
'N' Gravy	7.8-oz. serving	1250
Ham:		
Plain	3.7-oz. serving	1000
With egg	4.9-oz. serving	1050
With egg & cheese	5.3-oz. serving	1270
Rise 'N' Shine:		
Plain	2.9-oz. serving	740
Canadian bacon	5.7-oz. serving	1550
Sausage:		
Plain	4.2-oz. serving	1100
With egg	5.3-oz. serving	1150

Food and Description	Measure or Quantity	Sodium (milligrams)
Steak:		
Plain	5.2-oz. serving	1320
With egg	6.3-oz. serving	1370
Cheeseburger:		
Plain	4.4-oz. serving	710
Bacon	7.7-oz. serving	1030
Quarter-pound	6.4-oz. serving	1060
Chicken fillet sandwich	6.1-oz. serving	1060
Chicken, grilled, sandwich	6.8-oz. serving	890
Chicken Stix:		
6-piece	3½-oz. serving	680
9-piece	5.3-oz. serving	1020
Cool Twist:		
Cone:		
Chocolate	4.2-oz. serving	65
Vanilla	4.2-oz. serving	100
Vanilla/chocolate	4.2-oz. serving	80
Sundae:		
Caramel	6-oz. serving	290
Hot fudge	5.9-oz. serving	270
Strawberry	5.9-oz. serving	115
Fisherman's Fillet, sandwich	7.3-oz. serving	1030
Hamburger:		
Plain	3.9-oz. serving	490
Big Deluxe	7.6-oz. serving	760
Mushroom 'N' Swiss	6.6-oz. serving	940
Hot dog, all beef	4.2-oz. serving	710
Hot Ham 'N Cheese sandwich	5.3-oz. serving	1420
Margarine-butter blend	.2-oz. serving	40
Pancakes, three:		
Plain	4.8-oz. serving	15
With one sausage pattie	6.2-oz. serving	1290
With two bacon strips	5.3-oz. serving	1110
Potato:		
French fries	2½-oz. regular order	85
French fries	4-oz. large order	135
Hash Rounds	2.8-oz. serving	560
Roast beef:		
Regular	4-oz. serving	730

Food and Description	Measure or Quantity	Sodium (milligrams)
Big Roast Beef	4.7-oz. serving	880
Salad:		
Chef	10.4-oz. serving	930
Chicken & pasta	14.6-oz. serving	380
Garden	8½-oz. serving	270
Side	3.9-oz. serving	15
Shake:		
Chocolate	12 fl. oz.	340
Strawberry	12 fl. oz.	300
Vanilla	12 fl. oz.	300
Syrup	1½-oz. serving	25
Turkey club sandwich	7.3-oz. serving	1280
HAWAIIAN PUNCH, canned:		
Regular:		
Apple or grape	6 fl. oz.	13
Cherry or fruit juicy red	6 fl. oz.	17
Island fruit cocktail, orange or wild fruit	6 fl. oz.	19
Tropical fruit	6 fl. oz.	8
Very berry	6 fl. oz.	22
Dietetic, punch	6 fl. oz.	20
HAZELNUT (see **FILBERT**)		
HEADCHEESE (Oscar Mayer)	1-oz. serving	347
HEARTWISE, cereal (Kellogg's)	⅔ cup (1 oz.)	140
HERRING:		
Raw (USDA) Pacific, meat only	4 oz.	84
Smoked (USDA) Hard	4-oz. serving	7066
HOMINY, canned (Allen's)		
solids & liq.:		
Golden:		
Regular	½ cup	370
Mexican style	½ cup	430
White	½ cup	430
HOMINY GRITS:		
Dry:		
(USDA):		
Degermed	1 oz.	Tr.
Degermed	½ cup (2.8 oz.)	<1
(Albers)	¼ cup (1½ oz.)	<1
(Aunt Jemima)	3 T. (1 oz.)	<1

Food and Description	Measure or Quantity	Sodium (milligrams)
(Quaker):		
Regular	1 T. (.33 oz.)	Tr.
Instant:		
Regular	.8-oz. packet	385
With artificial cheese		
flavor	1-oz. packet	497
With imitation bacon bits	1-oz. packet	544
With imitation ham bits	1-oz. packet	544
(3-Minute Brand) quick,		
enriched	⅙ cup (1 oz.)	<1
Cooked (USDA) degermed	⅔ cup (5.6 oz.)	336
HONEY, strained:		
(USDA)	½ cup (5.7 oz.)	8
(USDA)	1 T. (.7 oz.)	1
HONEY BUNCHES OF OATS,		
cereal (Post):		
With almonds	⅔ cup (1 oz.)	157
Honey roasted	⅔ cup (1 oz.)	176
HONEYCOMB, cereal (Post)	1⅓ cups (1 oz.)	172
HONEYDEW, fresh (USDA):		
Whole	1 lb. (weighed whole)	34
Wedge	2″ × 7″ wedge (5.3 oz.)	11
Flesh only	4 oz.	14
Flesh only, diced	1 cup (5.9 oz.)	20
HONEY SMACKS, cereal		
(Kellogg's)	¾ cup	70
HOPPING JOHN, frozen (Green		
Giant) Southern recipe	⅓ of 10-oz. pkg.	419
HORSERADISH:		
Raw (USDA):		
Whole	1 lb. (weighed unpared)	26
Pared	1 oz.	2
Prepared (USDA)	1 oz.	27
HOT BITES (Banquet):		
Cheese, mozzarella nuggets	¼ of 10½-oz. pkg.	530

Food and Description	Measure or Quantity	Sodium (milligrams)
Chicken:		
Regular:		
Breast patties:		
Regular	¼ of 10½-oz. pkg.	460
Southern fried	¼ of 10½-oz. pkg.	620
Breast tenders:		
Regular	¼ of 10½-oz. pkg.	280
Southern fried	¼ of 10½-oz. pkg.	340
Drumsnackers	¼ of 10½-oz. pkg.	530
Nuggets:		
Plain	¼ of 10½-oz. pkg.	550
With cheddar	¼ of 10½-oz. pkg.	560
Hot 'N Spicy	¼ of 10½-oz. pkg.	380
Southern fried	¼ of 10½-oz. pkg.	530
Sticks	¼ of 10½-oz. pkg.	350
Microwave:		
Breast pattie:		
Regular, & bun	4-oz. pkg.	670
Southern fried, & biscuit	4-oz. pkg.	980
Breast tenders	4-oz. pkg.	560
Nuggets:		
Plain, with sweet & sour sauce	4½-oz. pkg.	770
Hot & Spicy, with barbecue sauce	4½-oz. pkg.	820
Southern fried breast nuggets with barbecue sauce	4½-oz. pkg.	930

Food and Description	Measure or Quantity	Sodium (milligrams)
HOT WHEELS, cereal		
(Ralston-Purina)	1 cup (1 oz.)	160
HULA COOLER DRINK,		
canned (Hi-C)	6 fl. oz.	17
HULA PUNCH DRINK,		
canned (Hi-C)	6 fl. oz.	17
HYACINTH BEAN (USDA)		
Young bean, raw:		
Whole	1 lb. (weighed untrimmed)	8
Trimmed	4 oz.	2

I

Food and Description	Measure or Quantity	Sodium (milligrams)
ICE CREAM and FROZEN CUSTARD:		
(USDA):		
10% fat	1 cup (4.7 oz.)	84
12% fat	1 cup (5 oz.)	57
12% fat, brick-type	2½-oz. slice	28
12% fat	small container (3½ fl. oz)	25
16% fat	1 cup (5.2 oz.)	49
Almond Amaretto (Baskin-Robbins)	4 fl. oz.	30
Almond supreme (Good Humor)	4 fl. oz.	64
Blueberry & cream (Häagen-Dazs)	4 fl. oz.	35
Bon-Bon (Carnation):		
Chocolate	1 piece	11
Vanilla	1 piece	8
Brittle bar (Häagen-Dazs)	1 bar	160

Food and Description	Measure or Quantity	Sodium (milligrams)
Bubble O'Bill bar (Good Humor)	3.5-fl.-oz. bar	28
Butter almond (Breyer's)	½ cup	125
Butter pecan:		
(Breyer's)	½ cup	125
(Häagen-Dazs)	4 fl. oz.	100
(Lady Borden)	½ cup	65
Cappuccino (Baskin-Robbins) chip	4 fl. oz.	40
Chip crunch bar (Good Humor)	3-fl.-oz. bar	40
Chocolate:		
(Baskin-Robbins):		
Regular	4 fl. oz.	128
Deluxe	4 fl. oz	160
Mousse Royale	4 fl. oz.	150
World Class	4 fl. oz.	145
(Borden) old fashioned or swirl	½ cup	65
(Bryer's)	½ cup	35
(Häagen-Dazs):		
Regular:		
Plain or mint	4 fl. oz.	50
Deep	4 fl. oz.	70
Bar, dark chocolate coating	1 bar	50
Chocolate chip:		
(Baskin-Robbins)	4 fl. oz.	110
(Breyer's) mint	½ cup	45
(Häagen-Dazs) chocolate	4 fl. oz.	40
(Nestlé):		
Bar	2.4-oz. bar	40
Sandwich	2.6-oz. bar	95
Chocolate Eclair bar (Good Humor)	3-fl.-oz. bar	54
Chocolate fudge cake (Good Humor)	3-fl.-oz. piece	50
Chocolate fudge (Häagen-Dazs) deep	4 fl. oz.	100
Chocolate malt bar (Good Humor)	3-fl.-oz. bar	50

Food and Description	Measure or Quantity	Sodium (milligrams)
Chocolate peanut butter (Häagen-Dazs) deep	4 fl. oz.	90
Chocolate raspberry truffle (Baskin-Robbins)	4 fl. oz.	115
Chocolate swirl (Borden)	½ cup	65
Coffee:		
(Breyer's)	½ cup	50
(Häagen-Dazs)	4 fl. oz.	55
Cookies & cream:		
(Breyer's)	½ cup	60
(Sealtest)	½ cup	75
Cookie sandwich (Good Humor)	2.7-fl.-oz. piece	195
Eskimo Pie:		
Chocolate fudge bar	1¾-fl.-oz. bar	30
Chocolate fudge bar	2½-fl.-oz. bar	45
Chocolate fudge bar	3-fl.-oz. bar	50
Dietary dairy bar, chocolate covered	2½-fl.-oz. bar	40
Old fashioned:		
Crispy	1 bar	70
Double chocolate	1 bar	150
Vanilla	1 bar	70
Pie:		
Regular:		
Chocolate	3-fl.-oz. bar	100
Crunch	3-fl.-oz. bar	55
Vanilla	3-fl.-oz. bar	45
Jr:		
Chocolate	1¾-fl.-oz. bar	60
Crunch	1¾-fl.-oz. bar	30
Vanilla	1¾-fl.-oz. bar	25
Original:		
Double chocolate	1 bar	75
Vanilla	1 bar	35
Thin mints	2-fl-oz. bar	30
Twin pop	1 bar	0
Fat Frog (Good Humor)	3-fl.-oz. pop	36
Fudge bar:		
(Good Humor)	2½-fl.-oz. bar	91

Food and Description	Measure or Quantity	Sodium (milligrams)
(Häagen-Dazs)	1 bar	50
Fudge cake (Good Humor)	6.3 fl. oz.	50
Grand Marnier (Baskin-Robbins)	4 fl. oz.	50
Halv bar (Good Humor)	2½-fl.-oz. bar	64
Honey (Häagen-Dazs)	4 fl. oz.	55
Jamora almond fudge (Baskin-Robbins)	4 fl. oz.	115
Jumbo Jet Star (Good Humor)	4½ fl. oz.	0
King Cone (Good Humor):		
Regular	5½ fl. oz.	119
Boysenberry	5 fl. oz.	151
Laser Blazer (Good Humor)	3 fl. oz.	71
Macadamia brittle (Häagen-Dazs)	4 fl. oz.	60
Macadamia nut (Häagen-Dazs)	4 fl. oz.	80
Maple walnut (Häagen-Dazs)	4 fl. oz.	55
Milky pop (Good Humor)	1½-fl.-oz. pop	23
Mocha double nut (Häagen-Dazs)	4 fl. oz.	85
Oreo, cookie & cream:		
Regular, any flavor	3 fl. oz.	100
Sandwich	1 sandwich	300
Stick	1 bar	100
Peach:		
(Breyer's)	½ cup	35
(Häagen-Dazs) elberta	4 fl. oz.	50
Peanut vanilla (Häagen-Dazs)	4 fl. oz.	120
Quik, bar (Nestlé)	3-fl.-oz. bar	40
Raspberry cream (Häagen-Dazs)	4 fl. oz.	30
Rocky road (Baskin-Robbins)	4 fl. oz.	123
Rum raisin (Häagen-Dazs)	4 fl. oz.	45
Shark Bar (Good Humor)	3-fl.-oz. pop	7
Strawberry:		
(Baskin-Robbins):		
Very berry	4 fl. oz.	95
Wild, light	4 fl. oz.	70
(Borden)	½ cup	55

Food and Description	Measure or Quantity	Sodium (milligrams)
(Breyer's) natural	½ cup	40
(Häagen-Dazs)	4 fl. oz.	40
Strawberry & cream (Borden)	½ cup	55
Strawberry shortcake (Good Humor)	3-fl.-oz. piece	88
Toasted almond bar (Good Humor)	3-fl.-oz. bar	33
Vanilla:		
(Baskin-Robbins):		
Regular	4 fl. oz.	91
Deluxe	4 fl. oz.	115
French	4 fl. oz.	90
(Borden)	½ cup	55
(Eagle Brand)	½ cup	55
(Häagen-Dazs)	4 fl. oz.	55
(Land O'Lakes)	4 fl. oz.	60
(Sealtest)	½ cup	50
Vanilla bar:		
(Good Humor) chocolate coated	3-fl.-oz. piece	44
(Häagen-Dazs):		
Regular bar:		
Dark chocolate coating	3.67-fl.-oz. bar	50
Milk chocolate coating	3½-fl.-oz. bar	60
Milk chocolate coating & almonds	3.72-fl.-oz. bar	65
Snack bar:		
Milk chocolate coated	1 bar	50
Semi-sweet chocolate coated	1 bar	45
Vanilla & caramel (Häagen-Dazs)	4 fl. oz.	100
Vanilla & caramel triple nuts (Häagen-Dazs)	4 fl. oz.	100
Vanilla-chocolate cup (Good Humor)	6 fl. oz.	80
Vanilla cup (Good Humor)	3 fl. oz.	35
Vanilla fudge (Häagen-Dazs)	4 fl. oz.	100
Vanilla & peanut butter swirl (Häagen-Dazs)	4 fl. oz.	120

Food and Description	Measure or Quantity	Sodium (milligrams)
Vanilla sandwich (Good Humor)	3 fl. oz.	155
Vanilla swiss almond (Häagen-Dazs)	4 fl. oz.	55
Whammy (Good Humor) assorted	1.6-oz. piece	17
ICE CREAM, SUBSTITUTE (See **FROZEN DESSERT**)		
ICE CREAM CONE (Baskin-Robbins):		
Sugar	1 cone	45
Waffle	1 cone	5
***ICE CREAM MIX** (Salada):		
Dutch chocolate	1 cup	75
Wild strawberry	1 cup	60
ICE MILK:		
(USDA):		
Hardened	1 cup (4.6 oz.)	89
Soft serve	1 cup (6.3 oz.)	119
(Borden):		
Chocolate	½ cup	80
Strawberry or vanilla	½ cup	65
(Land O'Lakes)	4 fl. oz.	55
Light N' Lively, coffee	½ cup	55
(Weight Watchers) *Grand Collection*, premium:		
Chocolate, chocolate chip, chocolate fudge, chocolate swirl, fudge marble, neapolitan, strawberries & cream, Swiss vanilla or vanilla	½ cup	75
Pecan praline & creme	½ cup	80
ICE TEASERS (Nestlé)	8 fl. oz.	0
ICING (See **CAKE ICING**)		
INSTANT BREAKFAST (See individual brand name or company listings)		
IRISH WHISKEY (See **DISTILLED LIQUORS**)		

Food and Description	Measure or Quantity	Sodium (milligrams)

J

JACKFRUIT, fresh (USDA):

Whole	1 lb. (weighed with seeds & skin)	3
Flesh only	4 oz.	2

JACK IN THE BOX:

Beef fajita pita sandwich	6.2-oz. serving	635
Breakfast Jack	4.4-oz. serving	871
Burger:		
Plain	3.6-oz. burger	556
Cheese:		
Regular	4-oz. burger	746
Bacon	8.1-oz. burger	1127
Ultimate	9.9-oz. burger	1176
Ham & Swiss	9.1-oz. burger	1217
Jumbo Jack:		
Regular	7.8-oz. burger	733
Cheese	8½-oz. burger	1090
Monterey	9.9-oz. burger	1124
Mushroom	6.4-oz. burger	910
Canadian crescent	4.7-oz. serving	851
Cheesecake	3½-oz. piece	208
Chicken fajita pita sandwich	6.7-oz. sandwich	703
Chicken strips	1 piece	177
Chicken supreme sandwich	8.1-oz. sandwich	1535
Club pita sandwich, excluding sauce	6.3-oz. sandwich	931
Egg, scrambled, platter	8.8-oz. serving	1188
Egg roll	1 piece	301
Fish supreme sandwich	8-oz. sandwich	1047

Food and Description	Measure or Quantity	Sodium (milligrams)
French fries	2.4-oz. regular order	164
Hot club supreme sandwich	7½-oz. sandwich	1467
Jelly, grape	1 T. (.5 oz.)	3
Ketchup	1 serving	99
Milk shake:		
Chocolate	10-oz. serving	270
Strawberry	10-oz. serving	240
Vanilla	10-oz. serving	230
Nachos:		
Cheese	6-oz. serving	1154
Supreme	11.9-oz. serving	2914
Onion rings	3.8-oz. serving	407
Pancake platter	8.1-oz. serving	888
Salad:		
Chef	11.7-oz. salad	900
Mexican chicken	15.2-oz. salad	1530
Side	3.9-oz. salad	84
Taco	14.8-oz. salad	1670
Salad dressing:		
Regular:		
Bleu cheese	1.2-oz. serving	459
Buttermilk	1.2-oz. serving	347
1000 Island	1.2-oz. serving	350
Dietetic, french	1.2-oz. serving	300
Sauce:		
A-1	1.8-oz. serving	809
BBQ	.9-oz. serving	300
Guacamole	.9-oz. serving	130
Mayo-mustard	.8-oz. serving	247
Mayo-onion	.8-oz. serving	140
Salsa	.9-oz. serving	129
Seafood cocktail	1-oz. serving	206
Sweet & sour	1-oz. serving	160
Sausage crescent	5½-oz. serving	1012
Shrimp	.3-oz. piece	67
Soft drink:		
Sweetened:		
Coca-Cola Classic	12 fl. oz.	14
Dr Pepper	12 fl. oz.	18

Food and Description	Measure or Quantity	Sodium (milligrams)
Sprite	12 fl. oz.	46
Dietetic, *Coke*	12 fl. oz.	26
Supreme crescent	5.1-oz. crescent	1053
Syrup, pancake	1½-oz. serving	6
Taco:		
Regular	2.9-oz. serving	406
Super	4.8-oz. serving	765
Turnover, hot apple	4.2-oz. piece	350
JAM, sweetened (See also individual listings by flavor):		
(USDA)	1 oz.	3
(USDA)	1 tsp.	2
JELL-O FRUIT & CREAM BAR:		
Blueberry, raspberry or strawberry	1.7-fl.-oz. bar	98
Peach	1.7-fl.-oz. bar	109
JELL-O GELATIN POPS	1.7-fl.-oz. pop	7
JELL-O PUDDING POP:		
Banana butterscotch or vanilla	2-fl.-oz. pop	63
Chocolate or chocolate fudge	2-fl.-oz. pop	99
Chocolate & caramel swirl	2-fl.-oz. pop	83
Chocolate & vanilla swirl	2-fl.-oz. pop	81
JELLY, sweetened (See also individual listings by flavor)		
(USDA)	1 T. (.6 oz.)	3
JORDAN ALMOND (See **CANDY**)		
JUICE (See individual flavors)		
JUJUBE or CHINESE DATE (USDA):		
Fresh, whole	1 lb. (weighed with seeds)	13
Fresh, flesh only	4 oz.	3
JUNIOR FOOD (See **BABY FOOD**)		
JUST RIGHT, cereal (Kellogg's):		
With fiber nuggets	⅔ cup (1 oz.)	200
With fruit & nuts	¾ cup (1.3 oz.)	190

Food and Description	Measure or Quantity	Sodium (milligrams)

K

KABOOM, cereal (General Mills)	1 cup (1 oz.)	290
KALE:		
Raw (USDA) leaves only	1 lb. (weighed untrimmed)	218
Boiled (USDA) leaves, including stems	½ cup (1.9 oz.)	24
Canned (Sunshine) chopped, solids & liq.	½ cup (4.1 oz.)	251
Frozen:		
(Birds Eye) chopped	⅓ of pkg.	14
(McKenzie) chopped	3.3 oz.	28
(Southland) chopped	⅕ of 16-oz. pkg.	15
KENMAI, cereal:		
Plain	¾ cup (1 oz.)	250
Almond & raisin	¾ cup (1.4 oz.)	240
KENTUCKY FRIED CHICKEN (KFC):		
Biscuit, buttermilk	2.3-oz. biscuit	655
Chicken:		
Lite 'N Crispy:		
Breast, center	3-oz. piece	416
Drumstick	1.7-oz. piece	196
Thigh	2.8-oz. piece	386
Original recipe:		
Breast:		
Center	4-oz. piece	672
Side	3.2-oz. piece	735
Drumstick	2-oz. piece	275
Thigh	3.7-oz. piece	619
Wing	1.9-oz. piece	372
Extra tasty crispy:		
Breast:		
Center	4.8-oz. piece	636
Side	3.1-oz. piece	646
Drumstick	2.4-oz. piece	292

Food and Description	Measure or Quantity	Sodium (milligrams)
Thigh	4.2-oz. piece	688
Wing	2.3-oz. piece	432
Chicken Littles, sandwich	1.7-oz. serving	331
Chicken nugget	.6-oz. piece	140
Chicken sandwich, *Colonel's*	5.9-oz. serving	1060
Cole slaw	3.2-oz. serving	197
Corn on the cob	5-oz. serving	<20
Hot wings	.7-oz. piece	113
Potatoes:		
French fries, regular order	2.7-oz. serving	139
Mashed, & gravy	3½-oz. serving	339
Sauce:		
Barbecue	1-oz. serving	450
Honey	.5-oz. serving	<15
Mustard	1-oz. serving	346
Sweet & sour	1-oz. serving	148
KETCHUP (See **CATSUP**)		
KIDNEY (USDA):	Beef:	
Raw	4 oz.	200
Braised	4 oz.	287
Hog, raw	4 oz.	130
Lamb, raw	4 oz.	257
KINGFISH, raw (USDA):		
Whole	1 lb. (weighed whole)	166
Meat only	4 oz.	94
KIPPERS (See **HERRING**)		
KIWIFRUIT (Calavo)	any quantity	0
KIX, cereal (General Mills)	1½ cups (1 oz.)	260
KOHLRABI (USDA):		
Raw:		
Whole	1 lb. (weighed with skin, without leaves)	26
Diced	1 cup (4.8 oz.)	11
Boiled, without salt:		
Drained	4 oz.	7
Drained	1 cup (5.5 oz.)	9

Food and Description	Measure or Quantity	Sodium (milligrams)
KOOL-AID (General Foods):		
Canned, *Kool-Aid Koolers:*		
Cherry, grape, mountainberry punch, rainbow punch, sharkleberry fin, strawberry or tropical punch	8.45-fl.-oz. can	3
Orange	8.45-fl.-oz. can	2
*Mix:		
Unsweetened, sugar to be added:		
Berry blue or purplesaurus rex	8 fl. oz.	6
Mount-berry punch	8 fl. oz.	15
Raspberry or strawberry	8 fl. oz.	27
Pre-sweetened:		
Regular, sugar sweetened:		
Grape	8 fl. oz.	24
Purplesaures rex	8 fl. oz.	6
Rainbow punch	8 fl. oz.	20
Surfin' berry punch	8 fl. oz.	27
Dietetic, sugar free:		
Berry blue or purplesaurus rex	8 fl. oz.	6
Cherry	8 fl. oz.	3
Grape, rainbow punch or sharkleberry fin	8 fl. oz.	Tr.
Mountain berry punch	8 fl. oz.	33
Raspberry	8 fl. oz.	24
Tropical punch	8 fl. oz.	8
KRISPIES, cereal (Kellogg's):		
Plain	1 cup (1 oz.)	290
Frosted	¾ cup (1 oz.)	220
Fruity marshmallow	1¼ cups (1.3 oz.)	210
KUMQUAT, fresh (USDA):		
Whole	1 lb. (weighed with seeds)	30
Flesh & skin	4 oz.	8

Food and Description	Measure or Quantity	Sodium (milligrams)

L

LAKE HERRING, raw
(USDA):

Whole	1 lb.	111
Meat only	4 oz.	53

LAMB, choice grade (USDA):
Chop, broiled:
Loin. One 5-oz. chop
(weighed before cooking
with bone) will give you:

Lean & fat	2.8 oz.	55
Lean only	2.3 oz.	46

Rib. One 5-oz. chop
(weighed before cooking
with bone) will give you:

Lean & fat	2.9 oz.	57
Lean only	2 oz.	39

Leg:

Raw, lean & fat	1 lb. (weighed with bone)	280
Roasted, lean & fat	4 oz.	79
Roasted, lean only	4 oz.	79

Shoulder:

Raw, lean & fat	1 lb. (weighed with bone)	270
Roasted, lean & fat	4 oz.	79
Roasted, lean only	4 oz.	79

LARD, See **SHORTENING**
LASAGNA:

Dry (Buitoni) precooked	1 sheet	4
Canned (Hormel) *Short Order*	7½-oz. can	1083

Food and Description	Measure or Quantity	Sodium (milligrams)
Frozen:		
(Armour) *Dining Lite*, cheese	10-oz. meal	800
(Buitoni):		
Regular	9-oz. serving	929
Al forno	8-oz. serving	1107
Meat sauce	5-oz. serving	499
Sorrentina, cheese	8-oz. serving	728
(Celentano):		
Regular	½ of 16-oz. pkg.	700
Regular	¼ of 25-oz. pkg.	310
Primavera	11-oz. pkg.	470
(Healthy Choice) with meat		
sauce	9-oz. meal	420
(Stouffer's):		
Regular:		
Plain	10½-oz. meal	1020
Vegetable	10½-oz. meal	970
Lean Cuisine:		
With meat sauce	10¼-oz. meal	970
Tuna, with spinach		
noodles & vegetables	9¾-oz. meal	890
Zucchini	11-oz. meal	950
(Swanson):		
Regular, 4-compartment		
dinner	13-oz. meal	800
Hungry Man, with		
meat	18¾-oz. dinner	1510
Main Course	13¼-oz. entree	1120
(Van de Kamp's):		
Beef & mushroom	11-oz. meal	970
Creamy spinach	11-oz. meal	840
Italian sausage	11-oz. meal	1190
(Weight Watchers):		
Garden	11-oz. meal	880
Italian cheese or with		
meat sauce	11-oz. meal	990
LATKES, frozen (Empire		
Kosher):		
Mini	3-oz. serving	400

Food and Description	Measure or Quantity	Sodium (milligrams)
Rounds	2½-oz. serving	305
Triangles	3-oz. serving	335
LEEKS, raw (USDA):		
Whole	1 lb. (weighed untrimmed)	12
Trimmed	4 oz.	6
LEMON, fresh (USDA) peeled	1 med. (2⅛″ dia.)	1
LEMONADE:		
Canned:		
Capri Sun, natural	6¾ fl. oz.	2
(Hi-C)	8.45-fl.-oz. can	73
Kool-Aid Koolers	8.45-fl.-oz. container	3
Ssips (Johanna Farms)	8.45-fl.-oz. container	25
Chilled (Minute Maid) regular or pink	6 fl. oz.	23
*Frozen:		
(USDA)	½ cup (4.4 oz.)	Tr.
(Minute Maid)	6 fl. oz.	<23
(Sunkist)	6 fl. oz.	Tr.
*Mix, regular:		
Country Time, regular or pink	8 fl. oz.	21
(4 C)	8 fl. oz.	0
(Funny Face)	8 fl. oz.	0
Kool-Aid (General Foods) unsweetened package, regular or pink	8 fl. oz.	8
Kool-Aid (General Foods) pre-sweetened package, regular or pink	8 fl. oz.	Tr.
(Wyler's)	8 fl. oz.	44
*Mix, dietetic:		
Country Time	8 fl. oz.	<1
Crystal Light	8 fl. oz.	<1
(Kool-Aid)	8 fl. oz.	<1
(Sunkist)	8 fl. oz.	35
LEMONADE BAR (Sunkist)	3-fl.-oz. bar	3

Food and Description	Measure or Quantity	Sodium (milligrams)
LEMONADE PUNCH, *Country Time*:		
Regular	8 fl. oz.	15
Fructose sweetened	8 fl. oz.	9
LEMON JUICE:		
Fresh:		
(USDA)	1 cup (8.6 oz.)	2
(USDA)	1 T. (.5 oz.)	<1
Bottled, unsweetened:		
(USDA)	1 cup (8.6 oz.)	2
(USDA)	1 T. (.5 oz.)	<1
Plastic container:		
(USDA)	¼ cup (2 oz.)	<1
ReaLemon	1 T. (.5 oz.)	5
Frozen, unsweetened:		
(USDA):		
Concentrate	½ cup (5.1 oz.)	7
Single strength	½ cup (4.3 oz.)	1
(Minute Maid) full strength, reconstituted	1 fl. oz.	<1
***LEMON-LIMEADE,** dietetic, *Crystal Light*	8 fl. oz.	<1
LEMON-LIME DRINK, canned, *Ssips* (Johanna Farms)	8.45-fl.-oz. container	15
LEMON & PEPPER SEASONING (Lawry's)	1 tsp. (3.6 g.)	340
LENTIL, whole, dry:		
(USDA)	½ lb.	68
(USDA)	1 cup (6.7 oz.)	57
LETTUCE (USDA):		
Bibb, untrimmed	1 lb. (weighed untrimmed)	30
Bibb, untrimmed	7.8-oz. head (4″ dia.)	15
Boston, untrimmed	1 lb. (weighed untrimmed)	30
Boston, untrimmed	7.8-oz. head (4″ dia.)	15

Food and Description	Measure or Quantity	Sodium (milligrams)
Butterhead varieties (See Bibb & Boston)		
Cos (See Romaine)		
Dark green (See Romaine)		
Grand Rapids	1 lb. (weighed untrimmed)	26
Grand Rapids	2 large leaves (1.8 oz.)	4
Great Lakes	1 lb. (weighed untrimmed)	39
Great Lakes, trimmed	1-lb. head (4¾" dia.)	41
Iceberg:		
Untrimmed	1 lb. (weighed untrimmed)	39
Trimmed	1-lb. head (4¾" dia.)	41
Leaves	1 cup (2.3 oz.)	6
Chopped	1 cup (2 oz.)	5
Chunks	1 cup (2.6 oz.)	7
Looseleaf varieties (See Salad Bowl)		
New York	1 lb. (weighed untrimmed)	39
New York	1-lb. head (4¾" dia.)	41
Romaine:		
Untrimmed	1 lb. (weighed untrimmed)	26
Trimmed, shredded & broken into pieces	½ cup (.8 oz.)	2
Salad Bowl	1 lb. (weighed untrimmed)	26
Salad Bowl	2 large leaves (1.8 oz.)	4
Simpson	1 lb. (weighed untrimmed)	26
Simpson	2 large leaves (1.8 oz.)	4

Food and Description	Measure or Quantity	Sodium (milligrams)
White Paris (See Romaine)		
LIFE, cereal (Quaker):		
Regular	⅔ cup (1 oz.)	163
Cinnamon	⅔ cup (1 oz.)	149
LIMA BEAN (See **BEAN, LIMA**)		
LIME, fresh (USDA):		
Whole	1 lb. (weighed with skin & seeds)	8
Whole	1 med (2″ dia., 2.4 oz.)	1
***LIMEADE,** frozen, sweetened: (USDA) diluted with 4⅓ parts water	½ cup (4.4 oz.)	Tr.
(Minute Maid)	6 fl. oz.	20
LIME JUICE:		
Fresh (USDA)	1 cup (8.7 oz.)	2
Canned or bottled, unsweetened:		
(USDA)	1 cup (8.7 oz.)	2
(USDA)	1 T. (.5 oz.)	<1
(Rose's)	1 fl. oz.	6
Plastic container, *ReaLime*	1 T. (.5 oz.)	5
LINGCOD, raw (USDA):		
Whole	1 lb. (weighed whole)	91
Meat only	4 oz.	67
LINGUINI:		
(Healthy Choice) with shrimp	9½-oz. meal	440
(Stouffer's) *Lean Cuisine*, with clam sauce	9⅝-oz. meal	890
(Weight Watchers) seafood	9-oz. meal	750
LITCHI NUT (USDA):		
Fresh:		
Whole	4 oz. (weighed in shell with seeds)	2
Flesh only	4 oz.	3
Dried:		
Whole	4 oz. (weighed in shell with seeds)	2

Food and Description	Measure or Quantity	Sodium (milligrams)
Flesh only	2 oz.	2
LIVER:		
Beef:		
(USDA):		
Raw	1 lb.	617
Fried	4 oz.	209
(Swift) packaged, *True-Tender*, sliced, cooked	⅕ of 1-lb. pkg.	70
Calf (USDA):		
Raw	1 lb.	331
Fried	4 oz.	134
Chicken (USDA):		
Raw	1 lb.	318
Simmered	4 oz.	69
Goose, raw (USDA)	1 lb.	635
Hog (USDA):		
Raw	1 lb.	331
Fried	4 oz.	126
Lamb (USDA):		
Raw	1 lb.	236
Broiled	4 oz.	96
Turkey, raw (USDA)	1 lb.	286
LIVER PÂTÉ (See PÂTÉ)		
LIVER SAUSAGE or LIVERWURST, spread (Underwood)	1 oz.	237
LOBSTER (USDA):		
Cooked, meat only	4 oz.	238
Canned, meat only	4 oz.	238
LOBSTER NEWBURG, home recipe (USDA)	4 oz.	572
LOBSTER SALAD, home recipe (USDA)	4 oz.	141
LOGANBERRY (USDA):		
Fresh:		
Untrimmed	1 lb. (weighed with caps)	4
Trimmed	1 cup (5.1 oz.)	1
Canned, solids & liq.:		
Extra heavy syrup	4 oz.	1

Food and Description	Measure or Quantity	Sodium (milligrams)
Heavy syrup	4 oz.	1
Juice pack	4 oz.	1
Light syrup	4 oz.	1
LONG JOHN SILVER'S:		
Catfish:		
Dinner	13.2-oz. meal	990
Filet	2½-oz. piece	310
Catsup	.4-oz. serving	170
Chicken plank:		
Dinner:		
3-piece	13-oz. meal	1340
4-piece	14.6-oz. meal	1660
Single piece	1.6-oz. piece	320
Children's meals:		
Chicken plank	7.1-oz. meal	730
Fish	6½-oz. meal	590
Fish & chicken plank	8.1-oz. meal	910
Chowder, clam	7 fl. oz.	590
Clams:		
Breaded	2.3-oz. serving	410
Dinner	12.8-oz. serving	1200
Cod entree:		
Baked:		
Regular	5.8-oz. serving	140
Delight	6-oz. serving	390
Supreme	6.2-oz. serving	250
Broiled	5.4-oz. serving	170
Cole slaw, drained on fork	3.4-oz. serving	260
Corn on the cob, with whirl	6.6-oz. ear	95
Cracker, *Club*	.2-oz. piece	85
Fish, battered	2.6-oz. piece	510
Fish & chicken entree	14-oz. meal	1520
Fish dinner, 3-piece	16.1-oz. serving	1890
Fish dinner, home-style:		
3-piece	13.1-oz. serving	980
4-piece	14.8-oz. serving	1180
6-piece	18.1-oz. serving	1590
Fish & fryer, entree:		
2-piece	10-oz. serving	1120
3-piece	12.6-oz. serving	1630

Food and Description	Measure or Quantity	Sodium (milligrams)
Fish, homestyle	1.6-oz. piece	200
Fish & More, entree	13.4-oz. entree	1390
Fish Sandwich, homestyle:		
Regular	6.9-oz. sandwich	780
Platter	13.4-oz. meal	1110
Flounder, broiled	5.1-oz. piece	490
Gumbo, with cod & shrimp		
boles	7 fl. oz.	740
Halibut steak, broiled	4.1-oz. piece	115
Hushpuppie	.8-oz. piece	25
Pie:		
Lemon meringue	4.2-oz. piece	270
Pecan	4.4-oz. piece	470
Potato:		
Baked, without topping	7.1-oz. serving	5
Fries	3-oz. serving	60
Rice pilaf	3-oz. serving	280
Roll, dinner, plain	.9-oz. piece	105
Salad:		
Garden	8.7-oz. serving	380
Ocean chef	11.3-oz. serving	1340
Seafood, entree	11.9-oz. serving	670
Side	4.3-oz. serving	20
Salad dressing:		
Regular:		
Bleu cheese	1.5-oz. packet	380
Ranch	1.5-oz. packet	350
Sea salad	1.6-oz. packet	260
Dietetic, Italian	1.6-oz. packet	670
Salmon, broiled	4.4-oz. piece	180
Sauce:		
Honey mustard	1.2-oz. packet	170
Seafood	1.2-oz. packet	530
Sweet & sour	1.2-oz. packet	125
Tartar	1-oz. packet	80
Seafood platter, entree	14.1-oz. serving	1540
Shrimp, battered	.5-oz. piece	120
Shrimp, breaded	2.2-oz. serving	470

Food and Description	Measure or Quantity	Sodium (milligrams)
Shrimp dinner, battered:		
6-piece	11.1-oz. serving	1110
9-piece	12.6-oz. serving	1470
Shrimp feast, breaded:		
13-piece	12.6-oz. serving	1320
21-piece	14.8-oz. serving	1790
Shrimp, fish & chicken dinner	13.4-oz. serving	1450
Shrimp & fish dinner	12.3-oz. serving	1250
Shrimp scampi, baked	5.7-oz. entree	660
Vegetables, mixed	4-oz. serving	330
Vinegar, malt	.4-oz. packet	20
LOX, (See **SALMON, SMOKED**)		
LUCKY CHARMS, cereal		
(General Mills)	1 cup (1 oz.)	180
LUNCHEON MEAT (See also		
individual listings e.g.,		
BOLOGNA, etc.):		
All meat (Oscar Mayer)	1-oz. slice	321
Banquet loaf (Eckrich)	¾-oz. slice	250
Bar B-Q-Loaf:		
(Eckrich)	1-oz. slice	370
(Oscar Mayer)	1-oz. slice	332
Beef, jellied loaf (Hormel)	1 slice	450
Gourmet loaf (Eckrich):		
Regular	1-oz. slice	390
Smorgas Pac	¾-oz. slice	300
Ham & cheese (See **HAM &**		
CHEESE)		
Ham roll sausage (Oscar		
Mayer)	1-oz. slice	329
Honey loaf:		
(Hormel)	1 slice	292
(Oscar Mayer)	1-oz. slice	379
Jalapeño loaf (Oscar Mayer)	1-oz. slice	464
Liver cheese (Oscar Mayer)	1.3-oz. slice	418
Liver loaf (Hormel)	1 slice	352
Macaroni-cheese loaf		
(Eckrich)	1-oz. slice	370

Food and Description	Measure or Quantity	Sodium (milligrams)
New England brand sausage		
(Oscar Mayer) 92% fat free	.8-oz. slice	292
Old fashioned loaf:		
(Eckrich):		
Regular	1-oz. slice	330
Smorgas Pac	¾-oz. slice	250
(Oscar Mayer)	1-oz. slice	337
Olive loaf:		
(Eckrich)	1-oz. slice	370
(Hormel)	1 slice	405
(Oscar Mayer)	1-oz. slice	393
Peppered loaf (Oscar Mayer)	1-oz. slice	366
Pickle loaf:		
(Eckrich):		
Regular or *Smorgas Pac*	1-oz. slice	320
Beef, *Smorgas Pac*	¾-oz. slice	260
(Hormel) regular	1 slice	376
(Ohse)	1 oz.	330
Pickle & pimiento loaf (Oscar Mayer)	1-oz. slice	403
Picnic loaf (Oscar Mayer)	1-oz. slice	333
Spiced (Hormel) regular	1 slice	351

M

MACARONI. The longer plain macaroni products are cooked, the more water is absorbed and this affects the nutritive values.
Dry:
  (USDA):
    Elbow-type   1 cup (4.8 oz.)   3

Food and Description	Measure or Quantity	Sodium (milligrams)
1-inch pieces	1 cup (3.8 oz.)	2
2-inch pieces	1 cup (3 oz.)	2
(Creamette) spinach, ribbons	2 oz.	70
(Pritikin) whole wheat	2 oz.	40
Cooked (USDA):		
8–10 minutes, firm	1 cup (4.6 oz.)	1
8–10 minutes, firm	4 oz.	1
14–20 minutes, tender	1 cup (4.9 oz.)	1
14–20 minutes, tender	4 oz.	1
Canned (Franco-American)		
*PizzO*s, in pizza sauce	7½-oz. can	980
MACARONI & BEEF:		
Canned:		
(Bounty) *Chili Mac,* in tomato sauce	7¾-oz. can	1209
(Franco-American) *BeefyO*s, in tomato sauce	7½-oz. can	1250
Frozen:		
(Stouffer's) with tomatoes	5¾-oz. serving	810
(Swanson)	12-oz. dinner	850
MACARONI & CHEESE:		
Home recipe (USDA) baked	1 cup (7.1 oz.)	1086
Canned:		
(USDA)	1 cup	730
(Franco-American):		
Regular	7⅜-oz. can	960
Elbow	7⅜-oz. can	910
(Hormel) *Short Orders*	7½-oz. can	917
Frozen:		
(Banquet):		
Casserole	8-oz. pkg.	930
Dinner	10-oz. pkg.	450
(Birds Eye):		
Classics	½ of 10-oz. pkg.	350
For One	5¾-oz. pkg.	456
(Celentano) baked	½ of 12-oz. pkg.	425
(Green Giant)	5½-oz. entree	590
(Stouffer's)	6-oz. serving	730

Food and Description	Measure or Quantity	Sodium (milligrams)
(Swanson) 3-compartment:		
Dinner	12¼-oz. dinner	970
Entree	12-oz. entree	824
(Swanson):		
Entree	12-oz. entree	1850
Dinner	12¼-oz. dinner	980
Mix:		
(Golden Gram)	¼ of pkg.	430
*(Kraft):		
Regular:		
Plain	¼ of pkg.	420
Spiral	⅓ of pkg.	400
Velveeta, shells	¼ of pkg.	720
MACARONI & CHEESE PIE,		
frozen (Swanson)	7-oz. pie	880
*MACARONI, SHELLS, AND SAUCE, mix (Lipton):		
Creamy garlic	½ cup	535
Herb tomato	½ cup	435
MACE (French's)	1 tsp. (1.8 grams)	1
MAGIC SHELL (Smucker's):		
Chocolate or chocolate fudge	1 T.	12
Chocolate nut	1 T.	20
MAI TAI COCKTAIL MIX (Holland House):		
Instant	.56-oz. packet	4
Liquid	1 oz.	60
MALTED MILK MIX:		
(USDA) dry powder	1 oz.	125
(Carnation):		
Chocolate	3 heaping tsps. (.7 oz.)	47
Natural	3 heaping tsps. (.7 oz.)	98
MALT EXTRACT, dried (USDA)	1 oz.	23
MALT LIQUOR:		
Colt 45, 4.35% alcohol	12 fl. oz.	8
Elephant, 7.1% alcohol	12 fl. oz	12
Kingsbury, non-alcoholic	12 fl. oz.	5

Food and Description	Measure or Quantity	Sodium (milligrams)
Mickey's	12 fl. oz.	14
MALT-O-MEAL, cereal:		
Regular	1 T. (.3 oz.)	<1
Chocolate flavored	1 T. (.3 oz.)	<1
MAMEY or MAMMEE		
APPLE, fresh (USDA)	1 lb. (weighed with skin & seeds)	42
MANDARIN ORANGE (See **TANGERINE**)		
MANGO, fresh (USDA):		
Whole	1 lb. (weighed with seeds & skin)	21
Whole	1 med. (7 oz.)	9
Flesh only, diced or sliced	½ cup (2.9 oz.)	6
MANGO NECTAR, canned (Libby's)	6 fl. oz.	5
MANHATTAN COCKTAIL:		
Canned (Mr. Boston)	3 fl. oz.	4
Mix (Holland House) liquid	1 oz.	5
MANICOTTI frozen:		
(Buitoni):		
Cheese	5½-oz. serving	432
Florentine	2 pieces (5½ oz.)	396
(Celentano):		
Without sauce	½ of 14-oz. pkg.	580
With sauce	½ of 16-oz. pkg.	690
(Weight Watchers) cheese, in tomato sauce	9¼-oz. meal	660
***MANWICH** (Hunt's):		
Original	1 sandwich	590
Extra thick & crunchy	1 sandwich	870
Mexican	1 sandwich	690
MAPLE SYRUP (See **SYRUP**)		
MARGARINE:		
Salted:		
Regular:		
(USDA)	1 lb.	4477
(USDA)	1 cup (8 oz.)	2239

Food and Description	Measure or Quantity	Sodium (milligrams)
(USDA)	1 T. (.5 oz.)	138
Autumn, soft or stick	1 T.	109
(Blue Bonnet) soft or stick	1 T. (.5 oz.)	95
Country Morning:		
Regular:		
Stick, lightly salted	1 T.	105
Tub, lightly salted	1 T.	75
Light, lightly salted:		
Stick	1 T.	90
Tub	1 T.	75
(Fleischmann's) soft or stick	1 T. (.5 oz.)	95
Heart Beat (GFA):		
Regular	1 T.	110
Nucanola 68% spread:		
Soft	1 T.	80
Stick	1 T.	90
Holiday	1 T. (.5 oz.)	165
I Can't Believe It's Not Butter:		
Stick	1 T.	95
Tub	1 T.	90
(Imperial) soft	1 T. (.5 oz.)	96
(Land O'Lakes)	1 T.	35
(Mazola) regular	1 T. (.5 oz.)	100
(Nucoa):		
Regular	1 T. (.5 oz.)	160
Soft	1 T. (.4 oz.)	150
(Promise) soft or stick	1 T. (.5 oz.)	90
(Shedd's)	1 T.	100
Unsalted, regular:		
(USDA)	1 T.	1
(Mazola)	1 T.	4
Imitation or dietetic:		
(Blue Bonnet)	1 T.	99
(Imperial) diet	1 T. (.5 oz.)	136
(Mazola)	1 T.	130
(Mazola)	½ cup	1066

Food and Description	Measure or Quantity	Sodium (milligrams)
Whipped:		
(USDA) salted	½ cup	750
(USDA) unsalted	½ cup	<8
(Blue Bonnet)	1 T. (9 g.)	99
(Fleischmann's) soft, unsalted	1 T.	7
(Imperial) spread	1 T. (9 g.)	70
(Parkay) cup	1 T.	74
MARGARITA COCKTAIL MIX (Holland House):		
Instant:		
Regular	.5-oz. packet	4
Strawberry	.56-oz. packet	<1
Liquid:		
Regular	1 oz.	92
Strawberry	1 oz.	3
MARINADE MIX:		
(Adolph's):		
Chicken	1-oz. pkg.	4105
Meat	.8-oz. pkg.	4636
(Durkee) meat	1-oz. pkg.	4104
(French's) meat	1-oz. pkg.	4320
(Kikkoman) meat	1-oz. pkg.	4000
MARJORAM (French's)	1 tsp. (1.2 g.)	1
MARMALADE:		
Sweetened:		
(USDA)	1 T. (.7 oz.)	3
(Home Brands)	1 T.	7
(Smucker's)	1 T. (.7 oz.)	0
Dietetic:		
(Estee)	1 T.	<3
(Featherweight)	1 T.	40–50
(Louis Sherry)	1 T.	<3
MARSHMALLOW FLUFF	1 heaping tsp. (.6 oz.)	5
MARSHMALLOW KRISPIES, cereal (Kellogg's)	1¼ cups	285
MASA HARINA (Quaker)	⅓ cup (1.3 oz.)	2
MASA TRIGO (Quaker)	⅓ cup (1.3 oz.)	294

Food and Description	Measure or Quantity	Sodium (milligrams)
MATZO:		
(Goodman's) *Diet-10*'s	1 sq.	<1
(Horowitz-Margareten) unsalted	1 matzo (1.2 oz.)	<1
(Manischewitz):		
Regular	1 piece (1 oz.)	<5
American	1 piece	175
Dietetic:		
Tam Tams, unsalted	1 piece	Tr.
Thins	1 piece (.8 oz.)	<5
Egg	1 piece	<5
Egg & onion	1 piece	180
Miniatures	1 piece	Tr.
Tam Tams:		
Regular	1 piece	17
Garlic or onion	1 piece	16
Wheat	1 piece	18
MATZO MEAL (Manischewitz)	1 cup (4.1 oz.)	2
MAYONNAISE:		
Real:		
(Bama)	1 T.	65
(Bennett's)	1 T.	65
(Hellmann's)	1 T. (.5 oz.)	80
(Hellmann's)	½ cup (3.9 oz.)	624
(Kraft)	1 T.	65
Dietetic or imitation:		
(Diet Delight) *Mayo-Lite*	1 T.	75
(Estee)	1 T.	80
Heart Beat (GFA)	1 T.	110
(Hellmann's):		
Light	1 T.	115
Cholesterol free	1 T.	80
(Kraft)	1 T.	90
(Weight Watchers):		
Regular	1 T.	100
Cholesterol free	1 T.	80
Low sodium	1 T.	35
(Featherweight) *Soyamaise*	1 T.	3
(Kraft) light	1 T.	90

Food and Description	Measure or Quantity	Sodium (milligrams)
McDONALD'S:		
Big Mac	1 hamburger	950
Biscuit:		
With bacon, egg & cheese	5.5-oz. sandwich	1230
With biscuit spread	2.6-oz. piece	730
With sausage	4.3-oz. sandwich	1080
With sausage & egg	6.2-oz. sandwich	1250
Cheeseburger	1 cheeseburger	750
Chicken McNuggets	1 serving (4 oz.)	520
Chicken McNugget sauce:		
Barbecue	1.1-oz. serving	340
Honey	.5-oz. serving	0
Hot mustard	1-oz. serving	250
Sweet & sour	1.1-oz. serving	190
Cookie:		
Chocolate chip	2-oz. pkg.	280
McDonaldland	2-oz. pkg.	300
Danish:		
Apple	4-oz. serving	370
Cheese, iced	3.9-oz. serving	420
Cinnamon raisin	3.9-oz. serving	430
Raspberry	4.1-oz. serving	310
Egg McMuffin	1 serving	740
Egg, scrambled	1 serving	290
English muffin, buttered	2.2-oz. muffin	270
Filet-o-Fish sandwich	1 sandwich	1030
Grapefruit juice	6 fl. oz.	0
Hamburger	1 hamburger	500
Hot cakes, with butter & syrup	1 serving	640
McD.L.T. sandwich	8¼-oz. serving	990
McLean Deluxe	1 burger	670
Orange juice	6 fl. oz.	0
Pie, apple	3-oz. pie	240
Potato:		
French fries	2.4-oz. order	110
Hash browns	1.9-oz. order	330
Quarter Pounder:		
Regular	1 burger	660

Food and Description	Measure or Quantity	Sodium (milligrams)
With cheese	1 burger	1150
Salad:		
Chef	10-oz. serving	490
Chicken, chunky	8.6-oz. serving	230
Garden	7½-oz. serving	160
Side	4.1-oz. serving	85
Salad dressing:		
Regular:		
Bleu cheese	.5-oz. serving	150
Caesar	.5-oz. serving	170
French	.5-oz. serving	180
Peppercorn	.5-oz. serving	85
Ranch	.5-oz. serving	130
1000 Island	.5-oz. serving	100
Dietetic:		
Red french	.5-oz. serving	110
Vinaigrette	.5-oz. serving	75
Sausage, pork	1.7-oz. serving	350
Sausage McMuffin:		
Plain	4.1-oz. sandwich	830
With egg	5.8-oz. sandwich	980
Shake:		
Chocolate	10.3-oz. serving	240
Strawberry	10.2-oz. serving	170
Vanilla	10.3-oz. serving	170
Soft drink:		
Sweetened:		
Coca-Cola Classic	12 fl. oz.	15
Coca-Cola Classic	16 fl. oz.	20
Coca-Cola Classic	22 fl. oz.	25
Orange drink	12 fl. oz.	10
Orange drink	16 fl. oz.	15
Orange drink	22 fl. oz.	18
Sprite	12 fl. oz.	15
Sprite	16 fl. oz.	20
Sprite	22 fl. oz.	25
Dietetic, Coke:		
Small	12 fl. oz.	30
Medium	16 fl. oz.	40

Food and Description	Measure or Quantity	Sodium (milligrams)
Large	22 fl. oz.	60
Sundae:		
Caramel, hot	6.1-oz. serving	160
Hot fudge	6-oz. serving	160
Strawberry	6-oz. serving	80
Vanilla soft-serve, with cone	3 fl. oz.	70
MEATBALL DINNER or ENTREE:		
*Canned (Hunt's) *Minute Gourmet*	7.6-oz. serving	942
Frozen (Swanson)	8½-oz. meal	900
MEATBALL, SWEDISH, frozen (Armour):		
Dining Lite, & sauce	9-oz. meal	660
Dinner Classics	11¼-oz. meal	720
(Stouffer's) with parsley noodles	11-oz. meal	1510
MEAT LOAF DINNER or ENTREE, frozen:		
(Armour) *Dinner Classics*	11¼-oz. meal	1170
(Banquet)	11-oz. dinner	770
(Morton) dinner	10-oz. dinner	1520
(Swanson):		
Dinner	11-oz. dinner	970
Entree, with tomato sauce	9-oz. entree	950
*MEAT LOAF SEASONING MIX (Bell's)	4½ oz. serving	700
MEAT, POTTED:		
(Hormel)	1 T.	145
(Libby's)	⅓ of 5-oz. can	297
MEAT TENDERIZER (French's) unseasoned or seasoned	1 tsp. (5 g.)	1760
MELBA TOAST (Old London):		
Garlic rounds	1 piece (2 g.)	22
Pumpernickel	1 piece (5 g.)	39
Rye:		
Regular	1 piece (5 g.)	39
Unsalted	1 piece (5 g.)	<1

Food and Description	Measure or Quantity	Sodium (milligrams)
Sesame rounds	1 piece (2 g.)	28
Wheat:		
Regular	1 piece (5 g.)	39
Unsalted	1 piece (5 g.)	<1
White:		
Regular	1 piece (5 g.)	39
Rounds	1 piece (2 g.)	22
Unsalted	1 piece (5 g.)	<1
MELON (See individual listings such as CANTALOUPE; WATERMELON; etc.)		
MELON BALLS (cantaloupe & honeydew) in syrup, frozen (USDA)	½ cup (4.1 oz.)	10
MENUDO, canned:		
(Hormel) *Casa Grande*	7½-oz. can	1097
(Old El Paso)	½ of can	770
MEXICALI DOGS, frozen (Hormel)	5 oz.	952
MEXICAN DINNER, frozen:		
(Banquet) dinner:		
Regular	12-oz. dinner	2000
Combination	12-oz. dinner	1980
(Morton)	10-oz. dinner	1390
(Patio):		
Regular	13¼-oz. meal	1940
Fiesta	12¼-oz. meal	2040
(Swanson):		
Regular	16-oz. dinner	1780
Hungry Man	22-oz. dinner	2430
MILK, CONDENSED (Carnation) sweetened, canned	1 cup (10.8 oz.)	392
MILK, DRY:		
Whole (USDA) packed cup	1 cup (5.1 oz.)	587
*Nonfat, instant:		
(Alba):		
Regular	8 fl. oz.	120
Chocolate flavor	8 fl. oz.	114
(Carnation)	8 fl. oz.	125

Food and Description	Measure or Quantity	Sodium (milligrams)
Sanalac (Sanna)	1 cup	<1
MILK, EVAPORATED, canned:		
Regular:		
(USDA) unsweetened	1 cup (8.9 oz.)	297
(Carnation)	1 fl. oz.	33
(Pet)	1 fl. oz.	35
Buttermilk (Borden) *Golden*		
Churn Brand	1 fl. oz.	31
Low fat (Carnation)	1 fl. oz.	34
Skimmed (Carnation)	1 fl. oz.	35
MILK, FRESH:		
Buttermilk, cultured, fresh:		
(Friendship) no salt added	8 fl. oz.	125
(Land O'Lakes)	8 fl. oz.	220
Chocolate milk drink, fresh:		
(USDA)	1 cup (8.8 fl. oz.)	118
(Borden) *Dutch Brand*	8 fl. oz.	180
(Hershey's) whole	1 cup	120
(Johanna):		
Regular	1 cup	200
Low fat	1 cup	210
(Land O'Lakes):		
½%	8 fl. oz.	170
With *Nutrasweet*	8 fl. oz.	200
Lowfat:		
(Borden):		
1% milkfat	8 fl. oz.	130
2% milkfat,		
Hi-Protein Brand	8 fl. oz.	150
(Johanna):		
Regular:		
1% milkfat	1 cup	125
2% milkfat:		
Regular	1 cup	125
Mighty Milk	1 cup	150
Buttermilk	1 cup	250
(Land O'Lakes)	8 fl. oz.	125
Skim:		
(USDA)	1 cup (8.6 oz.)	127

Food and Description	Measure or Quantity	Sodium (milligrams)
(Borden):		
Regular	8 fl. oz.	130
Skim-Line	8 fl. oz.	150
(Dean)	1 cup (8.2 oz.)	130
(Land O'Lakes)	8 fl. oz.	125
(Weight Watchers)	1 cup	140
Whole:		
(USDA)	1 cup (8.6 oz.)	122
(Borden) regular or hi-calcium	8 fl. oz.	130
(Dean)	1 cup (8.6 oz.)	112
(Land O'Lakes)	8 fl. oz.	125
MILK, GOAT (USDA)	1 cup (8.6 oz.)	83
MILK, HUMAN (USDA)	1 oz. (by wt.)	5
MILK MAKERS (Swiss Miss):		
Chocolate	8 fl. oz.	230
Malted	8 fl. oz.	220
Strawberry	8 fl. oz.	170
MILNOT, dairy vegetable blend	1 fl. oz.	35
MINCEMEAT (See **PIE FILLING**)		
MINERAL WATER		
(Schweppes)	6 fl. oz.	3
MINESTRONE SOUP (See **SOUP,** Minestrone)		
MINI-WHEATS, cereal (Kellogg's) brown-sugar cinnamon or sugar frosted	1 biscuit (.25 oz.)	0
MINT LEAVES (HHS/FAO):		
Raw, untrimmed	1 lb. (weighed with tough stems & branches)	1
Raw, trimmed	½ oz.	Tr.
MOLASSES:		
(USDA):		
Blackstrap	1 T. (.7 oz.)	18
Light	1 T. (.7 oz.)	3
Dark	1 T. (.7 oz.)	7
Medium	1 T. (.7 oz.)	8

Food and Description	Measure or Quantity	Sodium (milligrams)
(Grandma's) unsulphured:		
Gold label	1T. (.7 oz.)	28
Green label	1T. (.7 oz.)	57
MOUSSE:		
Frozen (Weight Watchers):		
Chocolate	½ of 5-oz. pkg.	190
Praline pecan	½ of 5.4-oz. pkg.	180
Raspberry	½ of 5-oz. pkg.	150
*Mix:		
Regular (Knorr):		
Unflavored	½ cup	45
Chocolate	½ cup	50
Dietetic:		
(Estee) any flavor	½ cup	50
Lite Whip (TKI Foods), any flavor, prepared with skim or whole milk	½ cup	55
(Weight Watchers):		
Cheesecake	½ cup	75
Chocolate:		
Regular	½ cup	45
White, almond	½ cup	50
Raspberry	½ cup	75
MUESLI, cereal (Ralston-Purina)	½ cup (1.45-oz.)	95
MÜESLIX, cereal (Kellogg's):		
Crispy blend	⅔ cup (1½ oz.)	150
Golden Crunch	½ cup (1.2 oz.)	170
MUFFIN (See also **MUFFIN MIX**):		
Blueberry:		
Home recipe (USDA)	3″ muffin (1.4 oz.)	253
(Pepperidge Farm)	1.9-oz. muffin	250
Bran:		
(USDA) home recipe	3″ muffin (1.4 oz.)	179
(Pepperidge Farm) with raisins	2.1-oz. muffin	295

Food and Description	Measure or Quantity	Sodium (milligrams)
Corn:		
Home recipe (USDA) prepared with whole-ground cornmeal	1.4-oz. muffin	198
(Pepperidge Farm)	1.9-oz. muffin	260
English:		
Millbrook:		
Regular or cinnamon raisin	2-oz. muffin	200
Sourdough or whole wheat	2-oz. muffin	220
(Pepperidge Farm):		
Regular	1 muffin	180
Cinnamon raisin	1 muffin	180
Pritikin	2.3-oz. muffin	160
Sun Maid, raisin	2.3-oz. muffin	220
(Thomas') regular	2-oz. muffin	207
Plain, home recipe (USDA)	1.4-oz. muffin (3" dia.)	176
Raisin (Arnold)	2½-oz. muffin	350
MUFFIN MIX:		
*Apple cinnamon (Betty Crocker)	¹⁄₁₂ of pkg.	140
*Applesauce, *Gold Medal*	¹⁄₁₆ of pkg.	240
*Apple streusel (Betty Crocker)	¹⁄₁₂ of pkg.	240
*Banana, *Gold Medal*	⅙ of pkg.	240
*Banana nut (Betty Crocker)	¹⁄₁₂ of pkg.	140
*Blueberry (Betty Crocker) wild	1 muffin	150
*Caramel, *Gold Medal*	⅙ of pkg.	250
*Carrot nut (Betty Crocker)	¹⁄₁₂ of pkg.	160
*Chocolate chip (Betty Crocker)	¹⁄₁₂ of pkg.	180
*Cinnamon streusel (Betty Crocker)	¹⁄₁₀ of pkg.	240
*Cinnamon swirl (Duncan Hines) bakery style	1 muffin	243
Corn:		
(USDA) prepared with egg & milk	1.4-oz. muffin	136
(USDA) prepared with egg & water	1.4-oz. muffin	138

Food and Description	Measure or Quantity	Sodium (milligrams)
*Gold Medal	⅙ of pkg.	250
Cranberry orange nut (Duncan Hines) bakery style	¹⁄₁₂ of pkg.	199
*Honey bran, Gold Medal	⅙ of pkg.	240
*Oat, Gold Medal	⅙ of pkg.	220
Oat bran:		
*(Betty Crocker)	⅛ of pkg.	240
(Duncan Hines):		
Blueberry	1 muffin	208
& honey	1 muffin	213
*(Estee) dietetic	1 muffin	65
*Oatmeal raisin (Betty Crocker)	¹⁄₁₂ of pkg.	125
Pecan nut (Duncan Hines) bakery style	1 muffin	231
*Strawberry crown (Betty Crocker)	¹⁄₁₀ of pkg.	170
MULLET, raw (USDA):		
Whole	1 lb. (weighed whole)	195
Meat only	4 oz.	92
MUNG BEAN SPROUT (See **BEAN SPROUT**)		
MUSCATEL WINE (Gold Seal)		
19% alcohol	3 fl. oz.	3
MUSHROOM:		
Raw (USDA):		
Whole	½ lb. (weighed untrimmed)	33
Trimmed, slices	½ cup (1.2 oz.)	5
Canned, solids & liq.:		
(USDA)	½ cup (4.3 oz.)	488
(Green Giant):		
Regular	¼ cup	290
B & B	¼ cup	240
(Shady Oak)	4-oz. can	452
Frozen:		
(Birds Eye) whole, deluxe	⅓ of 8-oz. pkg.	3
(Larsen)	3.5 oz.	15
(Ore-Ida) breaded	2⅔ oz.	515

Food and Description	Measure or Quantity	Sodium (milligrams)
MUSHROOM, CHINESE (HHS/FAO):		
Dried	1 oz.	11
Dried, soaked, drained	1 oz.	Tr.
MUSKMELON (See **CANTA-LOUPE; CASABA; HONEYDEW**)		
MUSSEL (USDA) Atlantic & Pacific, raw, meat only	4 oz.	328
MUSTARD, DRY or POWDERED (French's)	1 tsp.	Tr.
MUSTARD, PREPARED:		
Brown:		
(USDA)	1 tsp.	118
(French's) *'N Spicy*	1 tsp.	50
Chinese (La Choy) hot	1 tsp. (2. oz.)	130
Grey Poupon	1 tsp.	149
Horseradish (French's)	1 tsp.	93
Hot, *Mr. Mustard*	1 tsp.	90
Medford (French's)	1 tsp.	83
Onion (French's)	1 tsp.	67
Yellow (French's)	1 tsp.	60
MUSTARD GREENS:		
Raw (USDA) whole	1 lb. (weighed untrimmed)	102
Boiled (USDA) drained	1 cup (7.8 oz.)	40
Canned (Sunshine) chopped, solids & liq.	½ cup (4.1 oz.)	371
Frozen:		
(USDA) boiled, drained	½ cup (3.8 oz.)	11
(McKenzie) chopped	3.3 oz.	37
(Southland) chopped	⅕ of 16-oz. pkg.	20

Food and Description	Measure or Quantity	Sodium (milligrams)

N

NATHAN'S:
  French fries | 1 regular order | 151
  Hamburger | 4½-oz. sandwich | 203
  Hot dog | 1 order | 675

NATURAL CEREAL:
  Familia:
    Regular | ½ cup | 8
    Bran | ½ cup | 90
    Granola | ½ cup | 67
    No added sugar | ½ cup | 2
  Heartland (Pet) | ¼ cup | 80
  Nature Valley (General Mills):
    Cinnamon & raisin or
      toasted oat | ⅓ cup | 90
    Fruit & nut | ⅓ cup | 75
  (Quaker):
    100% natural:
      Regular | ¼ cup (1-oz.) | 11
      With apples & cinnamon | ¼ cup (1 oz.) | 15
      With raisins & dates | ¼ cup (1 oz.) | 11
      Whole wheat, hot | ⅓ cup (1 oz.) | 1

NATURE SNACKS (Sun-Maid):
  Carob crunch | 1-oz. serving | 13
  Carob peanut | 1¼-oz. serving | 16
  Carob raisin | 1¼-oz. serving | 21
  Raisin crunch | 1-oz. serving | 41
  Rocky road | 1-oz. serving | 4
  Sesame nut crunch | 1-oz. serving | 159
  Tahitian treat | 1-oz. serving | 7
  Yogurt crunch | 1-oz. serving | 28

Food and Description	Measure or Quantity	Sodium (milligrams)
Yogurt peanut	1¼-oz. serving	25
Yogurt raisin	1¼-oz. serving	20
NECTARINE, fresh (USDA):		
Whole	1 lb. (weighed with pits)	25
Flesh only	4 oz.	7
NEW ZEALAND SPINACH (USDA):		
Raw	1 lb.	721
Boiled, drained	4 oz.	104
NINTENDO CEREAL SYSTEM (Ralston-Purina)	1 cup (1 oz.)	70
NOODLE:		
Dry	1 oz.	1
Dry, 1½″ strips	1 cup (2.6 oz.)	4
Cooked	1 oz.	<1
NOODLE & CHICKEN (See also **CHICKEN & NOODLES**)		
Canned (Hormel) *Dinty Moore, Short Orders*	7½-oz. can	1144
Frozen (Banquet)	10-oz. dinner	460
NOODLE, CHOW MEIN, canned (La Choy)	½ cup (1. oz.)	230
NOODLE MIX:		
*(Betty Crocker):		
Fettucini Alfredo	¼ pkg.	490
Parisienne	¼ pkg.	540
Romanoff	¼ pkg.	705
Stroganoff	¼ pkg.	605
*(Lipton) & sauce:		
Regular:		
Beef	½ cup	595
Butter	½ cup	565
Butter & herb	½ cup	525
Cheese	½ cup	540
Chicken	½ cup	465
Sour cream & chive	½ cup	455
Deluxe:		
Alfredo	½ cup	560

Food and Description	Measure or Quantity	Sodium (milligrams)
Chicken Bombay	½ cup	515
Parmesano	½ cup	445
Stroganoff	½ cup	510
(Noodle Roni) parmesano	⅕ pkg.	270
*NOODLE, RAMEN, canned (La Choy):		
Beef	½ of 3-oz. pkg.	1040
Chicken	½ of 3-oz. pkg.	1159
Oriental	½ of 3-oz. pkg.	742
NOODLE, RICE, canned (La Choy)	⅓ of 3-oz. can	420
NOODLE ROMANOFF, frozen (Stouffer's)	4-oz. servng	840
NUT, MIXED (See also individual kinds):		
(Adams) All America Nut	1 oz.	85
(Eagle) roasted, regular or deluxe	1 oz.	130
(Fisher):		
Dry, salted	1 oz.	110
Honey roasted & cashews	1 oz.	90
Oil:		
Salted:		
Regular	1 oz.	85
Cashews & peanuts	1 oz.	80
No peanuts	1 oz.	70
Lightly salted	1 oz.	45
(Guy's) with peanuts	1 oz.	140
(Planters):		
Dry:		
Salted	1 oz.	270
Unsalted	1 oz.	0
Oil:		
Regular	1 oz.	130
Deluxe	1 oz.	135
Unsalted	1 oz.	0
NUT & HONEY CRUNCH, cereal (Kellogg's)	⅔ cup (1 oz.)	200

Food and Description	Measure or Quantity	Sodium (milligrams)
NUT & HONEY CRUNCH Os,		
cereal (Kellogg's)	⅔ cup (1 oz.)	190
NUTMEG (French's)	1 tsp.	Tr.
NUTRIFIC, cereal (Kellogg's)	1 cup (1.3 oz.)	240
NUTRI-GRAIN, cereal (Kellogg's):		
Almond raisin	⅔ cup (1.4 oz.)	220
Raisin bran	1 cup (1.4 oz.)	200
Wheat	⅔ cup (1 oz.)	170

O

OATBAKE, cereal (Kellogg's):		
Honey bran	⅓ cup	180
Raisin nut	⅓ cup	190
OAT FLAKES, cereal (Post)	⅔ cup (1 oz.)	127
OATMEAL:		
Regular, dry:		
(USDA)	1 T.	<1
(Elam's) Scotch style	1 oz.	3
(H-O):		
Old fashioned	1 T. (5 g.)	<1
Old fashioned	1 cup (2.6 oz.)	<1
(Quaker)	⅓ cup (1 oz.)	1
(Ralston Purina)	⅓ cup (1 oz.)	1
*Regular, cooked (USDA)	1 cup (8.5 oz.)	523
Instant, dry:		
(Harvest Brand):		
Regular	1 oz.	230
Apple & cinnamon	1¼ oz.	242
Cinnamon & spice	1⅝ oz.	307
Maple & brown sugar	1½ oz.	295
Peaches & cream	⅓ cup (1¼ oz.)	199

Food and Description	Measure or Quantity	Sodium (milligrams)
(General Mills) *Oatmeal Swirlers:*		
Apple cinnamon	1.7-oz. packet	120
Cherry	1.7-oz. packet	130
Cinnamon spice or maple brown sugar	1.6-oz. packet	100
Milk chocolate	1.7-oz. packet	100
Strawberry	1.6-oz. packet	120
(H-O):		
Regular, box	1 T. (4 g.)	Tr.
Regular	1-oz. packet	230
Apple cinnamon	1.2-oz. packet	220
Maple brown sugar	1½-oz. packet	285
Raisin & spice	1½-oz. packet	240
Sweet & mellow	1.3-oz. packet	270
(3-Minute Brand):		
Regular	1-oz. packet	280
Apple & cinnamon	1⅜-oz. packet	300
Cinnamon & spice	1½-oz. packet	380
Maple & brown sugar	1½-oz. packet	290
Total (General Mills):		
Regular	1.2-oz. packet	220
Apple cinnamon	1¼-oz. packet	105
Cinnamon raisin	1.8-oz. packet	130
Maple brown sugar	1.6-oz. packet	150
Quick, dry:		
(Harvest Brand)	⅓ cup (1 oz.)	<5
(H-O)	1 cup (2.5 oz.)	<10
OATS & FIBER, cereal (H-O) hot:		
Boxed, dry	⅓ cup (1 oz.)	5
Packets, plain, apple & bran or raisin & bran	1 packet	140
OCEAN PERCH, fresh (USDA):	Atlantic:	
Raw, whole	1 lb. (weighed whole)	111
Fried	4 oz.	174
Pacific:		
Raw, whole	1 lb. (weighed whole)	77

Food and Description	Measure or Quantity	Sodium (milligrams)
Raw, meat only	4 oz.	71
OIL, SALAD or COOKING	Any quantity	0
OKRA:		
Raw (USDA) whole	1 lb. (weighed untrimmed)	12
Boiled (USDA) drained:		
Whole	½ cup (3.1 oz.)	2
Pods	8 pods, 3″ × ⅝″ (3 oz.)	2
Slices	½ cup (2.8 oz.)	2
Frozen:		
(USDA) boiled, drained:		
Cut	½ cup (3.2 oz.)	2
Whole	½ cup (2.4 oz.)	1
(Frosty Acres)	3.3 oz.	0
(Larsen) cut or whole	3.3 oz.	5
(McKenzie)	3.3 oz.	19
(Ore-Ida) breaded	3 oz.	665
(Southland):		
Cut	⅕ of 16-oz. pkg.	0
Whole	⅕ of 16-oz. pkg.	0
OLD FASHIONED COCKTAIL MIX (Holland House) liquid	1 oz.	6
OLEOMARGARINE (See **MARGARINE**)		
OLIVE:		
Green style (USDA):		
With pits, drained	1 oz.	748
Pitted, drained	1 oz.	932
Green (USDA)	1 oz.	680
Ripe, by variety (USDA):		
Ascalano, any size, pitted & drained	1 oz.	230
Manzanilla, any size	1 oz.	230
Mission, any size	1 oz.	213
Mission	3 small or 2 large	75
Mission, slices	½ cup (2.2 oz.)	465
Sevillano, any size	1 oz.	235

Food and Description	Measure or Quantity	Sodium (milligrams)
ONION (See also **ONION, GREEN:**		
Raw, all varieties (USDA):		
Whole	1 lb. (weighed untrimmed)	41
Whole	3.9-oz. onion (2½″ dia.)	10
Chopped	½ cup (3 oz.)	9
Chopped	1 T. (.4 oz.)	1
Grated	1 T. (.5 oz.)	1
Slices	½ cup (2 oz.)	6
Boiled, drained (USDA):		
Whole	½ cup (3.7 oz.)	7
Whole, pearl onion	½ cup (3.7 oz.)	6
Halves or pieces	½ cup (3.2 oz.)	6
Canned, *O & C* (Durkee):		
Boiled	1-oz. serving	2
In cream sauce	1-oz. serving	2854
Dehydrated:		
Flakes:		
(USDA)	1 tsp. (1.3 g.)	1
(Gilroy)	1 tsp.	<1
Powder (Gilroy)	1 tsp.	1
Frozen:		
(Birds Eye):		
Chopped	1 oz.	2
Small, whole	⅓ of 12-oz. pkg.	9
Small, with cream sauce	⅓ of 9-oz. pkg.	333
(Frosty Acres) chopped	1 oz.	5
(Green Giant) cheese sauce	½ cup	400
(Larsen):		
Diced	1 oz.	Tr.
Whole	3.3 oz.	10
(McKenzie) chopped	1 oz.	2
(Mrs. Paul's) rings, breaded & fried	½ of 5-oz. pkg.	305
(Ore-Ida):		
Chopped	2 oz.	10

Food and Description	Measure or Quantity	Sodium (milligrams)
Onion Ringers, diced & battered	2 oz.	180
(Southland) chopped	⅕ of 10-oz. pkg.	0
ONION BOUILLON:		
(Herb-Ox):		
Regular	1 cube	560
Instant	1 packet	800
MBT	1 packet	795
(Wyler's) instant	1 tsp.	670
ONION, COCKTAIL (Vlasic) lightly spiced	1 oz.	371
ONION, GREEN, raw (USDA):		
Whole	1 lb. (weighed untrimmed)	22
Bulb & entire top	1 oz.	1
Bulb without green top	3 small onions (.9 oz.)	1
Slices, bulb & white portion of top	½ cup (1.8 oz.)	2
Tops only	1 oz.	1
ONION SOUP (See **SOUP,** Onion)		
ORANGE, fresh (USDA):		
California Navel:		
Whole	1 lb. (weighed with rind & seeds)	3
Fruit including peel	6.3-oz orange (2⅘″ dia.)	1
Sections	1 cup (8.5 oz.)	2
California Valencia:		
Whole	1 lb. (weighed with rind & seeds)	3
Fruit including peel	6.3-oz. orange (2⅝″ dia.)	4
Sections	1 cup (8.5 oz.)	2
Florida, all varieties:		
Whole	1 lb. (weighed with rind & seeds)	3

Food and Description	Measure or Quantity	Sodium (milligrams)
Fruit including peel	7.4-oz. orange (3″ dia.)	2
Sections	1 cup (8.5 oz.)	2
ORANGE-APRICOT JUICE DRINK, canned (USDA)		
40% fruit juices	1 cup (8.8 oz.)	Tr.
ORANGE DRINK:		
Canned:		
Bama (Borden)	8.45-fl.-oz. container	60
Capri Sun, natural	6¾ fl. oz.	2
(Hi-C)	6 fl. oz.	17
Ssips (Johanna Farms)	8.45-fl.-oz. container	<10
Chilled (Sealtest)	6 fl. oz.	Tr.
*Mix:		
Regular (Funny Face)	6 fl. oz.	22
Dietetic:		
Crystal Light	6 fl. oz.	<1
(Sunkist)	6 fl. oz.	52
ORANGE EXTRACT (Virginia Dare) 79% alcohol	1 tsp.	0
ORANGE FRUIT JUICE BLEND, canned (Mott's)	9.5-fl.-oz. can	6
ORANGE-GRAPEFRUIT JUICE:		
Canned, unsweetened:		
(USDA)	1 cup (8.7 oz.)	2
(Borden) *Sippin' Pak*	8.45-fl.-oz. container	25
(Del Monte)	6 fl. oz.	2
(Libby's)	6 fl. oz.	5
Canned, sweetened:		
(USDA)	1 cup (8.9 oz.)	3
(Del Monte)	6 fl. oz. (6.5 oz.)	2
*Frozen: (USDA) unsweetened	½ cup (4.4 oz.)	Tr.
ORANGE JUICE:		
Fresh (USDA):		
California Navel	½ cup (4.4 oz.)	1

Food and Description	Measure or Quantity	Sodium (milligrams)
California Valencia	½ cup (4.4 oz.)	1
Florida, early or midseason	½ cup (4.4 oz.)	1
Florida Temple	½ cup (4.4 oz.)	1
Florida Valencia	½ cup (4.4 oz.)	1
Canned, unsweetened:		
(USDA)	½ cup (4.4 oz.)	1
(Land O' Lakes)	6 fl. oz.	0
(Libby's)	6 fl. oz.	0
(Ocean Spray)	6 fl. oz.	5
(Texsun)	6 fl. oz.	2
Canned, sweetened:		
(USDA)	½ cup (4.4 oz.)	1
(Borden) *Sippin' Pak*	8.45-fl.-oz. container	25
(Del Monte)	6 fl. oz.	2
(Libby's)	6 fl. oz.	5
Chilled		
(Citrus Hill) regular or lite	6 fl. oz.	10
(Minute Maid) any style	6 fl. oz.	19
(Sunkist)	6 fl. oz.	2
*Dehydrated crystals (USDA)	½ cup (4.4 oz.)	1
*Frozen:		
(USDA)	½ cup (4.4 oz.)	1
(Citrus Hill)	6 fl. oz.	10
(Minute Maid)	6 fl. oz.	19
(Sunkist)	6 fl. oz.	2
ORANGE JUICE BAR, frozen (Sunkist)	3-fl.-oz. bar	<1
ORANGE JUICE DRINK, canned (General Mills) *Squeezit*	6¾-fl.-oz. can	5
ORANGE, MANDARIN (See **TANGERINE**)		
ORANGE, PINEAPPLE BANANA JUICE, canned (Land O' Lakes)	6 fl. oz.	0
ORANGE-PINEAPPLE JUICE, canned (Land O' Lakes)	6 fl. oz.	0
OREGANO, dried (French's)	1 tsp.	Tr.

Food and Description	Measure or Quantity	Sodium (milligrams)
OVEN FRY (General Foods):		
Chicken:		
Extra crispy	4.2-oz. pkg.	3300
Homestyle flour	3.2-oz. pkg.	3886
Pork, *Shake & Bake,* extra		
crispy	4.2-oz. pkg.	2754
Home style flour recipe	3.2-oz. envelope	3955
OYSTER:		
Raw (USDA) meat only:		
Eastern	13–19 med. oysters (1 cup, 8.5 oz.)	175
Eastern	4 oz.	83
Fried (USDA) dipped in egg, milk & breadcrumbs	4 oz.	234
OYSTER CRACKER (See **CRACKERS**)		
OYSTER STEW (USDA):		
Home recipe:		
1 part oysters to 2 parts milk by volume	1 cup (8.5 oz.)	814
1 part oysters to 3 parts milk by volume	1 cup (8.5 oz.)	487
*Frozen:		
Prepared with equal volume milk	1 cup (8.5 oz.)	878
Prepared with equal volume water	1 cup (8.5 oz.)	816

Food and Description	Measure or Quantity	Sodium (milligrams)

P

PANCAKE: (See also **PANCAKE & WAFFLE**)

Home recipe, plain (USDA)	4″ pancake (1 oz.)	115
Frozen (Pillsbury) microwave:		
Plain	1 pancake	183
Blueberry	1 pancake	180
Buttermilk	1 pancake	197
Harvest wheat	1 pancake	140

PANCAKE DINNER or ENTREE, frozen (Swanson):

& blueberry sauce	7-oz. meal	800
& sausage	6-oz. meal	940

PANCAKE & WAFFLE BATTER, frozen (Aunt Jemima):

Plain	4″ pancake	286
Blueberry	4″ pancake	233
Buttermilk	4″ pancake	244

PANCAKE & WAFFLE MIX:

Plain:

(USDA)	1 oz.	406
(USDA)	1 cup (4.8 oz.)	1935
*(USDA) prepared with milk	4″ pancake (1 oz.)	122
*(USDA) prepared with egg & milk	4″ pancake	152
*(Aunt Jemima):		
Complete	4″ pancake	290
Original	4″ pancake	183
*Bisquick Shake 'N Pour (General Mills):		
Regular	4″ pancake	283

Food and Description	Measure or Quantity	Sodium (milligrams)
Complete	1 waffle	465
*FastShake (Little Crow)	¼ of container	368
*Mrs. Butterworth's, old fashioned, butter flavor:		
Regular	4″ pancake	243
Complete	4″ pancake	270
*(Pillsbury) Hungry Jack:		
Extra Lights, regular	4″ pancake	163
Panshakes	4″ pancake	293
*Apple cinnamon, Bisquick Shake 'N Pour (General Mills)	4″ pancake	290
*Blueberry:		
Bisquick Shake 'N Pour (General Mills)	4″ pancake	287
FastShake (Little Crow)	¼ of 5-oz. container	342
(Pillsbury) Hungry Jack	4″ pancake	273
Buckwheat:		
(USDA)	1 cup (4.8 oz.)	1801
*(USDA) prepared with egg & milk	4″ pancake	125
Buttermilk:		
(USDA)	1 cup (4.8 oz.)	1935
*(USDA) prepared with egg & milk	4″ pancake	152
*(Aunt Jemima):		
Regular	4″ pancake	330
Complete	4″ pancake	290
*(Betty Crocker):		
Regular	4″ pancake	270
Complete	4″ pancake	167
*Bisquick Shake 'N Pour (General Mills)	4″ pancake	287
*FastShake (Little Crow)	¼ of 5-oz. container	385
*Gold Medal	⅛ of mix	280
*Mrs. Butterworth's	4″ pancake	270

Food and Description	Measure or Quantity	Sodium (milligrams)
*(Pillsbury) *Hungry Jack*, regular	4″ pancake	190
*Oat bran, *Bisquick Shake 'N Pour* (General Mills)	4″ pancake	193
*Whole wheat (Aunt Jemima)	4″ pancake	242
*Dietetic (Estee)	3″ pancake	45
PANCAKE & WAFFLE SYRUP (See **SYRUP**)		
PANCREAS, raw (USDA):		
Beef, lean only	4 oz.	76
Hog or hog sweetbread	4 oz.	50
PAPAYA, fresh (USDA):		
Whole	1 lb. (weighed with skin & seeds)	9
Cubed	1 cup (6.4 oz.)	5
PAPAYA JUICE, canned (HHS/FAO)	4 oz.	12
PAPRIKA, domestic (French's)	1 tsp.	Tr.
PARSLEY, fresh (USDA):		
Whole	½ lb.	102
Chopped	1 T. (4 g.)	2
PARSLEY FLAKES, dehydrated (French's)	1 tsp. (1.1 g.)	6
PARSNIP (USDA):		
Raw, whole	1 lb. (weighed unprepared)	46
Boiled, drained, cut in pieces	½ cup (3.7 oz.)	8
PASTA DINNER or ENTREE, frozen (See also **SHELLS, PASTA, STUFFED,** frozen):		
(Birds Eye):		
Continental style	½ of 10-oz. pkg.	347
Marinara, classics	½ of 10-oz. pkg.	415
Primavera, For One	5-oz. pkg.	444
(Celentano) & cheese, baked	½ of 12-oz. pkg.	395
(Green Giant):		
Regular:		
Dijon	9½-oz. pkg.	630

Food and Description	Measure or Quantity	Sodium (milligrams)
Florentine	9½-oz. pkg.	840
One Serving:		
Marinara	6-oz. pkg.	730
Parmesan, with sweet peas	5½-oz. pkg.	510
Pasta Accents:		
Creamy cheddar	⅙ of 16-oz. pkg.	310
Garden herb	⅙ of 16-oz. pkg.	220
Garlic	⅙ of 16-oz. pkg.	280
Primavera	⅙ of 16-oz. pkg.	180
(Stouffer's):		
Carbonara	9¾-oz. pkg.	780
Casino	9¼-oz. pkg.	800
Mexicali	10-oz. pkg.	1020
Oriental	9⅞-oz. pkg.	760
Primavera	10⅝-oz. pkg.	580
(Weight Watchers):		
Primavera	8½-oz. pkg.	800
Rigati	11-oz. pkg.	870
PASTA SALAD, frozen (Birds Eye) Classics, Italian style	½ of 10-oz. pkg.	183
***PASTA & SAUCE MIX** (Lipton):		
Cheddar broccoli with fusilli	¼ of pkg.	448
Cheese supreme	¼ of pkg.	406
Garlic, creamy	¼ of pkg.	545
Mushroom & chicken	¼ of pkg.	435
Mushroom, creamy	¼ of pkg.	424
Oriental, with fusilli	¼ of pkg.	506
Tomato, herb	¼ of pkg.	456
PASTINA, DRY (USDA) egg	1 oz.	1
PASTRAMI, packaged:		
(Carl Buddig)	1 oz.	320
(Eckrich)	1 oz.	360
PASTRY POCKETS (Pillsbury)	1 piece	520
PASTRY SHEET, PUFF, frozen (Pepperidge Farm)	1 sheet	1160
PASTRY SHELL (See also **PIE CRUST**):		
Home recipe (USDA) baked	1 shell (1.5 oz.)	260
Frozen (Pet-Ritz)	1 shell	150

Food and Description	Measure or Quantity	Sodium (milligrams)
PÂTÉ, liver (Sell's)	4.8-oz. can	1142
PEA, green:		
Raw (USDA):		
In pod	1 lb. (weighed in pod)	3
Shelled	1 lb.	9
Shelled	½ cup (2.4 oz.)	1
Boiled (USDA) drained	½ cup (2.9 oz.)	<1
Canned, regular pack:		
(USDA):		
Alaska, early or June:		
Solids & liq.	½ cup (4.4 oz.)	293
Solids only	½ cup (3 oz.)	203
Sweet:		
Solids & liq.	½ cup (4.4 oz.)	293
Solids only	½ cup (3 oz.)	203
Drained liquid	4 oz.	268
(Comstock) solids & liq.	½ cup	400
(Del Monte) solids & liq:		
Seasoned	½ cup	355
Sweet	½ cup	355
(Festal):		
Early garden, solids & liq.	½ cup	333
Seasoned, solids only	½ cup	226
Sweet, tiny size, solids only	½ cup	313
(Green Giant) solids & liq.:		
Early June	½ cup	330
Sweet:		
Regular	½ cup	320
Small	½ cup	340
With onion	½ cup	510
(Larsen) *Freshlike*	½ cup	370
(Libby's) sweet, solids & liq.	½ cup (4.2 oz.)	337
(Stokely-Van Camp) solids & liq.:		
Early	½ cup (4.4 oz.)	375

Food and Description	Measure or Quantity	Sodium (milligrams)
Sweet	½ cup (4.4 oz.)	375
Canned, dietetic or low calorie:		
(USDA):		
Alaska, early or June:		
Solids & liq.	4 oz.	3
Solids only	4 oz.	3
Sweet:		
Solids & liq.	4 oz.	3
Solids only	4 oz.	3
(Del Monte) no salt added, solids & liq.	½ cup	<10
(Diet Delight) solids & liq.	½ cup (4.3 oz.)	5
(Larsen) *Fresh-Lite,* sweet, solids & liq.	½ cup	10
(S&W) *Nutradiet,* sweet, solids & liq.	½ cup	<10
Frozen:		
(USDA) boiled, drained	½ cup (3 oz.)	97
(Birds Eye):		
With butter sauce	⅓ of 10-oz. pkg.	641
With cream sauce	⅓ of 8-oz. pkg.	446
Sweet, 5-minute style	⅓ of 10-oz. pkg.	131
Tender tiny, deluxe	⅓ of 10-oz. pkg.	121
(Frosty Acres):		
Regular	3.3 oz.	90
Tiny	3.3 oz.	130
(Green Giant):		
Early June:		
Butter sauce, one serving	4½-oz. pkg.	500
Harvest Fresh	½ cup (3 oz.)	170
Polybag	½ cup (2.7 oz.)	120
Sweet:		
Plain:		
Harvest Fresh	½ cup (3 oz.)	200
Polybag	½ cup (2.7 oz.)	95
Butter sauce	½ cup (4 oz.)	410
(Larsen)	3.3 oz.	75
(Le Sueur) early, in butter sauce	⅓ of 10-oz. pkg.	364

Food and Description	Measure or Quantity	Sodium (milligrams)
(McKenzie):		
Regular	3.3 oz.	122
Tiny	3.3 oz.	47
PEA & CARROT:		
Canned, regular pack, solids & liq.:		
(Comstock)	½ cup	430
(Del Monte)	½ cup (4 oz.)	355
(Larsen) *Freshlike*	½ cup	340
(Libby's) solids & liq.	½ cup (4.2 oz.)	315
(Veg-All)	½ cup	340
Canned, dietetic or low calorie, solids & liq.:		
(Blue Boy)	½ cup	4
(Diet Delight)	½ cup (4.3 oz.)	5
(Larsen) *Fresh-Lite*	½ cup	30
(S&W) *Nutradiet*	½ cup	<10
Frozen:		
(USDA) boiled, without salt, drained	½ cup (3.1 oz.)	73
(Birds Eye)	⅓ pkg.	92
(Frosty Acres)	3.3 oz.	75
(Green Giant)	3.3 oz.	60
(McKenzie)	3.3 oz.	75
PEA, CROWDER, frozen (Birds Eye)	⅕ of 16-oz. pkg.	6
PEA, MATURE SEED, dry (USDA):		
Whole	1 lb.	159
Whole	1 cup	70
Split	1 lb.	181
Split	1 cup (7.2 oz.)	81
Cooked, split, drained solids	½ cup (3.4 oz.)	13
PEA & ONION:		
Canned (Larsen) *Freshlike*	½ cup	440
Frozen:		
(Frosty Acres)	3.3 oz.	80
(Larsen)	3.3 oz.	100
PEA POD, frozen (La Choy)	6 oz.	<20

Food and Description	Measure or Quantity	Sodium (milligrams)
PEA PUREE, canned (Larsen)		
low sodium	½ cup	7
PEACH:		
Fresh (USDA):		
Whole	1 lb. (weighed unpeeled)	4
Whole	4-oz. peach (2″ dia.)	1
Diced	½ cup (4.7 oz.)	1
Sliced	½ cup (3 oz.)	1
Canned, regular pack, solids & liq.:		
(USDA):		
Extra heavy syrup	4 oz.	2
Heavy syrup	2 med. halves & 2 T. syrup (4.1 oz.)	2
Juice pack	4 oz.	2
Light syrup	4 oz.	2
(Del Monte):		
Cling halves or slices	½ cup	<10
Freestone, halves or slices	½ cup	<10
Spiced	½ of 7¼-oz. can	<10
(Hunt's)	4-oz.	7
(Libby's) heavy syrup:		
Halves	½ cup (4.5 oz.)	9
Slices	½ cup (4.5 oz.)	10
(Stokely-Van Camp):		
Halves	½ cup (4.4 oz.)	23
Slices	½ cup (4.5 oz.)	23
Canned, dietetic or low calorie, solids & liq.:		
(USDA) water pack	½ cup (4.3 oz.)	2
(Del Monte) *Lite*	½ cup	<10
(Diet Delight) Cling or Freestone, juice pack	½ cup (4.4 oz.)	7
(Featherweight):		
Cling or Freestone, halves or slices, juice pack	½ cup	<10

Food and Description	Measure or Quantity	Sodium (milligrams)
Cling, halves or slices, water pack	½ cup	<10
(Libby's) water pack, sliced	½ cup (4.3 oz.)	3
Dehydrated (USDA):		
Uncooked	1 oz.	6
Cooked, with added sugar, solids & liq.	½ cup (5.4 oz.)	8
Dried (USDA):		
Uncooked	½ cup	14
Cooked:		
Unsweetened	½ cup	7
Sweetened	½ cup (5.4 oz.)	6
Frozen:		
(USDA) unthawed, slices, sweetened	½ cup	2
(Birds Eye) quick thaw	½ of 10-oz. pkg.	9
PEACH DRINK, canned (Hi-C)	6 fl. oz.	18
PEACH JUICE, canned (Smucker's)	8 fl. oz.	10
PEACH NECTAR, canned (Libby's)	6 fl. oz.	5
PEACH PRESERVE or JAM:		
Sweetened (Smucker's)	1 T. (.7 oz.)	0
Dietetic (Tillie Lewis) *Tasti Diet*	1 T.	<1
PEACH, STRAINED, canned (Larsen) low sodium	½ cup	6
PEANUT:		
Raw (USDA):		
In shell	1 lb. (weighed in shell)	17
With skins	1 oz.	1
Without skins	1 oz.	1
Roasted:		
(USDA):		
Whole	1 lb. (weighed in shell)	25

Food and Description	Measure or Quantity	Sodium (milligrams)
Chopped	½ cup	288
Halves	½ cup	301
(Adams) *All American Nut*	1 oz.	85
(Beer Nuts)	1 oz.	60
(Eagle):		
Fancy Virginia	1 oz.	130
Honey Roast:		
Regular	1 oz.	130
Cinnamon or maple	1 oz.	90
Lightly salted	1 oz.	90
(Fisher):		
Dry roasted:		
Lightly salted	1 oz.	85
Salted	1 oz.	220
Unsalted	1 oz.	0
Honey roasted:		
Regular	1 oz.	100
Dry	1 oz.	90
Oil roasted, salted, blanched	1 oz.	125
Party	1 oz.	140
(Guy's) dry roasted	1 oz.	310
(Planters):		
In shell, roasted:		
Salted	1 oz.	160
Unsalted	1 oz.	0
Shelled:		
Dry roasted:		
Salted	1 oz.	250
Unsalted	1 oz.	0
Lite	1 oz.	180
Honey roasted	1 oz.	180
Oil roasted:		
Regular or cocktail:		
Salted	1 oz.	160
Unsalted	1 oz.	0
Sweet 'N Crunchy	1 oz.	20
Tavern nuts	1 oz.	65

Food and Description	Measure or Quantity	Sodium (milligrams)
(Tom's):		
In shell	1 oz.	3
Shelled:		
Dry roasted	1 oz.	170
Hot flavored	1 oz.	230
Redskin	1 oz.	130
Toasted	1 oz.	110
(Weight Watchers)	1 pouch	50
Spanish, roasted:		
(Adams) *All American Nut*	1 oz.	85
(Fisher):		
Raw	1 oz.	0
Oil roasted:		
Salted	1 oz.	115
Lightly salted	1 oz.	50
(Frito-Lay's)	1 oz.	161
(Planters):		
Raw, unsalted	1 oz.	0
Roasted:		
Dry	1 oz.	200
Oil	1 oz.	150
PEANUT BUTTER:		
(Algood):		
Crunchy	1 T.	65
Old fashioned:		
Crunchy	1 T.	57
Smooth	1 T.	62
Smooth	1 T.	75
(Bama):		
Creamy	1 T.	70
Crunchy	1 T.	57
Cap'n Kid:		
Crunchy	1 T.	65
Smooth	1 T.	75
(Holsum)	1 T. (.6 oz.)	82
(Home Brands) real	1 T.	56
(Jif):		
Creamy	1 T.	78
Extra crunchy	1 T.	66

Food and Description	Measure or Quantity	Sodium (milligrams)
(Peter Pan):		
Crunchy	1 T.	60
Smooth	1 T. (.6 oz.)	75
(Skippy):		
Creamy	1 T. (.6 oz.)	75
Super chunk	1 T.	65
(Smucker's) natural	1 T.	62
Low sodium:		
(Algood)	1 T.	5
(Estee) regular or chunky	1 T.	2.5
(Home Brands):		
Lightly salted or no added sugar	1 T.	62
Unsalted	1 T.	<4
(Peter Pan)	1 T.	0
(Smucker's)	1 T.	<10
PEANUT BUTTER AND JELLY (Bama)	1 T.	37
PEANUT BUTTER BAKING CHIPS (Nestlé)	3 T. (1 oz.)	60
PEAR:		
Fresh (USDA):		
Whole	1 lb. (weighed with stems & core)	8
Whole	6.4-oz. pear (3″ × 2½″ × 2½″dia.)	3
Quartered	1 cup (6.8 oz.)	4
Slices	½ cup (6.8 oz.)	2
Canned, regular pack, solids & liq.:		
(USDA):		
Extra heavy syrup	4 oz.	1
Heavy syrup	½ cup	1
Juice pack	4 oz.	1
Light syrup	4 oz.	<1
(Del Monte) Bartlett halves or slices, regular or chunky	½ cup (4 oz.)	<10
(Hunt's) halves	4 oz.	6

Food and Description	Measure or Quantity	Sodium (milligrams)
(Stokely-Van Camp):		
Halves	½ cup (4.5 oz.)	15
Slices	½ cup (4.5 oz.)	10
Canned, unsweetened or dietetic, solids & liq.:		
(USDA) water pack	½ cup (4.3 oz.)	1
(Del Monte) *Lite,* Bartlett halves	½ cup	<10
(Diet Delight)	½ cup (4.4 oz.)	5
(Libby's)	½ cup (4.3 oz.)	10
Dried (USDA):		
Uncooked	1 lb.	32
Cooked:		
Without added sugar	4 oz.	3
With added sugar, solids & liq.	4 oz.	3
PEAR NECTAR, canned		
(Ardmore Farms)	6 fl. oz.	Tr.
PEAR-PASSION FRUIT NECTAR, canned (Libby's)	6 fl. oz.	5
PEBBLES, cereal (Post):		
Cocoa	⅞ cup (1 oz.)	160
Fruity	⅞ cup (1 oz.)	156
PECAN:		
In shell (USDA)	1 lb. (weighed in shell)	Tr.
Shelled (USDA):		
Whole	1 lb.	Tr.
Chopped	½ cup (1.8 oz.)	Tr.
Chopped	1 T. (7 g.)	Tr.
Halves	12–14 halves (.5 oz.)	Tr.
Halves	½ cup (1.9 oz.)	Tr.
Oil dipped (Fisher) salted	¼ cup	126
Roasted:		
(Eagle) honey roast	1 oz.	130
(Fisher) salted	¼ cup (1.1 oz.)	110
(Flavor House)	1 oz.	32
(Planter's) salted	1 oz.	222

Food and Description	Measure or Quantity	Sodium (milligrams)
PECTIN, FRUIT:		
Certo	1 T.	<1
Certo	6-oz. pkg.	5
Sure-Jell:		
Regular	1¾-oz. pkg.	12
Light	1¾-oz. pkg.	5
PEP, cereal (Kellogg's)	¾ cup (1 oz.)	200
PEPPER, BLACK (French's):		
Regular	1 tsp. (2.3 g.)	Tr.
Seasoned	1 tsp. (2.9 g.)	5
PEPPER, HOT CHILI:		
Green:		
Canned:		
(Del Monte) whole or		
diced	1 oz.	172
(Old El Paso):		
Chopped	1 T.	35
Whole	1 pepper	105
(Ortega) diced, strips or		
whole	1 oz.	22
Jalapeño, canned:		
(Del Monte) whole or		
sliced	1 oz.	422
(La Victoria):		
Marinated	1 T. (.5 oz.)	251
Nacho	1 T. (.5 oz.)	335
(Ortega) diced or whole	1 oz.	6
(Vlasic)	1 oz.	380
PEPPER, STUFFED:		
Home recipe (USDA) with beef & crumbs	2¾″ × 2½″ pepper with 1⅛ cups stuffing (6.5 oz.)	581
Frozen (Stouffer's)	½ of 15½-oz. pkg.	940
PEPPER, SWEET:		
Raw (USDA):		

Food and Description	Measure or Quantity	Sodium (milligrams)
Whole	1 lb. (weighed untrimmed)	48
Without stems & seeds	1 med. pepper (2.6 oz.)	8
Chopped	½ cup (2.6 oz.)	10
Slices	½ cup (1.4 oz.)	5
Strips	½ cup (1.7 oz.)	6
Boiled (USDA):		
Strips, drained	½ cup (2.4 oz.)	6
Whole, drained	1 med. pepper (2.6 oz.)	8
PEPPER, BANANA (Vlasic)	1 oz.	465
PEPPER, CHERRY (Vlasic)	1 oz.	410
Frozen:		
(Frosty Acres) diced:		
Green	1 oz.	1
Red & green	1 oz.	22
(Larsen) green or red	1 oz.	0
(Southland) dried	2 oz.	0
PEPPERONCINI (Vlasic)		
Greek, mild	1 oz.	450
PEPPERONI (Hormel):		
Regular	1 oz.	462
Chub, chunk	1 oz.	423
Leoni Brand	1 oz.	508
Packaged, sliced	1 slice	140
Rosa	1 oz.	626
Rosa Grande	1 oz.	512
PEPPER STEAK DINNER:		
*Canned:		
(Chun King)	6 oz.	1003
(La Choy)	¾ cup	960
Frozen:		
(Armour):		
Classics Lite, beef	11¼-oz. meal	970
Dining Lite, oriental	9-oz. meal	1050
(Healthy Choice):		
Dinner	11-oz. dinner	530
Entree	9½-oz. entree	340

Food and Description	Measure or Quantity	Sodium (milligrams)
(La Choy)	10-oz. meal	1082
(Stouffer's) with rice	10½-oz. meal	1440
PERCH, yellow, raw (USDA):		
Whole	1 lb. (weighed whole)	120
Meat only	4 oz.	77
PERCH DINNER or ENTREE, frozen:		
(Gorton's) *Fishmarket Fresh*	5 oz.	100
(Mrs. Paul's) fillets, breaded & fried, crispy, crunchy	2-oz. fillet	240
(Van de Kamp's) *Today's Catch*	4 oz.	180
PERSIMMON (USDA):		
Japanese or Kaki, fresh:		
With seeds	1 lb. (weighed with skin, calyx & seeds)	22
With seeds	4.4-oz. persimmon	6
Seedless	1 lb. (weighed with skin & calyx)	23
Seedless	4.4-oz. persimmon (2½" dia.)	6
Native, fresh:		
Whole	1 lb. (weighed with seeds & calyx)	4
Flesh only	4 oz.	1
PICKLE:		
Chow chow (See **CHOW CHOW**)		
Cucumber, fresh or bread & butter:		
(USDA)	3 slices (¼" × 1½")	141
(Fanning's)	1 fl. oz.	189

Food and Description	Measure or Quantity	Sodium (milligrams)
(Featherweight) dietetic, slices	1 oz.	3
(Vlasic):		
Chips, sweet butter	1 oz.	160
Chunks, deli or old fashioned	1 oz.	120
Stix, sweet butter	1 oz.	110
Dill:		
(USDA)	4.8-oz. pickle	1928
(Featherweight) low sodium	1 oz.	<5
(Smucker's):		
Candied stick	4″ pickle (.8 oz.)	182
Hamburger	1 slice (.13 oz.)	<141
(Vlasic):		
Original	1 oz.	375
No garlic	1 oz.	210
Hamburger (Vlasic) chips, dill	1 oz.	175
Hot & Spicy (Vlasic) garden mix	1 oz.	380
Kosher dill:		
(Claussen):		
Halves	2 oz.	599
Whole	2 oz.	581
(Featherweight) low sodium	1 oz.	<5
(Smucker's) whole	2½″-long pickle	642
(Vlasic):		
Baby, crunchy or gherkins	1 oz.	210
Crunchy, half-the-salt	1 oz.	125
Deli	1 oz.	290
Spear:		
Regular	1 oz.	175
Half-the-salt	1 oz.	120
Sour:		
(USDA) cucumber	1¾″ × 4″ (4.8 oz.)	384
(Aunt Jane's)	2-oz. pickle	769
Sweet:		
(Aunt Jane's)	1.5-oz. pickle	420
(Smucker's) whole	2½″-long pickle (.4 oz.)	119
(Vlasic) butter chips, half-the-salt	1 oz.	80

Food and Description	Measure or Quantity	Sodium (milligrams)
Sweet & sour (Claussen) slices	1 slice	25
PIE:		
Commercial type, non-frozen:		
Apple:		
Home recipe (USDA)		
2-crust	⅙ of 9″ pie (5.6 oz.)	476
(Dolly Madison)	4½-oz. pie	500
Banana, home recipe		
(USDA) cream or custard,		
unenriched or enriched	⅙ of 9″ pie (5.4 oz.)	295
Blackberry, home recipe		
(USDA) 2-crust, made with		
vegetable shortening	⅙ of 9″ pie (5.6 oz.)	423
Blueberry:		
Home recipe (USDA)		
2-crust, made with lard	⅙ of 9″ pie (5.6 oz.)	423
(Dolly Madison)	4½-oz. pie	585
Boston cream, home recipe (USDA)	¹⁄₁₂ of 8″ pie (2.4 oz.)	128
Butterscotch, home recipe (USDA)	⅙ of 9″ pie (5.4 oz.)	325
Cherry:		
Home recipe (USDA)		
2-crust	⅙ of 9″ pie (5.6 oz.)	480
(Dolly Madison):		
Regular	4½-oz. pie	480
N'Cream	4½-oz. pie	455
Chocolate (Dolly Madison):		
Regular	4½-oz. pie	530
Pudding pie	4½-oz. pie	290
Chocolate chiffon, home recipe (USDA) made with lard	⅙ of 9″ pie (3.8 oz.)	353

Food and Description	Measure or Quantity	Sodium (milligrams)
Chocolate meringue, home recipe (USDA) made with vegetable shortening	⅙ of 9″ pie (4.9 oz.)	358
Coconut custard, home recipe (USDA)	⅙ of 9″ pie (5.4 oz.)	375
Custard, home recipe (USDA) enriched or unenriched	⅙ of 9″ pie (5.4 oz.)	436
Lemon:		
Chiffon, home recipe (USDA) made with lard or vegetable shortening	⅙ of 9″ pie	282
Meringue, home recipe, (USDA) 1-crust	⅙ of 9″ pie (4.9 oz.)	395
(Dolly Madison)	4½-oz. pie	510
Mince, home recipe (USDA) 2-crust, enriched or unenriched	⅙ of 9″ pie (5.6 oz.)	708
Peach:		
Home recipe (USDA) 2-crust	⅙ of 9″ pie (5.6 oz.)	423
(Dolly Madison)	4½-oz. pie	625
Pecan, home recipe (USDA) 1-crust, made with lard or vegetable shortening	⅙ of 9″ pie	305
Pineapple, home recipe (USDA) 2-crust, made with lard or vegetable shortening	⅙ of 9″ pie (5.6 oz.)	428
Pineapple custard, home recipe (USDA) made with lard or vegetable shortening	⅙ of 9″ pie (5.4 oz.)	283

Food and Description	Measure or Quantity	Sodium (milligrams)
Pumpkin, home recipe (USDA) 1 crust, made with lard or vegetable shortening	⅙ of 9″ pie (5.4 oz.)	325
Raisin, home recipe (USDA) 2-crust, made with lard or vegetable shortening	⅙ of 9″ pie (5.6 oz.)	450
Rhubarb, home recipe (USDA) 2-crust, made with lard or vegetable shortening	⅙ of 9″ pie (5.6 oz.)	427
Strawberry, home recipe (USDA) made with lard or vegetable shortening	⅙ of 9″ pie (5.6 oz.)	307
Vanilla (Dolly Madison)	4½-oz. pie	310
Frozen:		
Apple:		
(USDA) baked	5-oz. serving	302
(Banquet)	⅙ of 20-oz. pie	290
(Mrs. Smith's):		
Regular:		
Plain	⅛ of 8″ pie	200
Plain	⅛ of 10″ pie	330
Dutch	⅛ of 8″ pie	180
Dutch	⅛ of 10″ pie	280
Natural Juice:		
Plain	⅛ of 9″ pie	350
Dutch	⅛ of 9″ pie	250
Pie In Minutes	⅛ of 25-oz. pie	250
(Pet-Ritz)	⅙ of 26-oz. pie	385
(Weight Watchers)	3½ oz.	290
Banana:		
(Banquet) cream	⅙ of 14-oz. pie	150
(Pet-Ritz) cream	⅙ of 14-oz. pie	155
Blackberry (Banquet)	⅙ of 20-oz. pie	350
Blueberry:		
(Banquet)	⅙ of 20-oz. pie	350

Food and Description	Measure or Quantity	Sodium (milligrams)
(Mrs. Smith's):		
Regular	⅛ of 8″ pie (3¼ oz.)	210
Natural Juice	⅛ of 9″ pie (4.6 oz.)	300
Pie In Minutes	⅛ of 25-oz. pie	240
(Pet-Ritz)	⅙ of 26-oz. pie	330
Cherry:		
(Banquet) family size	⅙ of 20-oz. pie	260
(Mrs. Smith's):		
Regular	⅛ of 26-oz. pie	210
Regular	⅛ of 46-oz. pie	350
Natural Juice	⅛ of 36.8-oz. pie	300
Pie In Minutes	⅛ of 25-oz. pie	200
(Pet-Ritz)	⅙ of 26-oz. pie	330
Chocolate cream:		
(Banquet)	⅙ of 14-oz. pie	106
(Pet-Ritz)	⅙ of 14-oz. pie	145
Chocolate mocha (Weight Watchers)	2¾-oz. serving	150
Coconut cream:		
(Banquet)	⅙ of 14-oz. pie	120
(Pet-Ritz)	⅙ of 14-oz. pie	145
Coconut custard (Mrs. Smith's):		
8″ pie	⅛ of 25-oz. pie	190
10″ pie	⅛ of 44-oz. pie	300
Custard (Morton) *Great Little Desserts*	6½-oz. pie	495
Lemon, cream:		
(Banquet)	⅙ of 14-oz. pie	120
(Pet-Ritz)	⅙ of 14-oz. pie	150
Lemon meringue (Mrs. Smith's)	⅛ of 8″ pie (3 oz.)	130
Mince:		
(Banquet)	⅙ of 20-oz. pie	370
(Mrs. Smith's):		
26-oz. pie	⅛ of pie (3¼ oz.)	260
46-oz. pie	⅛ of pie (5¾ oz.)	460
Neapolitan (Pet-Ritz)	⅙ of 14-oz. pie	185

Food and Description	Measure or Quantity	Sodium (milligrams)
Peach:		
(Banquet) family size	⅙ of 20-oz. pie	280
(Mrs. Smith's):		
Regular	⅛ of 26-oz. pie	200
Regular	⅛ of 46-oz. pie	340
Natural Juice	⅛ of 36.8-oz pie	300
Pie In Minutes	⅛ of 25-oz. pie	190
(Pet-Ritz)	⅙ of 26-oz. pie	320
Pecan (Mrs. Smith's):		
Regular	⅛ of 24-oz. pie	200
Regular	⅛ of 36-oz. pie	370
Pie In Minutes	⅛ of 24-oz. pie	200
Pumpkin:		
(Banquet)	⅙ of 20-oz. pie	350
(Mrs. Smith's) *Pie In*		
Minutes	⅛ of 25-oz. pie	230
Pumpkin custard (Mrs. Smith's):		
26-oz. pie	⅛ of pie (3¼ oz.)	200
46-oz. pie	⅛ of pie (5¾ oz.)	310
Raspberry (Mrs. Smith's) red	⅛ of 26-oz. pie	200
Strawberry cream:		
(Banquet)	⅙ of 14-oz. pie	120
(Pet-Ritz)	⅙ of 14-oz. pie	145
Strawberry rhubarb (Mrs. Smith's)	⅛ of 26-oz. pie	250
Sweet potato (Pet-Ritz)	⅙ of 20-oz. pie	110
PIE CRUST (See also **PASTRY SHELL**):		
Home recipe (USDA) baked	9″ pie crust (6.3 oz.)	1100
Frozen:		
(Mrs. Smith's):		
8″ shell	⅛ of 10-oz. shell	105
9″ shell:		
Regular	⅛ of 12-oz. shell	125
Shallow	⅛ of 10-oz. shell	105
9⅝″ shell	⅛ of 15-oz. shell	160

Food and Description	Measure or Quantity	Sodium (milligrams)
(Oronoque):		
Regular	⅙ of 7.4-oz. shell	170
Deep dish	⅙ of 8½-oz. shell	200
(Pet-Ritz):		
Regular	⅙ of 5-oz. shell	110
Deep dish:		
Regular	⅙ of 6-oz. shell	120
All vegetable shortening	⅙ of 6-oz. shell	65
Graham cracker	⅙ of 5-oz. shell	80
Mix:		
(USDA) dry	10-oz. pkg.	1968
(USDA) prepared with water, baked	4 oz.	922
(Betty Crocker):		
Regular	⅟₁₆ of pkg.	140
Stick	⅛ of stick	140
*(Flako)	⅙ of 9″ pie shell	314
*(Pillsbury) mix or stick	⅙ of 2-crust pie	420
Refrigerated (Pillsbury) 2-crust shell	2 shells	2220
PIE FILLING (See also **PUDDING or PIE FILLING**)		
Apple:		
(Comstock)	21-oz. can	900
(Thank You Brand)	3½-oz.	94
(White House)	½ cup (4.8 oz.)	60
Apricot (Comstock)	21-oz. can	1500
Banana cream (Comstock)	21-oz. can	3600
Blueberry (White House)	½ cup	65
Cherry:		
(Comstock)	21-oz. can	2400
(Thank You Brand):		
Regular	3½ oz.	15
Sweet	3½ oz.	20
(White House)	½ cup (4.8 oz.)	75
Chocolate cream (Comstock)	21-oz. can	3600
Coconut cream (Comstock)	21-oz. can	3900
Lemon (Comstock)	21-oz. can	1800
Peach (White House)	½ cup	45

Food and Description	Measure or Quantity	Sodium (milligrams)
Pineapple (Comstock)	21-oz. can	900
Pumpkin (See also **PUMPKIN,** canned) (Comstock)	4½-oz. serving	3600
Raisin (Comstock)	21-oz. can	1200
Strawberry (Comstock)	21-oz. can	1200
Dietetic (Thank You Brand):		
Apple	3½ oz.	42
Cherry	3⅓ oz.	9
*PIE MIX:		
(Betty Crocker) Boston cream	⅛ of pie	405
(Royal) *No Bake,* chocolate mint	⅛ of pie	280
PIEROGIES, frozen:		
(Empire Kosher):		
Cheese	1½ oz.	120
Onion	1½ oz.	158
(Mrs. Paul's) potato & cheese	1.7-oz. piece	260
PIGEONPEA (USDA):		
Raw, immature seeds in pods	1 lb.	9
Dry seeds	1 lb.	118
PIKE, raw (USDA) walleye:		
Whole	1 lb. (weighed whole)	132
Meat only	4 oz.	58
PILI NUT (USDA):		
In shell	1 lb. (weighed in shell)	2
Shelled	4 oz.	3
PIMIENTO, canned (Sunshine) diced or sliced, drained	1 T. (.6 oz.)	3
PINA COLADA COCKTAIL:		
Canned (Mr. Boston)	3 fl. oz.	29
*Frozen (Bacardi)	4 fl. oz.	14
Mix:		
*(Bar-Tender's)	5 fl. oz.	45
(Holland House):		
Instant	.56-oz. packet	<1
Liquid	1 oz.	4
PINEAPPLE:		
Fresh (USDA):		

Food and Description	Measure or Quantity	Sodium (milligrams)
Whole	1 lb. (weighed untrimmed)	2
Diced	½ cup (2.8 oz.)	<1
Sliced	¾″ × 3½″ slice (3 oz.)	<1
Canned, regular pack, solids & liq.:		
(USDA):		
Heavy syrup:		
Crushed	½ cup (5.6 oz.)	1
Slices	1 large slice & 2 T. syrup (4.3 oz.)	1
Tidbits	½ cup (4.6 oz.)	1
Juice pack	4 oz.	1
Light syrup	5 oz.	1
(Del Monte):		
Chunks	½ cup	<10
Crushed	½ cup (4 oz.)	<10
Slices:		
Medium	½ cup	2
Large	½ cup	3
Tidbits	½ cup	2
(Dole) heavy syrup, chunks, crushed, slices or tidbits	½ cup	10
Canned, dietetic or low calorie, solids & liq.:		
(USDA)	4 oz.	1
(Libby's) *Lite*	½ cup	10
PINEAPPLE-GRAPEFRUIT JUICE, canned (Texsun)	6 fl. oz.	2
PINEAPPLE & GRAPEFRUIT JUICE DRINK, canned:		
(USDA) 40% fruit juices	½ cup (4.4 oz.)	Tr.
(Del Monte):		
Regular	6 fl. oz.	50
Pink	6 fl. oz.	50
(Dole) pink	6 fl. oz.	20

Food and Description	Measure or Quantity	Sodium (milligrams)
PINEAPPLE JUICE:		
Canned, unsweetened:		
(Ardmore Farms)	6 fl. oz.	Tr.
(Del Monte)	6 fl. oz.	<10
(Dole)	6 fl. oz.	10
(Minute Maid):		
Regular	8.45-fl.-oz. container	27
On The Go	10-fl.-oz. bottle	31
(Mott's)	9½-fl.-oz. can	0
(Tree Top)	6 fl. oz.	0
Chilled (Minute Maid)	6 fl. oz.	19
*Frozen, unsweetened:		
(USDA)	½ cup (4.4 oz.)	1
(Dole)	6 fl. oz.	5
(Minute Maid)	6 fl. oz.	19
PINEAPPLE & ORANGE JUICE DRINK:		
Canned:		
(USDA) 40% fruit juices	½ cup (4.4 oz.)	Tr.
(Del Monte)	6 fl. oz.	6
(Hi-C)	6 fl. oz.	<1
Tree Ripe (Johanna Farms)	8.45-fl.-oz. container	3
*Frozen (Minute Maid)	6 fl. oz.	2
PINEAPPLE PRESERVE, unsweetened (Smucker's)	1 T.	0
PISTACHIO NUT, roasted:		
(Dole) natural	1 oz.	250
(Fisher) salted:		
In shell	1 oz.	50
Shelled	1 oz.	100
(Flavor House) dry roasted	1 oz.	32
(Frito-Lay's)	1 oz.	213
(Planters)	1 oz.	250
PIZZA PIE (See also **PIZZA PIE MIX** and *SHAKEY'S*):		
Regular, non-frozen:		

Food and Description	Measure or Quantity	Sodium (milligrams)
Domino's:		
Cheese:		
Plain:		
Small	⅛ of 12″ pizza	255
Large	¹⁄₁₂ of 16″ pizza	335
Double:		
Small	⅛ of 12″ pizza	318
Large	¹⁄₁₂ of 16″ pizza	421
Double with pepperoni:		
Small	⅛ of 12″ pizza	429
Large	¹⁄₁₂ of 16″ pizza	561
Mushroom & sausage:		
Small	⅛ of 12″ pizza	301
Large	¹⁄₁₂ of 16″ pizza	396
Pepperoni:		
Plain:		
Small	⅛ of 12″ pizza	365
Large	¹⁄₁₂ of 16″ pizza	474
With sausage:		
Small	⅛ of 12″ pizza	411
Large	¹⁄₁₂ of 16″ pizza	534
Sausage:		
Small	⅛ of 12″ pizza	300
Large	¹⁄₁₂ of 16″ pizza	395
Godfather's:		
Cheese:		
Original:		
Mini	¼ of pizza	260
Small	⅙ of pizza	400
Large:		
Regular	¹⁄₁₀ of pizza	494
Hot slice	⅛ of pizza	620
Stuffed:		
Small	⅙ of pizza	560
Medium	⅛ of pizza	610
Large	¹⁄₁₀ of pizza	677
Thin crust:		
Small	⅙ of pizza	370

Food and Description	Measure or Quantity	Sodium (milligrams)
Medium	⅛ of pizza	410
Large	⅒ of pizza	464
Combo:		
Original:		
Mini	¼ of pizza	450
Small	⅙ of pizza	830
Medium	⅛ of pizza	930
Large:		
Regular	⅒ of pizza	1019
Hot Slice	⅛ of pizza	1270
Stuffed:		
Small	⅙ of pizza	1000
Medium	⅛ of pizza	1105
Large	⅒ of pizza	1205
Thin crust:		
Small	⅙ of pizza	710
Medium	⅛ of pizza	790
Large	⅒ of pizza	870
Frozen:		
Bacon (Totino's)	½ of 10-oz. pie	1030
Canadian-style bacon:		
(Jeno's) crisp 'n tasty	½ of 7.7-oz. pie	880
(Stouffer's) french bread	½ of 11⅝-oz. pkg.	960
(Totino's) party	½ of 10.2-oz. pkg.	1150
Cheese:		
(Banquet) *Zap*, french bread	4½-oz. serving	800
(Celentano):		
Mini slice	2.7-oz. slice	390
Thick crust	⅓ of 13-oz. pizza	700
(Jeno's):		
Crisp 'n tasty	½ of 7.4-oz. pizza	770
4-pack	¼ of 8.9-oz. pkg.	460
(Kid Cuisine)	6½-oz. serving	390
(Pappalo's) french bread	5.7-oz. piece	830
(Pillsbury) microwave:		
Regular	½ of 7.1-oz. pkg.	540
French bread	5.7-oz. serving	680

Food and Description	Measure or Quantity	Sodium (milligrams)
(Stouffer's) french bread pizza:		
Regular:		
Regular	½ of 10⅜-oz. pkg.	840
Double cheese	½ of 11¾-oz. pkg.	950
Lean Cuisine:		
Regular	5⅛-oz. serving	750
Extra cheese	5½-oz. serving	850
(Tortino's):		
Microwave, small	3.9-oz. serving	760
My Classic, deluxe	⅙ of pkg. (3.1-oz.)	420
Pan, three cheese	⅙ of pkg. (3.9-oz.)	510
Party	½ of 9.8-oz pkg.	1000
Slices	2½-oz. slice	350
(Weight Watchers):		
Regular	5¾-oz. serving	910
French bread	5.12-oz. serving	680
Combination:		
(Jeno's):		
Crisp 'n tasty	½ of 7.8-oz. pie	840
4-pack	¼ of 9.6-oz. pkg.	470
(Pappalo's):		
French bread	6½-oz. serving	1120
Pan	⅙ of 26½-oz. pizza	700
Thin crust	⅙ of 22-oz. pizza	590
(Pillsbury) microwave	½ of 9-oz. pie	780
(Totino's):		
My Classic, deluxe	⅙ of 22½-oz. pkg.	630
Party	½ of 10½-oz. pkg.	1230
Slices	2.7-oz. slice	630
(Weight Watchers) deluxe	6¾-oz. pkg.	760
Deluxe:		
(Banquet) *Zap,* french bread	4.8-oz. serving	890
(Stouffer's) french bread:		
Regular	½ of 12⅜-oz. pkg.	1130
Lean Cuisine	6⅛-oz. serving	990
(Weight Watchers) french bread	6.12-oz. serving	780

Food and Description	Measure or Quantity	Sodium (milligrams)
Golden topping (Fox Deluxe)	½ of 6.8-oz. pizza	600
Hamburger:		
(Fox Deluxe)	½ of 7.6-oz. pizza	700
(Jeno's):		
Crisp 'n tasty	½ of 8.1-oz. pizza	810
4-pack	¼ of 10-oz. pkg.	500
(Pappalo's):		
Pan	⅙ of 26.3-oz. pizza	580
Thin crust	⅙ of 22-oz. pizza	470
(Stouffer's) french bread	½ of 12¼-oz. pkg.	1010
(Totino's) party	½ of 10.6-oz. pkg.	1060
Mexican (Totino's) party	½ of 10.2-oz. pkg.	970
Pepperoni:		
(Banquet) *Zap*, french bread	4½-oz. serving	1040
(Fox Deluxe)	½ of 7-oz. pizza	640
(Jeno's):		
Crisp 'n tasty	½ of 7.6-oz. pizza	760
4-pack	¼ of 9.2-oz. pkg.	460
(Pappalo's):		
French bread	6-oz. piece	1130
Pan	⅙ of 25.2-oz. pizza	710
Thin crust	⅙ of 22-oz. pizza	600
(Pillsbury) microwave:		
Regular	½ of 8½-oz. pkg.	790
French bread	6-oz. serving	940
(Stouffer's) french bread:		
Regular	½ of 11¼-oz. pkg.	1120
Lean Cuisine	5½-oz. serving	970
(Totino's):		
Microwave, small	4-oz. pizza	880

Food and Description	Measure or Quantity	Sodium (milligrams)
My Classic	⅙ of 21.1-oz. pizza	630
Pan	⅙ of 25.2-oz. pizza	730
Party	½ of 10.2-oz. pizza	1310
Slices	2.6-oz. slice	530
(Weight Watchers):		
Regular	5.87-oz. serving	870
French bread	5¼-oz. serving	850
Pepperoni & mushrooms (Stouffer's)		
french bread	½ of 12¼-oz. pkg.	1340
Sausage:		
(Fox Deluxe)	½ of 7.2-oz. pie	630
(Jeno's):		
Crisp 'n tasty	½ of 7.8-oz. pizza	850
4-pack	¼ of 7.6-oz. pkg.	460
(Pappalo's):		
French bread	6.3-oz. piece	1000
Pan	⅙ of 26.3-oz. pizza	550
Thin crust	⅙ of 22-oz. pizza	490
(Pillsbury) microwave:		
Regular	½ of 8¾-oz. pizza	680
French bread	6.3-oz. piece	860
(Stouffer's) french bread:		
Regular	½ of 12-oz. pkg.	1110
Lean Cuisine	6-oz. serving	960
(Totino's):		
Microwave, small	4.2-oz. pizza	870
Pan	⅙ of 26.3.-oz. pizza	630
Party	½ of 10.6-oz. pizza	1180
Slices	2.7-oz. slice	540
(Weight Watchers)	6¼-oz. pkg.	810

Food and Description	Measure or Quantity	Sodium (milligrams)
Sausage & mushroom (Stouffer's) french bread	½ of 12½-oz. pkg.	1050
Sausage & pepperoni:		
(Fox Deluxe)	½ of 7.2-oz. pie	640
(Pillsbury) microwave	6½-oz. serving	950
(Stouffer's) french bread	½ of 12½-oz. pkg.	1350
(Totino's):		
Microwave, small	4.2-oz. serving	970
Pan	⅙ of 26.6-oz. pizza	720
Vegetable:		
(Stouffer's) french bread	½ of 12¾-oz. pkg.	830
(Totino's) party	½ of 10.7-oz. pkg.	910
PIZZA PIE CRUST:		
*Mix, *Gold Medal*	⅙ of pkg.	220
Refrigerated (Pillsbury)	⅛ of crust	170
PIZZA PIE MIX (Ragú)		
Pizza Quick:		
Crust only	1/12 of pkg.	360
*Pizza, cheese	¼ of pie	810
PIZZA ROLL, frozen (Jeno's):		
Cheese	½ of 6-oz. pkg.	350
Hamburger	½ of 6-oz. pkg.	280
Pepperoni & cheese:		
Regular	½ of 6-oz. pkg.	390
Microwave	⅓ of 9-oz. pkg.	440
Sausage & pepperoni:		
Regular	½ of 6-oz. pkg.	380
Microwave	⅓ of 9-oz. pkg.	440
PIZZA SAUCE, canned:		
(Contadina):		
Regular	½ cup	790
With cheese	½ cup	760
With pepperoni	½ cup	720
With tomato chunks	½ cup	600
(Ragú)		
Regular, with extra tomatoes	¼ of 15½-oz. jar	475
Pizza Quick:		
Chunky	⅓ of 14-oz. jar	786

Food and Description	Measure or Quantity	Sodium (milligrams)
Mushroom, sausage or traditional	⅓ of 14-oz. jar	824
Pepperoni	⅓ of 14-oz. jar	906
PIZZA SEASONING SPICE (French's)	1 tsp. (.1 oz.)	390
PLANTAIN, raw (USDA):		
Whole	1 lb. (weighed with skin)	16
Flesh only	4 oz.	6
PLUM:		
Fresh (USDA):		
Damson:		
Whole	1 lb. (weighed with pits)	8
Flesh only	4 oz.	2
Japanese & hybrid:		
Whole	1 lb. (weighed with pits)	4
Whole	2.1-oz. plum (2″ dia.)	<1
Diced	½ cup (2.9 oz.)	<1
Halves	½ cup (3.1 oz.)	<1
Slices	½ cup (3 oz.)	<1
Prune type:		
Whole	1 lb. (weighed with pits)	4
Halves	½ cup (2.8 oz.)	<1
Canned, purple, regular pack, solids & liq.:		
(USDA):		
Extra heavy syrup	4 oz.	1
Light syrup	4 oz.	1
(Stokely-Van Camp)	½ cup	28
(Thank You Brand):		
Heavy syrup	½ cup (4.8 oz.)	14
Light syrup	½ cup (4.7 oz.)	13
Canned, unsweetened or low calorie, solids & liq.:		
(Diet Delight) purple, juice pack	½ cup (4.4 oz.)	5

Food and Description	Measure or Quantity	Sodium (milligrams)
(Featherweight) purple:		
Juice pack	½ cup	<10
Water pack	½ cup	<10
(Thank You Brand) water pack	½ cup (4.8 oz.)	<5
PLUM JELLY, sweetened:		
(Home Brands)	1 T.	15
(Smucker's)	1 T. (.7 oz.)	<10
PLUM PRESERVE or JAM, sweetened (Smucker's)	1 T. (.7 oz.)	0
PLUM PUDDING, canned (Richardson & Robbins)	2″ wedge (3.6 oz.)	150
POLISH-STYLE SAUSAGE (See **SAUSAGE**)		
POLYNESIAN STYLE DINNER, frozen (Swanson)	12-oz. dinner	1430
POMEGRANATE, raw (USDA):		
Whole	1 lb. (weighed whole)	8
Pulp only	4 oz.	3
POMPANO, raw (USDA):		
Whole	1 lb. (weighed whole)	119
Meat only	4 oz.	53
PONDEROSA RESTAURANT:		
A-1 Sauce	1 tsp.	82
Beef, chopped (patty only):		
Regular	3½ oz.	58
Double Deluxe	5.9 oz.	99
Junior (*Square Shooter*)	1.6 oz.	27
Steakhouse Deluxe	2.96 oz.	50
Beverages:		
Coca-Cola	8 fl. oz.	1
Coffee	6 fl. oz.	26
Dr. Pepper	8 fl. oz.	18
Milk, chocolate	8 fl. oz.	149
Orange drink	8 fl. oz.	12
Root beer	8 fl. oz.	18
Sprite	8 fl. oz.	31
Tab	8 fl. oz.	18

Food and Description	Measure or Quantity	Sodium (milligrams)
Bun:		
Regular	2.4-oz. bun	334
Hot dog	1 bun	263
Junior	1.4-oz. bun	197
Steakhouse deluxe	2.4-oz bun	334
Chicken strips:		
Adult portion	2¾ oz.	420
Child	1.4 oz.	210
Cocktail sauce	1½ oz.	143
Filet mignon	3.8 oz. (edible portion)	82
Filet of sole, fish only (See also Bun above)	3-oz. piece	46
Fish, baked	4.9-oz. serving	363
Gelatin dessert	½ cup	55
Gravy, au jus	1 oz.	125
Ham & cheese:		
Bun (See Bun above)		
Cheese, Swiss	2 slices (.8 oz.)	310
Ham	2½ oz.	724
Hot dog, child's, meat only (See also Bun above)	1.6-oz. hot dog	542
Margarine:		
Pat	1 tsp.	49
On potato, as served	½ oz.	138
New York strip steak	6.1 oz. (edible portion)	79
Onion, chopped	1 T.	1
Pickle, dill	3 slices (.7 oz.)	279
Potato:		
Baked	7.2-oz. potato	6
French fries	3-oz. serving	5
Prime ribs:		
Regular	4.2 oz. (edible portion)	71
Imperial	8.4 oz. (edible portion)	141
King	6 oz. (edible portion)	101

Food and Description	Measure or Quantity	Sodium (milligrams)
Pudding, chocolate	4½ oz.	177
Ribeye	3.2 oz. (edible portion)	271
Ribeye & shrimp:		
Ribeye	3.2 oz.	271
Shrimp	2.2 oz.	114
Roll, kaiser	2.2-oz. roll	311
Salad bar:		
Beets	1 oz.	56
Broccoli	1 oz.	4
Cabbage, red	1 oz.	7
Carrots	1 oz.	13
Cauliflower	1 oz.	4
Celery	1 oz.	36
Chickpeas (garbanzos)	1 oz.	7
Cucumber	1 oz.	2
Mushrooms	1 oz.	4
Onion, white	1 oz.	3
Pepper, green	1 oz.	4
Radish	1 oz.	5
Tomato	1 oz.	Tr.
Salad dressing:		
Blue cheese	1 oz.	265
Italian, creamy	1 oz.	419
Low calorie	1 oz.	220
Oil & vinegar	1 oz.	Tr.
1000 Island	1 oz.	170
Shrimp dinner	7 pieces (3½ oz.)	182
Sirloin:		
Regular	3.3 oz. (edible portion)	372
Super	6½ oz. (edible portion)	695
Tips	4 oz. (edible portion)	375
Steak sauce	1 oz.	329
Tartar sauce	1.5 oz.	300
T-bone	4.3 oz. (edible portion)	545

Food and Description	Measure or Quantity	Sodium (milligrams)
Tomato (See also Salad Bar above):		
Slices	2 slices (.9 oz.)	7
Whole, small	3.5 oz.	3
Topping, whipped	¼ oz.	4
POPCORN:		
Unpopped (USDA)	1 oz.	<1
Popped, fresh:		
(USDA):		
Plain	1 oz.	<1
Plain, large kernel	1 cup (6 g.)	<1
Butter or oil & salt added	1 oz.	550
Butter or oil & salt added	1 cup (9 g.)	175
Sugar coated	1 cup (1.2 oz.)	<1
(Jiffy Pop):		
Plain	½ pkg. (2½ oz.)	936
Buttered	½ pkg. (2½ oz.)	936
(Jolly Time):		
Air popped, white or yellow	1 cup	Tr.
Butter flavor:		
Regular	1 cup (.2 oz.)	32
Light	1 cup	30
Natural:		
Regular	1 cup (.3 oz.)	33
Light	1 cup	27
(Orville Reddenbacher's)		
Gourmet:		
Original, plain	1 cup	0
Caramel crunch	1 oz.	100
Hot air corn	1 cup	0
Microwave:		
Regular:		
Butter flavored:		
Salted	1 cup	50
Without salt	1 cup	0
Natural:		
Salted	1 cup	65
Without salt	1 cup	0

Food and Description	Measure or Quantity	Sodium (milligrams)
Flavored:		
Caramel	1 cup	36
Cheese:		
Cheddar	1 cup	93
Nacho	1 cup	133
Sour cream & onion	1 cup	87
(Pillsbury) microwave popcorn:		
Butter flavor:		
Regular	1 cup	137
Frozen	1 cup	160
Original flavor:		
Regular	1 cup	137
Frozen	1 cup	140
Salt free, frozen	1 cup	0
Pop•Secret (General Mills):		
Regular, butter or natural	1 cup	57
Light:		
Butter flavor	1 cup	38
Natural	1 cup	53
Pops-Rite, microwave:		
Butter flavor:		
Regular	1 cup	47
Light	1 cup	23
Natural flavor:		
Regular	1 cup	63
Light	1 cup	23
(Weight Watchers) microwave	1-oz. serving	5
Packaged:		
(Cape Cod):		
Regular or cheese flavored	1 oz.	300
Light	1 oz.	95
Cracker Jack (Borden)	1 oz.	85
(Eagle) regular	1 oz.	300
(Tom's):		
Regular	1 oz.	300
Cheese flavored	1 oz.	460
(Snyder's) cheese flavored	1 oz.	250
(Weight Watchers):		
Lightly salted	.66-oz. pkg.	65

Food and Description	Measure or Quantity	Sodium (*milligrams*)
White cheddar cheese	.66-oz. pkg.	85
(Wise) butter flavored	1 oz.	440
POPCORN POPPING OIL		
(Orville Reddenbacher's)		
Gourmet, buttery flavor	1 T. (.5 oz.)	0
POPOVER:		
Home recipe (USDA)	1 average popover (2 oz.)	125
*Mix (Flako)	1 popover	355
POPPY SEED (French's)	1 tsp.	Tr.
PORGY, raw (USDA):		
Whole	1 lb. (weighed whole)	117
Meat only	4 oz.	71
PORK, medium-fat:		
Fresh (USDA):		
Boston butt:		
Raw	1 lb. (weighed with bone & skin)	260
Roasted, lean & fat	4 oz.	74
Roasted, lean only	4 oz.	74
Chop:		
Broiled, lean & fat	1 chop (4 oz., weighed with bone)	49
Broiled, lean & fat	1 chop (3 oz., weighed with bone)	55
Broiled, lean only	1 chop (3 oz., weighed without bone)	55
Ham (See also **HAM**):		
Raw	1 lb. (weighed with bone & skin)	320
Roasted, lean & fat	4 oz.	74
Roasted, lean only	4 oz.	74
Loin:		
Raw	1 lb. (weighed with bone)	260

Food and Description	Measure or Quantity	Sodium (milligrams)
Roasted, lean only	4 oz.	74
Picnic:		
Raw	1 lb. (weighed with bone & skin)	260
Simmered, lean & fat	4 oz.	74
Simmered, lean only	4 oz.	74
Spareribs:		
Raw, with bone	1 lb. (weighed with bone)	775
Braised, lean & fat	4 oz.	74
Cured, light commercial cure:		
Bacon (See **BACON**)		
Bacon butt (USDA), roasted, lean only	4 oz.	1055
Ham (See also **HAM**) roasted, lean only (USDA)	4 oz.	1055
Picnic:		
Raw (Wilson) smoked	4 oz.	1247
Roasted, lean only (USDA)	4 oz.	1055
PORK, CANNED, chopped luncheon meat (USDA):		
Regular	1 oz.	350
Chopped	1 cup (4.8 oz.)	1678
Diced	1 cup	1740
PORK, PACKAGED (Eckrich) slender sliced	1 oz.	350
PORK & BEANS (See **BEAN, BAKED**)		
PORK DINNER:		
*Canned (Hunt's) *Minute Gourmet Microwave Entree Maker,* Cajun	6.6 oz.	1270
Frozen (Swanson) loin of	11¼-oz. dinner	710
PORK RINDS, fried (Tom's):		
Regular	.6 oz.	220
BBQ	.6 oz.	260

Food and Description	Measure or Quantity	Sodium (milligrams)
PORK SAUSAGE (See **SAUSAGE**)		
PORK, SWEET & SOUR,		
frozen (La Choy)	½ of 15-oz. entree	1586
PORT WINE:		
(Gold Seal)	3 fl. oz.	3
(Great Western) Solera, Tawny	3 fl. oz.	34
POSTUM, cereal beverage (General Foods)	6 fl. oz.	3
POTATO (See also **POTATO CHIPS; POTATO MIX; POTATO SALAD; POTATO STICK;** etc.):		
Raw (USDA):		
Whole	1 lb. (weighed unpared)	11
Pared, chopped	1 cup (5.2 oz.)	4
Pared, diced	1 cup (5.5 oz.)	5
Pared, sliced	1 cup (5.2 oz.)	4
Cooked (USDA):		
Au gratin or scalloped, with cheese	½ cup (4.3 oz.)	433
Au gratin or scalloped, without cheese	½ cup (4.3 oz.)	545
Baked, peeled after baking	2½"-dia. potato (3 raw to 1 lb.)	4
Boiled, peeled after boiling	1 med. (3 raw to 1 lb.)	2
Boiled, peeled before boiling:		
Whole	1 med. (3 raw to 1 lb.)	2
Diced	½ cup (2.8 oz.)	2
Mashed	½ cup (3.7 oz.)	2
Riced	½ cup (4 oz.)	2
Sliced	½ cup (2.8 oz.)	2
French fried in deep fat	10 pieces (2" × ½" × ½", 2 oz.)	3

Food and Description	Measure or Quantity	Sodium (milligrams)
Hash browned, after holding overnight	½ cup (3.4 oz.)	281
Mashed, milk added	½ cup (3.5 oz.)	295
Mashed, milk & butter added	½ cup (3.4 oz.)	324
Pan fried from raw	½ cup (3 oz.)	190
Scalloped (See Au gratin above)		
Canned, solids & liq.:		
(USDA) solids & liq.	1 cup (8.8 oz.)	2
(Allen's) *Butterfield*	½ cup (4 oz.)	360
(Del Monte) white, sliced or whole	½ cup	355
(Hunt's)	4 oz.	230
(Larsen) *Freshlike*	½ cup (4½ oz.)	260
(Stokely-Van Camp) whole	½ cup (4.4 oz.)	335
(Sunshine) whole	½ cup	377
Dehydrated, mashed (see also **POTATO MIX**) (USDA):		
Flakes, dry, without milk	½ cup (.8 oz.)	20
*Flakes, prepared with water, milk & fat	½ cup (3.8 oz.)	247
Granules, dry, without milk	½ cup	84
*Granules, prepared with water, milk & butter	½ cup (3.7 oz.)	256
Frozen (See also **POTATO, STUFFED**):		
(USDA):		
French-fried, heated	10 pieces (2″ × ½″, 2 oz.)	2
Mashed, heated	4 oz.	407
(Birds Eye):		
Cottage fries	⅕ of 14-oz. pkg.	14
Crinkle cuts:		
Regular	⅓ of 9-oz. pkg.	36
Deep Gold	¼ of 12-oz. pkg.	12
Farm style wedge	⅛ of 24-oz. pkg.	25
French fries:		
Regular	3-oz. serving	23
Deep Gold	3-oz. serving	280

Food and Description	Measure or Quantity	Sodium (milligrams)
Hash browns:		
Regular	4-oz. serving	54
Shredded	3-oz. serving	21
Shoestring	3-oz. serving	45
Steak fries	3-oz. serving	25
Tasti Fries	2½-oz. serving	268
Tasti Puffs	2½-oz. serving	401
Tiny Taters	3.2-oz. serving	282
Triangles	1½-oz. piece	167
Whole, peeled	¹⁄₁₀ of 32-oz. pkg.	5
(Empire Kosher) french fries	3 oz.	35
(Green Giant) One Serving:		
Au gratin	5½-oz. serving	560
& broccoli, in cheese sauce	5½-oz. serving	720
(Larsen) diced	4 oz.	40
(McKenzie) whole, white, boiled	3.5-oz. serving	20
(Ore-Ida):		
Cheddar Browns	3-oz. serving	420
Cottage fries	3-oz. serving	25
Country Style Dinner Fries	3-oz. serving	15
Crinkle cuts:		
Deep fries	3-oz. serving	30
Microwave	3½-oz. serving	35
Crispers!	3-oz. serving	535
Crispy Crowns	3-oz. serving	500
Golden Crinkles	3-oz. serving	25
Golden Fries	3-oz. serving	30
Golden Patties	2½-oz. serving	280
Golden Twirls	3-oz. serving	55
Hash browns:		
Microwave	2-oz. serving	180
Shredded	3-oz. serving	40
Southern style	3-oz. serving	30
Toaster	1¾-oz. serving	285
Home Style Potato Wedges	3-oz. serving	25
Lite crinkle cuts	3-oz. serving	35
Pixie crinkles	3-oz. serving	45

Food and Description	Measure or Quantity	Sodium (milligrams)
Potatoes O'Brien	3-oz. serving	25
Shoestrings	3-oz. serving	25
Tater Tots:		
Regular	3-oz. serving	535
Microwave	4-oz. serving	695
With onions	3-oz. serving	795
Whole, small, peeled	3-oz. serving	40
(Stouffer's) au gratin	⅓ of 11½-oz. pkg.	510
POTATO & BACON, canned		
(Hormel) *Short Orders*	7½-oz. can	942
POTATO CHIP:		
(USDA)	1 oz.	284
(Cape Cod):		
Regular:		
Salted	1 oz.	120
No salt	1 oz.	0
Dill & sour cream:		
Regular	1 oz.	160
No salt	1 oz.	15
Waves:		
Regular	1 oz.	120
No salt	1 oz.	0
(Cottage Fries) no salt added	1 oz.	5
Delta Gold:		
Regular or dip style	1 oz.	160
Mesquite flavored Bar-B-Q	1 oz.	240
(Eagle):		
BBQ:		
Crunchy or Louisiana style	1 oz.	140
Thins	1 oz.	220
Extra crunchy or Idaho russet	1 oz.	180
Ridged or thins	1 oz.	220
Sour cream & onion	1 oz.	240
(Laura Scudder's):		
Barbecue	1 oz.	200
Sour cream & onion	1 oz.	170
Lay's:		
Regular	1 oz.	200
Bar-B-Q	1 oz.	310

Food and Description	Measure or Quantity	Sodium (milligrams)
Italian cheese	1 oz.	210
Jalapeño & cheddar	1 oz.	290
Salt & vinegar	1 oz.	460
Sour cream & onion	1 oz.	250
Unsalted	1 oz.	10
(New York Deli)	1 oz.	120
O'Grady's:		
Regular	1 oz.	210
Au gratin cheese	1 oz.	330
(Old Dutch):		
Regular	1 oz.	160
Au gratin or sour cream & onion	1 oz.	220
BBQ	1 oz.	360
Dill	1 oz.	340
Onion & garlic	1 oz.	420
Rip-L	1 oz.	150
Pringle's:		
Regular	1 oz.	170
Cheez-Ums	1 oz.	200
Light, regular	1 oz.	118
Rippled, original	1 oz.	150
Ruffles:		
Regular, bacon & sour cream or light	1 oz.	190
Bar-B-Q	1 oz.	320
Cajun Spice or sour cream & onion	1 oz.	240
Cheddar & sour cream	1 oz.	260
Cottage Fries:		
Regular	1 oz.	240
Unsalted	1 oz.	10
Ridgies:		
Natural flavor	1 oz.	150
Sour cream & onion	1 oz.	240
(Tom's):		
Regular	1 oz.	200
BBQ, sour cream & onion or vinegar & salt	1 oz.	280

Food and Description	Measure or Quantity	Sodium (milligrams)
Hot	1 oz.	310
(Wise):		
Barbecue	1 oz.	240
Garlic & onion	1 oz.	250
Lightly salted	1 oz.	100
Natural	1 oz.	150
Salt & vinegar	1 oz.	350
POTATO & HAM canned		
(Hormel) *Short Orders*	7½-oz. can	1189
POTATO MIX:		
*Au gratin:		
(Betty Crocker)	½ cup (⅙ of pkg.)	600
(French's) tangy	½ cup	460
(Lipton) & sauce	¼ pkg.	537
Beef & mushroom (Lipton)	½ cup	385
*Casserole (French's) cheddar		
cheese & bacon	½ cup	390
*Cheddar bacon (Betty Crocker)	⅙ of pkg.	520
Cheddar broccoli (Lipton)	½ cup	491
*Hash brown, (Betty Crocker)		
with onion	½ cup (⅙ of pkg.)	460
*Julienne (Betty Crocker)	½ cup (⅙ of pkg.)	580
*Mashed:		
(Betty Crocker) *Buds*	½ cup	360
(French's):		
Regular	½ cup	320
Spuds	½ cup	380
(Pillsbury) *Hungry Jack,*		
flakes	½ cup	380
*Scalloped:		
(Betty Crocker) plain	½ cup	580
(French's):		
Cheese	½ cup	540
Crispy top	½ cup	520
*Sour cream & chive (Betty		
Crocker)	½ cup (⅙ of pkg.)	520
*POTATO PANCAKE MIX		
(French's)	3″ pancake	130

Food and Description	Measure or Quantity	Sodium (milligrams)
POTATO SALAD, home recipe (USDA):		
With cooked salad dressing & seasonings	4 oz.	599
With mayonnaise & French dressing, hard-cooked eggs, seasonings	4 oz.	544
POTATO STICK, *O&C* (Durkee)	1½-oz. can	383
POTATO, STUFFED, BAKED, frozen:		
(Ore-Ida):		
Butter flavor	5-oz. serving	395
Cheddar cheese	5-oz. serving	635
Sour cream & chive	5-oz. serving	370
(Weight Watchers):		
Broccoli & cheese	10½-oz. serving	770
Chicken divan	11-oz. serving	820
POT ROAST DINNER or ENTREE, frozen:		
(Armour) *Dinner Classics*	10-oz. meal	670
(Healthy Choice)	11-oz. meal	310
(Stouffer's) *Right Course*	9¼-oz. meal	550
PRETZEL:		
(Eagle) regular	1 oz.	570
(Estee) unsalted	1 piece	0
(Nabisco) *Mister Salty:*		
Regular:		
Dutch	1 piece	220
Logs	1 piece	57
Mini	1 piece	28
Nuggets	1 piece	26
Rings, regular	1 piece	23
Rods	1 piece (.5 oz.)	250
Sticks, regular	1 piece	7
Twists	1 piece	118
Juniors	1 piece	18
(Pepperidge Farm):		
Nuggets	1½ oz.	497
Sticks, thin	1¼ oz.	492
Twist, tiny	1 oz.	366

Food and Description	Measure or Quantity	Sodium (milligrams)
(Planters)	1 oz.	700
Rold Gold:		
Rods	1 oz.	550
Sticks	1 oz.	760
Tiny Tim	1 oz.	610
Twists	1 oz.	470
(Seyfert's) rods, butter	1 oz.	530
(Snyder's) hard:		
Hard	1 oz.	548
Stix	1 oz.	386
Thins	1 oz.	655
(Tom's) twists	1 oz.	430
(Wise) nugget	1 oz.	600
PRICKLY PEAR, fresh (USDA):		
Whole	1 lb. (weighed with rind & seeds)	4
Flesh only	4 oz.	2
PRODUCT 19, cereal (Kellogg's)	1 cup (1 oz.)	320
PROSCIUTTO (Hormel) boneless	1 oz.	502
PRUNE:		
Canned, regular pack (Sunsweet) stewed	½ cup	2
Canned, dietetic (Featherweight) stewed, water pack, solids & liq.	½ cup	<10
Dried:		
(USDA) dried, cooked, with sugar	1 cup (16–18 prunes & ⅔ cup liq.)	9
(Del Monte)	2 oz.	<10
(Sunsweet):		
With pits	2 oz.	5
Pitted	2 oz.	3
PRUNE JUICE, canned:		
(USDA)	½ cup (4.5 oz.)	2
(Del Monte)	6 fl. oz.	<10
Lady Betty (Algood):		
Regular	6 fl. oz.	20
With pulp	6 fl. oz.	25

Food and Description	Measure or Quantity	Sodium (milligrams)
(Sunsweet):		
Regular	6 fl. oz.	4
Home style, with pulp	6 fl. oz.	12
PRUNE WHIP, home recipe		
(USDA)	1 cup (4.8 oz.)	221
PUDDING or PIE FILLING		
(See also **PIE FILLING or**		
PUDDING:		
Home recipe (USDA):		
Rice, made with raisins	½ cup (4.7 oz.)	94
Tapioca:		
Apple	½ cup (4.4 oz.)	64
Cream	½ cup (2.9 oz.)	128
Vanilla, with starch base	½ cup (4.5 oz.)	83
Canned, regular pack:		
Banana:		
(Del Monte) *Pudding Cup*	5-oz. container	277
(Hunt's) *Snack Pack*	4¼-oz. container	180
(Thank You Brand)	½ cup (4.6 oz.)	182
Butterscotch:		
(Del Monte) *Pudding Cup*	5-oz. container	277
(Hunt's) *Snack Pack*	4¼-oz. container	200
Swiss Miss	4-oz. container	210
(Thank You Brand)	½ cup (4.6 oz.)	221
Chocolate:		
(Betty Crocker)	½ cup (5 oz.)	260
(Del Monte) *Pudding Cup:*		
Regular	5-oz. container	327
Fudge	5-oz. container	297
(Hunt's) *Snack Pack:*		
Regular, German or		
marshmallow	4¼-oz. container	135
Fudge	4¼-oz. container	140
Swiss Miss:		
Regular:		
Plain	4-oz. container	200
Fudge	4-oz. container	190
Fruit on bottom:		
Black cherry	4-oz. container	150

Food and Description	Measure or Quantity	Sodium (milligrams)
Strawberry	4-oz. container	160
(Thank You Brand):		
Regular	½ cup (4.6 oz.)	117
Fudge	½ cup (4.6 oz.)	130
Lemon:		
(Hunt's) *Snack Pack*	4¼-oz. container	70
(Thank You Brand)	½ cup (4.6 oz.)	195
Rice:		
(Betty Crocker)	½ cup (4¼ oz.)	150
(Comstock)	½ of 7½-oz. can	450
(Hunt's) *Snack Pack*	4¼-oz. container	200
(Menner's)	½ of 7½-oz. can	450
Tapioca:		
(Betty Crocker)	½ cup (4¼ oz.)	170
(Del Monte) *Pudding Cup*	5-oz. container	253
(Hunt's) *Snack Pack*	4¼-oz. container	140
Swiss Miss	4-oz. container	190
(Thank You Brand)	½ cup (4.6 oz.)	169
Vanilla:		
(Del Monte) *Pudding Cup*	5-oz. container	320
(Hunt's) *Snack Pack*	4¼-oz. container	160
Swiss Miss	4-oz. container	200
(Thank You Brand)	½ cup (4.6 oz.)	182
Canned, dietetic (Estee):		
Butterscotch	½ cup	80
Chocolate or vanilla	½ cup	75
Chilled, *Swiss Miss:*		
Butterscotch	4-oz. container	175
Chocolate:		
Regular	4-oz. container	176
Malt	4-oz. container	175
Sundae	4-oz. container	166
Double rich	4-oz. container	173
Rice	4-oz. container	296
Tapioca	4-oz. container	170
Vanilla:		
Regular	4-oz. container	175
Sundae	4-oz. container	166

Food and Description	Measure or Quantity	Sodium (milligrams)
Frozen (Rich's):		
Banana	3-oz. container	118
Butterscotch	4½-oz. container	192
Chocolate	4½-oz. container	205
Vanilla	4½-oz. container	243
*Mix, regular pack:		
Banana:		
(Jell-O) cream:		
Regular	½ cup	257
Instant	½ cup	445
(Royal) cream:		
Regular	½ cup	210
Instant	½ cup	390
Butter pecan (Jell-O) instant	½ cup	442
Butterscotch:		
(Jell-O):		
Regular	½ cup	247
Instant	½ cup	483
(Royal):		
Regular	½ cup	210
Instant	½ cup	390
Chocolate:		
(Jell-O):		
Regular:		
Plain	½ cup	170
Fudge	½ cup	171
Milk	½ cup	173
Instant:		
Plain or milk	½ cup	507
Fudge	½ cup	482
(Royal):		
Regular, plain or *Dark N' Sweet*	½ cup	150
Instant, plain, chocolate chip mint or *Dark N' Sweet*	½ cup	390
Coconut:		
(Jell-O) cream:		
Regular	⅙ of 8″ pie (excluding crust)	140

Food and Description	Measure or Quantity	Sodium (milligrams)
Regular	½ cup	216
Instant	½ cup	358
(Royal) instant	½ cup	350
Custard:		
Jell-O Americana, golden egg	½ cup	222
(Royal) regular	½ cup	115
Flan:		
(Knorr):		
Without sauce	½ cup	65
With sauce	½ cup	70
(Royal)	½ cup	115
Lemon:		
(Jell-O):		
Regular	⅙ of 9″ pie (excluding crust)	91
Regular	½ cup	94
Instant	½ cup	397
(Royal):		
Regular	½ cup	120
Instant	½ cup	350
Lime (Royal) regular, key lime	½ cup	120
Pineapple (Jell-O) cream, instant	½ cup	400
Pistachio:		
(Jell-O) instant	½ cup	445
(Royal) instant	½ cup	350
Raspberry (Salada) *Danish Dessert*	½ cup	5
Rice, *Jell-O Americana*	½ cup	158
Strawberry (Salada) *Danish Dessert*	½ cup	5
Tapioca:		
Jell-O Americana chocolate or vanilla	½ cup	170
(Royal) Vanilla	½ cup	150
Vanilla:		
(Jell-O):		

Food and Description	Measure or Quantity	Sodium (milligrams)
Regular:		
Plain	½ cup	198
French	½ cup	201
Instant, French	½ cup	442
(Royal):		
Regular	½ cup	210
Instant	½ cup	390
*Mix, dietetic pack:		
Butterscotch:		
(D-Zerta)	½ cup	115
(Royal) instant	½ cup	470
(Weight Watchers)	½ cup	420
Chocolate:		
(D-Zerta)	4-oz. serving	116
(Estee) instant	½ cup	75
(Royal) instant	½ cup	470
(Weight Watchers)	½ cup	460
Vanilla:		
(D-Zerta)	½ cup	105
(Estee) instant	½ cup	75
(Royal) instant	½ cup	470
(Weight Watchers)	½ cup	510
PUDDING SUNDAE (Swiss Miss):		
Caramel, mint or peanut butter	4-oz. container	180
Chocolate or vanilla	4-oz. container	200
PUFFED CORN, cereal (USDA) with added nutrients	1 oz.	301
PUFFED OAT, cereal (USDA):		
Plain, added nutrients	1 oz.	359
Sugar coated, added nutrients	1 oz.	167
PUFFED RICE, cereal:		
(Malt-O-Meal)	1 cup (½ oz.)	0
(Quaker)	1 cup (½ oz.)	1
PUFFED WHEAT, cereal:		
(Malt-O-Meal)	1 cup (½ oz.)	Tr.
(Quaker)	1 cup (½ oz.)	1

Food and Description	Measure or Quantity	Sodium (milligrams)
PUMPKIN:		
Fresh (USDA):		
Whole	1 lb. (weighed with rind & seeds)	3
Flesh only	4 oz.	1
Canned:		
(USDA) salted	½ cup (4.3 oz.)	288
(Del Monte)	½ cup (4.3 oz.)	<10
(Festal)	½ cup	6
(Libby's) solid pack	½ cup	5
PUMPKIN BUTTER		
(Smucker's) *Autumn Harvest*	1 T.	42
PUNCH DRINK (Minute Maid):		
Canned:		
Concord, regular	8.45 fl. oz.	25
Tropical	8.45 fl. oz.	24
Chilled or frozen	6 fl. oz.	18
PURE & LIGHT, fruit juice		
(Dole)	6 fl. oz.	10

Q

QUAIL, raw (USDA) meat & skin only	4 oz.	45
QUIK (Nestlé):		
Regular:		
Chocolate	1 T.	18
Strawberry	1 T.	0
Sugar free	1 T.	40
QUINCE, fresh (USDA):		
Untrimmed	1 lb. (weighed with skin & seeds)	11

Food and Description	Measure or Quantity	Sodium (milligrams)
Flesh only	4 oz.	5
QUINCE JELLY		
(Smucker's)	1 T.	<10

R

RABBIT (USDA) domesticated:
Raw, ready-to-cook	1 lb. (weighed with bones)	154
Stewed, flesh only	4 oz.	46

RADISH (USDA) common, raw:
Without tops	½ lb. (weighed untrimmed)	36
Trimmed, whole	4 small radishes (1.4 oz.)	7
Trimmed, sliced	½ cup (2 oz.)	10

RAISIN:
Dried:
(USDA):
Whole, pressed down	½ cup (2.9 oz.)	22
Chopped	½ cup (2.9 oz.)	22
Ground	½ cup (4.7 oz.)	36

(Del Monte):
Golden	3 oz.	<10
(Dole)	¼ cup (1.5 oz.)	25
(Sun-Maid) seedless, natural,	3 oz.	15
Thompson	½ cup (3 oz.)	12

Cooked (USDA) added sugar,
solids & liq.	½ cup (4.3 oz.)	16

RASPBERRY:
Black (USDA):
Fresh:
Whole	1 lb. (weighed with caps & stems)	2

Food and Description	Measure or Quantity	Sodium (milligrams)
Without caps & stems	½ cup (2.4 oz.)	<1
Canned, water pack, un-sweetened, solids & liq.	4 oz.	1
Red:		
Fresh (USDA):		
Whole	1 lb. (weighed with caps & stems)	2
Without caps & stems	½ cup (2.5 oz.)	<1
Canned, water pack, un-sweetened or low calorie, solids & liq. (USDA)	4 oz.	1
Frozen (Birds Eye) quick thaw	½ of 10-oz. pkg.	1
*RASPBERRY DRINK, mix (Funny Face)	8 fl. oz.	0
RASPBERRY JELLY, sweetened:		
(Home Brands)	1 T.	15
(Smucker's) black or red	1 T.	<10
RASPBERRY JUICE, canned (Smucker's)	8 fl. oz.	10
RASPBERRY PRESERVE or JAM sweetened (Smucker's) black or red	1 T.	2
RATATOUILLE, frozen (Stouffer's)	5 oz.	1320
RAVIOLI:		
Canned, regular pack (Franco-American) beef:		
In meat sauce	7½-oz. serving	1090
In meat sauce, RavioliOs	7½-oz. serving	890
Canned, dietetic or low calorie:		
(Dia-Mel) beef, in sauce	8-oz. can	75
(Estee)	7½-oz. can	110
(Featherweight)	8-oz. can	68
Frozen:		
(Buitoni):		
Cheese:		
Ravioletti	2.6 oz.	217
Square	4.8 oz.	237

Food and Description	Measure or Quantity	Sodium (milligrams)
Meat:		
Ravioletti	2.6 oz.	244
Square	4.8 oz.	371
(Celentano) cheese:		
Regular	½ of 13-oz. pkg.	510
Mini	½ of 8-oz. box	210
(Kid Cuisine) cheese, mini	8¾-oz. meal	730
(Weight Watchers) cheese,		
baked	9-oz. serving	550
RED LOBSTER RESTAURANT		
(lunch portion refers to cooked 5-oz. portion, weighed raw, before cooking unless otherwise noted):		
Calamari, breaded & fried	lunch portion	1150
Catfish	lunch portion	50
Chicken breast	4-oz. serving	60
Crab legs:		
King	16-oz. serving	900
Snow	16-oz. serving	1630
Flounder	lunch portion	95
Grouper	lunch portion	70
Hamburger, without bun	5.3-oz. burger	70
Lobster, tail	1 tail	1090
Monkfish	lunch portion	95
Munch	3 oz.	150
Oyster	6 raw oysters	90
Salmon	lunch portion	60
Shrimp	8–12 pieces	110
Steak:		
Porterhouse	18-oz. serving	150
Sirloin	7-oz. serving	85
Strip	7-oz. serving	70
RELISH:		
Dill (Vlasic)	1 oz.	415
Hamburger (Vlasic)	1 oz.	255
Hot dog (Vlasic)	1 oz.	255
Sweet:		
(USDA) finely chopped	1 T. (.5 oz.)	107
(Aunt Jane's)	1 rounded tsp. (.4 oz.)	71

Food and Description	Measure or Quantity	Sodium (milligrams)
(Smucker's)	1 T. (.6 oz.)	158
(Vlasic)	1 oz.	220
RENNET MIX (Junket):		
*Powder:		
Chocolate:		
Made with skim milk	½ cup	70
Made with whole milk	½ cup	65
Raspberry or strawberry:		
Made with skim milk	½ cup	65
Made with whole milk	½ cup	60
Vanilla:		
Made with skim milk	½ cup	70
Made with whole milk	½ cup	65
Tablet	1 tablet	165
RHINE WINE:		
(Gold Seal) 12% alcohol	3 fl. oz.	3
(Great Western):		
Regular, 12% alcohol	3 fl. oz.	25
Dutchess, 12% alcohol	3 fl. oz.	27
RHUBARB (USDA):		
Fresh:		
Partly trimmed	1 lb. (weighed with part leaves, ends & trimmings)	7
Trimmed	4 oz.	2
Diced	½ cup (2.2 oz.)	1
Cooked, sweetened, solids & liq.	½ cup (4.2 oz.)	2
Frozen, sweetened, cooked, added sugar	½ cup (4.4 oz.)	4
RICE:		
Brown:		
Raw (USDA)	½ cup (3.7 oz.)	9
Dry, parboiled (Uncle Ben's) long-grain	1 oz.	4
*(Uncle Ben's) parboiled:		
No added butter or salt	⅔ cup	5
Added butter & salt	⅔ cup (4.2 oz.)	458
White:		
Dry:		

Food and Description	Measure or Quantity	Sodium (milligrams)
(USDA) long grain, instant or precooked	1 oz.	<1
(USDA) regular	½ cup (3.3 oz.)	5
*Cooked:		
(USDA) long grain	⅔ cup (3.3 oz.)	254
(Minute Rice) no butter:		
With salt	⅔ cup	268
Without salt	⅔ cup	2
(Uncle Ben's):		
Converted, no butter or salt	⅔ cup (4.6 oz.)	2
Converted, with butter & salt		
Long grain, no added butter or salt	⅔ cup (4.2 oz.)	13
Long grain, with butter or salt	⅔ cup (4.3 oz.)	233
RICE BRAN (USDA)	1 oz.	Tr.
RICE CAKE:		
(Hain):		
Regular:		
Plain:		
Regular	1 cake	10
No salt added	1 cake	<5
5-grain	1 cake	10
Sesame:		
Regular	1 cake	10
No salt added	1 cake	<5
Mini:		
Plain:		
Regular	½-oz. serving	75
No salt added	½-oz. serving	5
Apple cinnamon	½-oz. serving	5
Barbecue	½-oz. serving	70
Cheese or teriyaki	½-oz. serving	80
Honey nut	½-oz. serving	15
Nacho cheese or ranch	½-oz. serving	90
Heart Lovers (TKI Foods) plain or sesame	.3-oz. cake	30

Food and Description	Measure or Quantity	Sodium (milligrams)
(Pritikin):		
Regular:		
Plain	1 cake	30
Sesame or 7-grain	1 cake	35
Low sodium, any flavor	1 cake	0
RICE, FRIED:		
*Canned, (La Choy)	¾ cup	930
Frozen:		
(Birds Eye)	⅓ of 11-oz. pkg.	432
(Chun King):		
Chicken	8-oz. serving	1460
Pork	8-oz. serving	1210
(Green Giant) *Boil 'N Bag*	10-oz. entree	1130
(La Choy) meat	8-oz. entree	1770
*Seasoning mix (Durkee)	1 cup	1597
RICE, FRIED, & PORK		
ENTREE, frozen (La Choy)	½ of 12-oz.	
	entree	1716
RICE KRISPIES, cereal		
(Kellogg's):		
Regular	1 cup (1 oz.)	285
Cocoa	¾ cup (1 oz.)	195
Frosted	¾ cup (1 oz.)	200
Marshmallow	1¼ cups	285
Strawberry	¾ cup (1 oz.)	200
RICE MIX:		
Beef:		
*(Lipton) & sauce	½ cup	571
*(Minute Rice) rib roast	½ cup	720
*Cajun (Lipton) & sauce	¼ of pkg.	596
Chicken:		
*(Lipton) & sauce	½ cup	442
*(Minute Rice) drumstick	½ cup	694
*Fried (Minute Rice)	½ cup	549
*Herb & butter (Lipton) &		
sauce	½ cup	442
*Long grain & wild:		
(Lipton) & sauce, original	½ cup	530
(Minute Rice)	½ cup	578

Food and Description	Measure or Quantity	Sodium (milligrams)
Milanese (Knorr) risotto	½ cup	420
*Mushroom (Lipton) & sauce	½ cup	497
*Pilaf (Lipton) & sauce	½ cup	403
Spanish:		
*(Minute Rice)	½ cup	839
(Rice-A-Roni)	⅐ of pkg.	720
*Tomato (Knorr) risotto	½ cup	460
RICE PUDDING (See PUDDING or PIE FILLING)		
***RICE SEASONING** (French's)		
Spice Your Rice:		
Beef flavor & onion	½ cup	560
Buttery herb	½ cup	430
Cheese & chives	½ cup	400
Chicken flavor & herb or parmesan	½ cup	440
RICE, SPANISH:		
Home recipe (USDA)	4 oz.	358
Canned, regular pack:		
(Comstock)	½ of 7½-oz. can	850
(Libby's)	½ of 15-oz. can	1108
(Old El Paso)	½ cup	400
RICE & VEGETABLES:		
Frozen:		
(Birds Eye):		
For One:		
& broccoli, au gratin	5-oz. pkg.	309
With green beans & almonds	5½-oz. pkg.	667
Mexican, with corn	5½-oz. pkg.	392
Pilaf	5½-oz. pkg.	706
Internationals:		
Country style	⅓ of 10-oz. pkg.	381
French style	⅓ of 10-oz. pkg.	609
Spanish style	⅓ of 10-oz. pkg.	539
(Green Giant):		
One serving:		
& broccoli, in cheese sauce	4½-oz. pkg.	550

Food and Description	Measure or Quantity	Sodium (milligrams)
& peas & mushrooms	5½-oz. pkg.	410
Rice Originals:		
& broccoli, in cheese sauce	½ cup	510
Italian blend & spinach	½ cup	400
Medley	½ cup	310
Pilaf	½ cup	530
& wild rice	½ cup	540
*Mix:		
(Knorr) risotto:		
Mushrooms	½ cup	430
With onions	½ cup	390
With peas & corn	½ cup	470
(Lipton):		
Asparagus, with hollandaise sauce	½ cup	462
& broccoli, with cheddar	½ cup	418
RIGATONI, frozen (Healthy Choice) & meat sauce	9½-oz. meal	470
ROCKFISH (USDA):		
Raw, meat only	1 lb.	272
Oven steamed, with onion	4 oz.	77
ROE, baked or broiled, cod & shad, prepared with butter or margarine & lemon juice or vinegar (USDA)	4 oz.	83
ROLL or BUN (See also **ROLL DOUGH; ROLL MIX**):		
Apple (Dolly Madison)	2-oz. piece	190
Brown & serve:		
(USDA) browned	1-oz. roll	159
Merita	1-oz. roll	130
(Pepperidge Farm) club	1.3-oz. roll	220
(Roman Meal) original	1-oz. roll	144
Cherry (Dolly Madison)	2-oz. piece	165
Cinnamon (Dolly Madison)	1¾-oz. piece	220
Cloverleaf (USDA) home recipe	1 cloverleaf (1.2 oz.)	98

Food and Description	Measure or Quantity	Sodium (milligrams)
Crescent, butter (Pepperidge Farm)	1 roll	160
Croissant (Pepperidge Farm):		
Almond	2-oz. roll	260
Butter	2-oz. roll	310
Chocolate	2.4-oz. roll	325
Cinnamon	2-oz. roll	280
Honey sesame	2-oz. roll	270
Raisin	2-oz. roll	265
Walnut	2-oz. roll	275
Danish (Dolly Madison)		
Danish Twirls:		
Apple, cherry or cinnamon raisin	2-oz. piece	210
Cheese, cream	3½-oz. piece	490
Dinner:		
Butternut	1-oz. roll	170
Eddy's	1½-oz. roll	330
Mrs. Karl's	2-oz. roll	340
(Roman Meal)	1-oz. roll	140
Egg bun, *Weber's*	1-oz. bun	180
Frankfurter:		
(USDA)	1.4-oz. roll	202
(Arnold)	1.3-oz. roll	290
(Pepperidge Farm)	1¾-oz. roll	240
(Roman Meal)	1.5-oz. roll	212
French:		
(Arnold) Francisco, sourdough	1.1-oz. roll	160
(Pepperidge Farm):		
Regular	1.3-oz. roll	250
Sourdough	1 roll	240
Golden twist (Pepperidge Farm)	1 roll	160
Hamburger:		
(USDA)	1.4-oz. roll	202
(Pepperidge Farm)	1½-oz. roll	260
(Roman Meal)	1.6-oz. roll	227
Hard (USDA) round or rectangular	1.8-oz. roll	312

Food and Description	Measure or Quantity	Sodium (milligrams)
Honey (Dolly Madison)	3½-oz. piece	325
Kaiser:		
Dutch Hearth	1½-oz. piece	400
Sweetheart	2-oz. piece	500
Lemon (Dolly Madison)	2-oz. piece	280
Old fashioned (Pepperidge Farm)	.6-oz. roll	95
Parkerhouse:		
(Arnold) *Dinner Party*	.7-oz. roll	63
(Pepperidge Farm)	1 roll	90
Party pan (Pepperidge Farm)	1 roll	50
Plain (USDA)	1-oz. roll	143
Raisin (USDA)	1-oz. roll	109
Raspberry (Dolly Madison)	2-oz. piece	250
Sandwich:		
(Arnold):		
Francisco	2-oz. roll	325
Soft, plain	1.3-oz. roll	260
Soft, sesame seeds	1.3-oz. roll	260
(Pepperidge Farm):		
Regular with poppy or sesame seeds	1.6-oz. roll	210
Onion, with poppy seeds	1.9-oz. roll	240
Sourdough, French (Pepperidge Farm)	1.3-oz. roll	255
Sweet (USDA)	1.5-oz. bun	167
Whole wheat (USDA)	1⅓-oz. roll	214
ROLL DOUGH:		
*Frozen (Rich's) homestyle	1 roll	168
Refrigerated:		
(Pillsbury):		
Butterflake	1 piece	520
Caramel danish with nuts	1 piece	240
Cinnamon:		
Regular	1 piece	260
With icing	1 piece	260
& raisins	1 piece	230
Crescent	1 piece	230
Orange danish with icing	1 piece	240

Food and Description	Measure or Quantity	Sodium (milligrams)
(Roman Meal) biscuit:		
Regular	1.2-oz. piece	228
Honey nut oat bran	1½-oz. piece	278
White	1½-oz. piece	308
*ROLL MIX (Pillsbury) hot roll	1 roll	215
ROMAN MEAL CEREAL, hot:		
Regular, 2- or 5-minute	⅓ cup (1 oz.)	2
Regular:		
Cream of rye	⅓ cup (1.3 oz.)	0
Multi-bran with cinnamon apples	⅓ cup (1.2 oz.)	14
Oat bran	¼ cup (1 oz.)	3
Oats, wheat, dates, raisins & almonds	⅓ cup (1.3 oz.)	4
Original, plain or with oats	⅓ cup	<1
Instant, oats, wheat, honey, coconut & almonds	⅓ cup (1.3 oz.)	7
With oats, 5-minute	⅓ cup (1 oz.)	6
ROSEMARY LEAVES		
(French's)	1 tsp.	<1
ROSÉ WINE (Great Western)		
12% alcohol:		
Regular	3 fl. oz.	38
Isabella	3 fl. oz.	<1
ROY ROGERS:		
Bar Burger, R.R.	1 burger	1252
Biscuit	1 biscuit	575
Breakfast crescent sandwich:		
Regular	4.5-oz. sandwich	820
With bacon	4.7-oz. sandwich	982
With ham	5.8-oz. sandwich	1245
With sausage	5.7-oz. sandwich	1145
Cheeseburger:		
Regular	1 burger	830
With bacon	1 burger	1025
Chicken:		
Breast	1 piece	609
Breast & wing	6.9-oz. serving	894
Leg	1 piece	190

Food and Description	Measure or Quantity	Sodium (milligrams)
Thigh	1 piece	406
Wing	1 piece	285
Chicken nuggets	1 piece	91
Coleslaw	3⅝-oz. serving	261
Drinks:		
Coffee, black	6 fl. oz.	2
Coke:		
Regular	12 fl. oz.	22
Diet	12 fl. oz.	52
Hot chocolate	6 fl. oz.	124
Milk	8 fl. oz.	120
Orange juice:		
Regular	7 fl. oz.	2
Large	10 fl. oz.	3
Shake:		
Chocolate	1 shake	290
Vanilla	1 shake	261
Strawberry	1 shake	282
Tea, iced, plain	8 fl. oz.	Tr.
Egg & biscuit platter:		
Regular	1 meal	1020
With bacon	1 meal	1236
With ham	1 meal	1442
With sausage	1 meal	1345
Hamburger	1 burger	607
Pancake platter, with syrup & butter:		
Plain	1 order	547
With bacon	1 order	763
With ham	1 order	969
With sausage	1 order	872
Potato fries	3-oz. serving	122
Potato salad	3½-oz. order	696
Roast beef sandwich:		
Plain:		
Regular	1 sandwich	732
Large	1 sandwich	840
With cheese:		
Regular	1 sandwich	954

Food and Description	Measure or Quantity	Sodium (milligrams)
Large	1 sandwich	1062
Salad bar:		
Bacon bits	1 T.	189
Beets, sliced	¼ cup	162
Broccoli	½ cup	12
Carrot, shredded	¼ cup	7
Cheese, cheddar	¼ cup	195
Croutons	1 T.	130
Cucumber	1 slice	Tr.
Egg, chopped	1 T.	21
Lettuce	1 cup	7
Macaroni salad	1 T.	155
Mushrooms	¼ cup	3
Noodle, Chinese	¼ cup	100
Pea, green	¼ cup	66
Pepper, green	1 T.	1
Potato salad	1 T.	175
Sunflower seeds	1 T.	4
Tomato	1 slice	1
Salad dressing:		
Regular:		
Bacon & tomato	1 T.	75
Bleu cheese	1 T.	76
Ranch	1 T.	50
1,000 Island	1 T.	75
Low calorie, Italian	1 T.	50
Strawberry shortcake	7.2-oz. serving	674
Sundae:		
Caramel	1 sundae	193
Hot fudge	1 sundae	230
Strawberry	1 sundae	99
RUM (See DISTILLED LIQUOR)		
RUTABAGA:		
Raw (USDA):		
Without tops	1 lb. (weighed with skin)	19
Diced	½ cup (2.5 oz.)	4
Boiled (USDA) drained, diced	½ cup (3 oz.)	3

Food and Description	Measure or Quantity	Sodium (milligrams)
Canned (Sunshine) solids & liq.	½ cup (4.2 oz.)	393
Frozen (Southland)	4 oz.	20
RYE, whole grain (USDA)	1 oz.	<1
RYE FLOUR (See **FLOUR**)		
RYE WHISKEY (See **DISTILLED LIQUOR)**		

S

SABLEFISH, raw (USDA):		
Whole	1 lb. (weighed whole)	107
Meat only	4 oz.	64
SAGE (French's)	1 tsp. (.9 grams)	<1
SALAD DRESSING (See also **SALAD DRESSING MIX):**		
Regular:		
Bacon & tomato (Henri's)	1 T.	140
Blue or bleu cheese:		
(USDA)	1 T. (.5 oz.)	164
(Henri's)	1 T.	220
Boiled, home recipe (USDA)	1 T. (.6 oz.)	116
Buttermilk (Hain)	1 T.	100
Caesar:		
(Hain) creamy	1 T.	220
(Wish-Bone)	1 T.	234
Cheddar & bacon (Wish-Bone)	1 T.	110
Cucumber (Wish-Bone)	1 T.	125
Cucumber dill (Hain)	1 T.	210
Dijon vinaigrette:		
(Hain)	1 T.	180

Food and Description	Measure or Quantity	Sodium (*milligrams*)
(Wish-Bone)	1 T.	191
French:		
Home recipe (USDA)		
made with corn or		
cottonseed oil	1 T. (.6 oz.)	105
(USDA) commercial type	1 T. (.6 oz.)	219
(Hain) creamy	1 T.	80
(Henri's):		
Hearty	1 T.	95
Original	1 T.	110
Sweet & Saucy Frontier	1 T.	95
(Wish-Bone):		
Deluxe	1 T.	73
Garlic or Sweet & Spicy	1 T.	158
French mustard (Hain) spicy	1 T.	190
Garden tomato vinaigrette		
(Hain) with canola oil	1 T.	150
Garlic (Wish-Bone) creamy	1 T.	157
Garlic & sour cream (Hain)	1 T.	100
Honey & sesame (Hain)	1 T.	210
Italian:		
(USDA)	1 T. (.5 oz.)	314
(Hain):		
Canola oil	1 T.	150
& cheese vinaigrette	1 T.	130
Creamy	1 T.	100
Traditional	1 T.	330
(Henri's):		
Authentic	1 T.	300
Creamy garlic	1 T.	150
(Wish-Bone):		
Creamy	1 T. (.5 oz.)	146
Herbal	1 T.	228
Robusto	1 T. (.5 oz.)	258
Mayonnaise-type (Luzianne)		
Blue Plate	1 T. (.5 oz.)	105
Ranchhouse (Henri's)		
Chef's Recipe	1 T.	125

Food and Description	Measure or Quantity	Sodium (milligrams)
Russian:		
(USDA)	1 T. (.5 oz.)	130
(Henri's)	1 T.	95
(Wish-Bone)	1 T.	147
Swiss cheese vinaigrette		
(Hain)	1 T.	160
Tangy citrus (Hain)	1 T.	75
Tas-Tee (Henri's)	1 T.	105
1000 Island:		
(USDA)	1 T. (.6 oz.)	112
(Hain)	1 T.	85
(Henri's)	1 T.	120
(Wish-Bone)	1 T.	162
Dietetic or low calorie:		
Bleu or blue cheese:		
(USDA)	1 T. (.6 oz.)	177
(Estee)	1 T. (.5 oz.)	50
(Henri's)	1 T.	230
(Walden Farms) chunky	1 T.	270
(Wish-Bone) chunky	1 T. (.5 oz.)	190
Caesar:		
(Hain) creamy, low salt	1 T.	16
(Weight Watchers)	¾-oz. pouch	270
Catalina (Kraft)	1 T.	125
Chef's Recipe Ranchouse		
(Henri's)	1 T.	115
Cucumber, creamy:		
Herb Magic (Luzianne		
Blue Plate)	1 T.	100
(Kraft)	1 T.	210
French:		
(USDA)	1 T. (.6 oz.)	126
(Estee)	1 T.	10
(Henri's):		
Original	1 T.	135
Hearty	1 T.	105
(Pritikin)	1 T.	0
(Wish-Bone)	1 T.	70
Garlic (Estee) creamy	1 T.	10

Food and Description	Measure or Quantity	Sodium (milligrams)
Herb (Hain) savory, no salt added	1 T.	25
Herb basket, *Herb Magic* (Luzianne *Blue Plate*)	1 T.	170
Italian:		
(USDA)	1 T.	118
(Estee) creamy	1 T. (.5 oz.)	10–15
(Hain) no salt added:		
Creamy	1 T.	25
Traditional	1 T.	20
(Henri's):		
Authentic	1 T.	270
Creamy	1 T.	230
Herb Magic (Luzianne *Blue Plate*)	1 T.	125
(Kraft) zesty	1 T.	210
(Pritikin) regular or creamy	1 T.	0
(Weight Watchers):		
Regular, creamy	1 T. (.5 oz.)	80
Single serving packet	¾-oz. packet	430
(Wish-Bone)	1 T.	237
Mayonnaise, imitation (USDA)	1 T. (.6 oz.)	19
Olive oil vinaigrette (Wish-Bone) lite	1 T.	126
Onion & chive (Wish-Bone)	1 T.	163
Ranch:		
(Henri's):		
Chef's Recipe	1 T.	150
Parmesan	1 T.	130
Herb Magic (Luzianne *Blue Plate*)	1 T.	110
(Pritikin)	1 T.	0
(Weight Watchers)	¾-oz. pouch	110
(Wish-Bone)	1 T.	148
Red wine vinegar (Estee)	1 T.	10
Russian:		
(Pritikin)	1 T.	20

Food and Description	Measure or Quantity	Sodium (milligrams)
(Weight Watchers)	1 T.	80
Sweet & sour, *Herb Magic* (Luzianne *Blue Plate*)	1 T.	80
1000 Island:		
(USDA)	1 T. (.5 oz.)	105
(Estee)	1 T.	30
(Henri's)	1 T.	160
Herb Magic (Luzianne *Blue Plate*)	1 T.	45
(Weight Watchers)	1 T.	80
(Wish-Bone)	1 T.	107
Tomato (Pritikin) zesty	1 T.	0
Vinaigrette (Pritikin)	1 T.	0
Whipped (Weight Watchers)	1 T.	100
SALAD DRESSING MIX:		
*Regular (Good Seasons):		
Bleu or blue cheese & herb	1 T.	148
Buttermilk, farm style	1 T.	137
Classic dill	1 T.	147
French, old fashioned	1 T.	185
Garlic, with cheese	1 T.	167
Garlic & herbs	1 T.	187
Italian:		
Regular	1 T.	172
Cheese	1 T.	127
Mild	1 T.	192
Zesty	1 T.	121
Lemon & herbs	1 T.	143
Ranch	1 T.	112
Dietetic or low calorie:		
*Blue cheese (Hain)	1 T.	190
*Buttermilk (Hain) no oil	1 T.	150
*Caesar (Hain) no oil	1 T.	200
*French (Hain) no oil	1 T.	340
*Garlic & cheese (Hain) no oil	1 T.	180
*Herb (Hain) no oil	1 T.	140
*Italian:		
(Good Seasons) lite:		

Food and Description	Measure or Quantity	Sodium (milligrams)
Regular	1 T.	177
Zesty	1 T.	133
(Hain) no oil	1 T.	170
*Ranch (Good Seasons) lite	1 T.	115
*1000 Island (Hain) no oil	1 T.	150
*Russian (Weight Watchers)	1 T.	128
*Thousand Island (Weight Watchers)	1 T.	265
SALAMI:		
(Eckrich):		
For beer	1-oz. slice	350
Cooked, chub	1 oz.	360
Cotto:		
Beef	.7-oz. slice	240
Meat	1-oz. slice	340
Hard	1 oz.	600
(Hormel):		
Beef	1 slice	110
Cotto:		
Chub	1 oz.	385
Sliced, regular	1 slice	375
Genoa:		
Regular	1 oz.	456
Di Lusso	1 oz.	443
Gran Valore	1 oz.	453
San Remo	1 oz.	544
Hard:		
Packaged, whole	1 slice	169
Whole:		
Regular	1 oz.	468
National	1 oz.	463
Party, sliced	1 oz.	399
(Ohse) cooked	1 oz.	330
(Oscar Mayer):		
For beer:		
Regular	.8-oz. slice	286
Beef	.8-oz. slice	281
Cotto:		
Regular	.8-oz. slice	290

Food and Description	Measure or Quantity	Sodium (milligrams)
Beef	.5-oz. slice	189
Beef	.8-oz. slice	302
Genoa	.3-oz. slice	162
Hard, all meat	.3-oz. slice	169
SALISBURY STEAK:		
Canned (Morton House)	⅓ of 12½-oz. can	512
Frozen:		
(Armour):		
Classics Lite	11½-oz. meal	980
Dining Lite	9-oz. meal	1000
Dinner Classics:		
Regular	11¼-oz.meal	1430
Parmigiana	11½-oz. meal	1120
(Banquet) dinner:		
Regular	11-oz. dinner	600
Extra Helping	18-oz. dinner	740
(Healthy Choice)	11½-oz. meal	480
(Morton)	10-oz. dinner	1420
(Stouffer's):		
Regular, with gravy	9⅞-oz. meal	1070
Lean Cuisine	9½-oz. meal	840
(Swanson):		
Regular:		
Dinner	11-oz. dinner	1050
Entree	5½-oz. entree	650
Hungry Man:		
Dinner:	16½-oz. dinner	1630
Entree	11¾-oz. entree	1340
Main course	8½-oz. entree	1400
(Weight Watchers) beef,		
Romana	8¾-oz.	910
SALMON:		
Raw:		
Chinook or king (USDA):		
Steak	1 lb. (weighed whole)	180
Meat only	4 oz.	51
Canned, solids & liq., including bones	4 oz.	51

Food and Description	Measure or Quantity	Sodium (milligrams)
Chum, canned (USDA) solids & liq., including bones	4 oz.	60
Coho, canned (USDA) solids & liq., including bones, no salt added	4 oz.	54
Keta, canned (Demings) solids & liq.	½ cup	450
Pink or humpback (USDA):		
Raw:		
Steak	1 lb. (weighed whole)	255
Meat only	4 oz.	73
Canned, solids & liq.:		
(USDA) including bones, not salted	4 oz.	73
(USDA) salted	4 oz.	439
(Deming's) skinless & boneless, chunk style	2 oz.	180
(Double "Q") skinless & boneless	½ of 6½-oz. can	420
(Peter Pan)	½ cup	450
Sockeye or red or blueback, canned, solids & liq.:		
(USDA) not salted	4 oz.	54
(Double "Q") red sockeye	½ cup	450
Unspecified kind of salmon		
(USDA) baked or broiled with vegetable shortening	4.2-oz. steak (approx. 4″ × 3″ × ½″)	139
Dietetic, canned (S&W) *Nutradiet*	½ cup	45
SALT:		
Regular:		
Butter-flavored (French's) imitation	1 tsp. (3.6 g.)	1090
Hickory smoke (French's)	1 tsp. (4 g.)	1170
Seasoned (French's)	1 tsp.	1230
Table:		
(USDA)	1 tsp. (5.5 g.)	2132

Food and Description	Measure or Quantity	Sodium (milligrams)
(Morton) iodized	1 tsp. (6.5 g.)	2544
Lite Salt (Morton) iodized	1 tsp. (6 g.)	1188
Substitute:		
(Adolph's):		
Regular	1 tsp. (6 g.)	<1
Packet	8-g. packet	Tr.
Seasoned	1 tsp.	<1
(Estee) *Salt-It*	1 tsp.	0
(Morton):		
Regular	1 tsp. (6 g.)	<1
Seasoned	1 tsp. (6 g.)	<1
SALT PORK, raw (USDA):		
With skin	1 lb. (weighed with skin)	5278
Without skin	1 oz.	344
SAND DAB, raw (USDA):		
Whole	1 lb. (weighed whole)	117
Meat only	4 oz.	88
SANDWICH SPREAD:		
Regular:		
(USDA)	1 T. (.5 oz.)	94
(Best Foods/Hellmann's)	1 T. (.5 oz.)	175
(Best Foods/Hellmann's)	½ cup (4.2 oz.)	1405
(Oscar Mayer)	1-oz. serving	268
Dietetic or low calorie (USDA)	1 T. (.5 oz.)	94
SARDINE:		
Raw (HHS/FAO):		
Whole	1 lb. (weighed whole)	249
Meat only	4 oz.	113
Canned:		
Atlantic:		
(USDA) in oil:		
Solids & liq.	3¾-oz. can	541
Drained solids, with skin & bones	3¾-oz. can	757
(Del Monte) in tomato sauce, solids & liq.	7½-oz. can	827

Food and Description	Measure or Quantity	Sodium (milligrams)
Imported (Underwood):		
In mustard sauce	3¾-oz. can	850
In tomato sauce	3¾-oz. can	850
Norwegian:		
(Granadaisa Brand) in tomato sauce	3¾-oz. can	434
(King David Brand) in olive oil	3¾-oz. can	842
(Queen Helga Brand) in sild oil	3¾-oz. can	603
(Underwood) in oil	3¾-oz. can	800
Pacific (USDA) in brine or mustard, solids & liq.	4 oz.	862
SAUCE (See also **SAUCE MIX**):		
A-1	1 T. (.6 oz.)	275
Barbecue:		
(USDA)	1 T. (.6 oz.)	130
(Estee) dietetic	1 T.	3
(French's):		
Regular or hot	1 T. (.6 oz.)	250
Smoky	1 T. (.6 oz.)	280
(Hunt's):		
Country style	1 T. (.5 oz.)	140
Hickory or original	1 T. (.5 oz.)	160
Homestyle or western	1 T. (.5 oz.)	170
Kansas City	1 T. (.5 oz.)	85
Open Pit:		
Regular	1 T. (.6 oz.)	236
Hot & spicy	1 T.	163
Hickory smoked flavor	1 T.	232
With minced onions	1 T.	252
Burrito (Del Monte)	¼ cup	355
Caramel (Knorr)	1 T. (.7 oz.)	5
Cheese (Snow's) welsh rarebit	½ cup	460
Chili (See **CHILI SAUCE**)		
Cocktail (See Seafood below)		
Grilling & broiling (Knorr):		
Chardonnay	⅛ of 12.8-oz. container	630

Food and Description	Measure or Quantity	Sodium (milligrams)
Spicy plum	⅛ of 13.6-oz. container	790
Tequila lime	⅛ of 12.8-oz. container	690
Tuscan herb	⅛ of 12.8-oz. container	605
Hollandaise (Knorr) microwave	1 fl. oz.	190
Hot (Gebhardt)	1 tsp.	90
Hot dog, *Just Right*	2 oz.	220
Mandarin ginger (Knorr) microwave	⅛ of 12.8-oz. container	690
Mexican (Pritikin) dietetic	1 oz.	9
Newburgh (Snow's)	⅓ cup	520
Orange (LaChoy) mandarin	1 T. (.6 oz.)	38
Parmesano (Knorr) microwave	⅛ of 12.8 oz. container	680
Picante (Old El Paso):		
Salsa	1 T.	80
Sauce:		
Regular	1 T.	155
Chunky	1 T.	135
Plum (LaChoy) tangy	1 oz.	17
Salsa Brava (La Victoria)	1 T.	100
Salsa Casera (La Victoria)	1 T.	80
Salsa Jalapeño (La Victoria):		
Green	1 T.	105
Red	1 T.	95
Salsa Mexicana (Contadina)	4 fl. oz.	570
Salsa Picante (La Victoria)	1 T.	80
Salsa Ranchera (La Victoria)	1 T.	85
Salsa Suprema (La Victoria)	1 T.	95
Salsa Verde (Old El Paso)	1 T.	67
Salsa Victoria (La Victoria)	1 T.	80
Seafood (Del Monte) cocktail	1 T. (.6 oz.)	228
Soy:		
(USDA)	1 oz.	2077
(USDA)	1 T. (.6 oz.)	1246
(Kikkoman):		
Regular	1 T.	938

Food and Description	Measure or Quantity	Sodium (milligrams)
Lite	1 T.	564
(La Choy) regular	1 T. (.5 oz.)	974
Stir-fry (Kikkoman)	1 tsp.	369
Sweet & sour:		
(Chun King)	1.8 oz.	234
(Kikkoman)	1 T.	97
(La Choy)	1 T.	320
Tabasco	¼ tsp.	9
Taco:		
(El Molino) red, mild	1 T.	85
(La Victoria) green or red	1 T.	85
(Old El Paso):		
Can	1 T.	150
Jar	1 T.	65
(Ortega) hot	1 oz.	207
Tartar:		
(USDA)	1 T. (.5 oz.)	99
Hellmann's (Best Foods)	1 T. (.5 oz.)	190
Teriyaki (Kikkoman)	1 T. (.6 oz.)	626
Tomato (See **TOMATO SAUCE**)		
Vera Cruz (Knorr) microwave	¼ of pkg.	580
White (USDA) medium	1 cup (9 oz.)	966
Worcestershire:		
(French's) regular or smoke	1 T.	200
(Lea & Perrins)	1 T. (.6 oz.)	175
SAUCE MIX:		
*Au jus (Knorr)	2 fl. oz.	160
Bearnaise (Knorr)	2 fl. oz.	340
*Cheese (French's)	½ cup	850
*Demi-glace (Knorr)	2 fl. oz.	310
*Hollandaise (Knorr)	2 fl. oz.	310
*Hunter (Knorr)	2 fl. oz.	340
*Italian (Knorr) Napoli	2 fl. oz.	960
*Lyonnaise (Knorr)	2 fl. oz.	360
*Mushroom (Knorr)	2 fl. oz.	240
*Pepper (Knorr)	2 fl. oz.	380
*Sour cream (French's)	2½ T.	130
*Stroganoff (French's)	⅓ cup	490

Food and Description	Measure or Quantity	Sodium (milligrams)
*Sweet & sour:		
(Durkee)	½ cup	526
(French's)	½ cup	135
(Kikkoman)	1 T.	63
*Teriyaki (French's)	1 T.	590
SAUERKRAUT, canned:		
(USDA) solids & liq.	1 cup (8.3 oz.)	1755
(Claussen) drained	½ cup (2.7 oz.)	491
(Comstock) solids, & liq.:		
Regular	½ cup	800
Bavarian	½ cup	600
(Del Monte) solids & liq.	1 cup (8 oz.)	1550
(Frank's) regular or Bavarian	½ cup	780
(Snow Floss)	½ cup	780
(Vlasic) old fashioned, solids & liq.	1 oz.	284
SAUERKRAUT JUICE, canned		
(USDA)	½ cup (4.3 oz.)	952
SAUSAGE:		
Brown & serve:		
*(Hormel)	1 link	215
*(Swift):		
Bacon & sausage	.7-oz. link	173
Beef	.7-oz. link	169
Kountry Kured	.7-oz. link	171
Original flavor	.7-oz. link	169
Knockwurst (Hebrew National) beef	3 oz.	724
Links (Ohse) hot	1 oz.	310
Patty (Hormel):		
Hot	1 pattie	549
Mild	1 pattie	541
Polish-style:		
(Eckrich) meat:		
Regular	1 oz.	260
Skinless	1 oz.	250
(Hormel):		
Regular	1 sausage	287
Kielbasa	½ link	826

Food and Description	Measure or Quantity	Sodium (milligrams)
Kolbase	3 oz.	904
(Ohse):		
Regular	1 oz.	290
Hot	1 oz.	270
Pork:		
(USDA) link or bulk:		
Uncooked	1-oz. serving	210
Cooked	1-oz. serving	272
*(Hormel) *Little Sizzlers*	1 sausage	96
(Jimmy Dean) uncooked	2-oz. serving	338
*(Oscar Mayer)		
Little Friers	1 link	194
Roll (Eckrich)	1 oz.	340
Smoked:		
(Eckrich):		
Beef:		
Regular	2 oz.	520
Smok-Y-Links	.8-oz. link	200
Cheese	2 oz.	500
Ham, *Smok-Y-Links*	.8 oz.	280
Maple flavor, *Smok-Y-Links*	.8 oz.	200
Meat	2 oz.	530
Meat, skinless	2 oz.	490
(Hormel) *Smokies:*		
Regular	1 sausage	298
Cheese	1 sausage	311
(Ohse)	1 oz.	320
(Oscar Mayer):		
Regular	1½-oz. link	425
Beef	1½-oz. link	430
Cheese	1½-oz. link	451
Little Smokies	.3-oz. link	91
Thuringer or summer (See **THURINGER**)		
Turkey (Ohse)	1 oz.	180
Vienna:		
(Hormel) regular	1 sausage	120
(Libby's) in beef broth:		
5-oz. can	1 link	94
9-oz. can	1 link	86

Food and Description	Measure or Quantity	Sodium (milligrams)
SAUTERNE:		
(B&G) 13% alcohol	3 fl. oz.	3
SAVORY (French's)	1 tsp. (1.4 grams)	Tr.
SCALLION (See **ONION, GREEN**)		
SCALLOP:		
Raw (USDA) meat only	4 oz.	289
Steamed (USDA)	4 oz.	301
Frozen:		
(Mrs. Paul's):		
breaded & fried	½ of 7-oz. pkg.	545
Mediterrean	11-oz. entree	775
(Stouffer's) *Lean Cuisine*,		
oriental	11-oz. meal	1325
SCALLOP & SHRIMP MARINER, frozen (Stouffer's)		
with rice	10¼-oz. meal	1120
SCOTCH (See **DISTILLED LIQUOR**)		
SCREWDRIVER COCKTAIL		
(Mr. Boston)	3 fl. oz.	104
SCROD, frozen (Gorton's)		
microwave entree, baked	1 pkg.	420
SEAFOOD DINNER or ENTREE, frozen (Armour)		
Classics Lite	10-oz. meal	1020
SEAFOOD NEWBURGH, frozen:		
(Healthy Choice)	8-oz. meal	440
(Mrs. Paul's)	8½-oz. entree	610
SEAFOOD PLATTER, frozen		
(Mrs. Paul's) combination,		
breaded & fried	9-oz. pkg.	1340
SEGO DIET FOOD, canned:		
Regular:		
Very banana, strawberry & vanilla	1 can	360
Very chocolate, chocolate malt & Dutch chocolate	1 can	445

Food and Description	Measure or Quantity	Sodium (milligrams)
Lite:		
Chocolate, chocolate jamocha almond, chocolate malt, double chocolate & Dutch chocolate	1 can	475
French vanilla, strawberry & vanilla	1 can	390
SESAME NUT MIX, canned (Planters) oil roasted	1 oz.	220
SESAME SEED, dry (USDA) whole	1 oz.	17
7-GRAIN CEREAL (Loma Linda):		
Crunchy	1 oz.	90
No sugar	1 oz.	75
SHAD (USDA):		
Raw:		
Whole	1 lb. (weighed whole)	118
Meat only	4 oz.	61
Cooked, home recipe:		
Baked with butter or margarine & bacon slices	4 oz.	90
Creole	4 oz.	83
SHAKE 'n BAKE:		
Chicken:		
Regular	5½-oz. pkg.	3609
Barbecue style	7-oz. pkg.	6731
Crispy country mild	4¾-oz. pkg.	4005
Fish	5¼-oz. pkg.	3246
Pork or ribs:		
Original	6-oz. pkg.	4816
Barbecue	5¾-oz. pkg.	5623
Extra crispy, *Oven Fry*	4.2-oz. pkg.	2754
SHAKEY'S:		
Chicken & potatoes:		
3-piece meal	1 order	2293
5-piece meal	1 order	5327
Ham & cheese, hot	1 sandwich	2135

Food and Description	Measure or Quantity	Sodium (milligrams)
Pizza:		
Thick:		
Cheese	13" pie	5740
Onion, green pepper, olive,		
mushroom	13" pie	3950
Pepperoni	13" pie	4940
Sausage, mushroom	13" pie	4450
Sausage, pepperoni	13" pie	6260
Special	13" pie	6060
Thin:		
Cheese	13" pie	3160
Onion, green pepper,		
olive, mushroom	13" pie	3950
Pepperoni	13" pie	4550
Sausage, mushroom	13" pie	4160
Sausage, pepperoni	13" pie	5870
Special	13" pie	5670
Potatoes	15-piece order	3703
Spaghetti with meat sauce &		
garlic bread	1 order	1904
Super hot hero	1 order	2688
SHALLOT, raw (USDA):		
With skin	1 oz.	3
With skin removed	1 oz.	3
SHARK BITES (General Mills)		
Fruit Corners	.9-oz. pouch	20
SHELLS, PASTA, STUFFED,		
frozen:		
(Buitoni) jumbo:		
Cheese	5½ oz.	483
Florentine	5½ oz.	323
(Celentano):		
Broccoli & cheese	13½-oz. pkg.	580
Cheese:		
Without sauce	½ of 12½-oz. box	420
With sauce	½ of 16-oz. box	340
SHERBET or SORBET:		
Lemon (Häagen-Dazs)	4 fl. oz.	5

Food and Description	Measure or Quantity	Sodium (milligrams)
Orange:		
(Baskin-Robbins)	4 fl. oz.	46
(Borden)	½ cup	40
(Dole)	½ cup	9
(Häagen-Dazs)	4 fl. oz.	7
Peach (Dole)	½ cup	11
Pineapple (Dole)	½ cup	10
Rainbow (Baskin-Robbins)	4 fl. oz.	85
Raspberry:		
(Baskin-Robbins)	4 fl. oz.	25
(Dole)	½ cup	12
(Häagen-Dazs)	4 fl. oz.	7
(Sealtest)	½ cup	30
Strawberry (Dole)	½ cup	11
SHERBET or SORBET & ICE CREAM (Häagen-Dazs):		
Bar, orange & cream	2.6-fl.-oz. bar	25
Bulk:		
Blueberry & cream, orange & cream or raspberry & cream	4 fl. oz.	35
Key lime & cream	4 fl. oz.	30
SHERBET SHAKE, mix (Weight Watchers) orange	1 envelope	210
SHERRY:		
Regular:		
(Gold Seal) 19% alcohol	3 fl. oz.	3
(Great Western) Solera, 18% alcohol	3 fl. oz.	31
Cocktail (Gold Seal) 19% alcohol	3 fl. oz.	3
Cream:		
(Gold Seal) 19% alcohol (Great Western) Solera, 18% alcohol	3 fl. oz.	32
Dry (Great Western) Solera, 18% alcohol	3 fl. oz.	34
SHORTENING	any quantity	0
SHREDDED WHEAT:		
(USDA):		
Plain, without salt	1 oz.	<1

Food and Description	Measure or Quantity	Sodium (milligrams)
With malt, salt & sugar	1 oz.	198
(Kellogg's) *Squares*:		
Apple cinnamon, blueberry or strawberry	½ cup (1 oz.)	5
Raisin	½ cup (1 oz.)	0
(Nabisco)	Any amount	0
(Quaker)	.7-oz. biscuit	<1
(Sunshine) regular or bite size	Any quantity	0
SHRIMP:		
Raw (USDA):		
Whole	1 lb. (weighed in shell)	438
Meat only	4 oz.	159
Cooked, french fried (USDA) dipped in egg, breadcrumbs and flour or in batter	4 oz.	211
Frozen (Sau-Sea) cooked	5 oz.	330
SHRIMP COCKTAIL (Sau-Sea) canned or frozen	4 oz.	1020
SHRIMP DINNER or ENTREE, frozen:		
(Armour) *Classics Lites*:		
Baby bay	9¾-oz. pkg.	890
Creole	11¼-oz. meal	900
(Gorton's):		
Crunchy, whole	5-oz. serving	870
Scampi	1 pkg.	720
(Healthy Choice):		
Creole	11¼-oz. meal	560
Marinara	10½-oz. meal	320
(La Choy) Fresh & Lite, with lobster sauce	10-oz. meal	946
(Mrs. Paul's):		
Oriental	11-oz. meal	940
Parmesan	11-oz. meal	1185
(Stouffer's) Newburgh	6½-oz. serving	555
SLIMER & THE REAL GHOSTBUSTERS, cereal (Ralston-Purina)	1 cup (1 oz.)	115

Food and Description	Measure or Quantity	Sodium (milligrams)
SLOPPY JOE:		
Canned:		
(Hunt's) *Manwich*	1 sandwich	620
(Libby's) beef	⅓ cup (2½ oz.)	190
(Morton House) barbecue sauce with beef	⅓ of 15-oz. can	919
Frozen (Banquet) *Cookin' Bag*	5-oz. pkg.	730
SLOPPY JOE SAUCE (Ragú)		
Joe Sauce	3½ oz.	645
SLOPPY JOE SEASONING MIX:		
*(Durkee):		
Regular	1¼ cup	1788
Pizza flavor	1¼ cup	1515
(French's)	1½-oz. pkg.	3040
*(Hunt's) *Manwich*	5.9-oz. serving	590
SMOKED SAUSAGE (See **SAUSAGE**)		
SMURF BERRY CRUNCH, cereal (Post)	1 cup (1 oz.)	65
SNACK (See **CRACKERS; POPCORN; POTATO CHIP;** etc.)		
SNACK MIX, *Chex* (Ralston-Purina):		
Barbecue	⅔ cup (1 oz.)	480
Cool sour cream & onion or golden cheddar	⅔ cup (1 oz.)	300
Traditional	⅔ cup (1 oz.)	320
SNAPPER, RED & GRAY, raw (USDA):		
Whole	1 lb. (weighed whole)	158
Meat only	4 oz.	76
SOFT DRINK:		
Sweetened:		
Aspen	6 fl. oz.	5
Birch beer (Canada Dry)	6 fl. oz.	14

Food and Description	Measure or Quantity	Sodium (milligrams)
Bitter lemon:		
(Canada Dry)	6 fl. oz.	13
(Schweppes)	6 fl. oz.	2
Bubble Up	6 fl. oz.	16
Cactus Cooler (Canada Dry)	6 fl. oz.	16
Cherry:		
(Canada Dry) wild	6 fl. oz.	16
(Shasta) black	6 fl. oz.	13
Cherry-Lime (Spree)	6 fl. oz.	1
Chocolate (Yoo-Hoo)	6 fl. oz.	87
Citrus mist (Shasta)	6 fl. oz.	9
Club:		
(Canada Dry)	6 fl. oz.	39
(Schweppes)	6 fl. oz.	25
(Shasta)	6 fl. oz.	23
Cola:		
(Canada Dry) *Jamaica*	6 fl. oz.	Tr.
Coca-Cola:		
Regular or caffeine free	6 fl. oz.	3
Cherry or classic	6 fl. oz.	7
Pepsi-Cola, regular or no caffeine	6 fl. oz.	1
(Royal Crown)	6 fl. oz.	<1
(Shasta) regular or cherry	6 fl. oz.	22
(Slice) cherry	6 fl. oz.	2
(Spree)	6 fl. oz.	Tr.
Cream:		
(Canada Dry)	6 fl. oz.	14
(Shasta)	6 fl. oz.	12
Dr. Diablo	6 fl. oz.	7
Dr. Nehi	6 fl. oz.	13
Dr Pepper	6 fl. oz.	9
Fruit punch:		
(Nehi)	6 fl. oz.	8
(Shasta)	6 fl. oz.	16
Ginger ale:		
(Canada Dry):		
Regular	6 fl. oz.	5

Food and Description	Measure or Quantity	Sodium (milligrams)
Golden	6 fl. oz.	18
(Fanta)	6 fl. oz.	13
(Nehi)	6 fl. oz.	Tr.
(Schweppes)	6 fl. oz.	10
(Shasta)	6 fl. oz.	11
(Spree)	6 fl. oz.	Tr.
Ginger beer (Schweppes)	6 fl. oz.	30
Grape:		
(Canada Dry) concord	6 fl. oz.	16
(Fanta)	6 fl. oz.	7
(Hi-C)	6 fl. oz.	6
(Nehi)	6 fl. oz.	8
(Patio)	6 fl. oz.	21
(Schweppes)	6 fl. oz.	15
(Shasta)	6 fl. oz.	23
Grapefruit:		
(Schwepps)	6 fl. oz.	28
(Spree)	6 fl. oz.	Tr.
Half & half (Canada Dry)	6 fl. oz.	13
Hi Spot (Canada Dry)	6 fl. oz.	19
Island Lime (Canada Dry)	6 fl. oz.	14
Kick (Royal Crown)	6 fl. oz.	25
Lemon (Hi-C)	6 fl. oz.	6
Lemon-lime (Shasta)	6 fl. oz.	9
Lemon sour (Spree)	6 fl. oz.	12
Lemon tangerine (Spree)	6 fl. oz.	Tr.
Mandarin lime (Spree)	6 fl. oz.	Tr.
Mello Yello	6 fl. oz.	13
Mr. PiBB	6 fl. oz.	11
Mt. Dew	6 fl. oz.	16
Orange:		
(Canada Dry) *Sunripe*	6 fl. oz.	16
(Fanta)	6 fl. oz.	7
(Hi-C)	6 fl. oz.	7
(Minute Maid)	6 fl. oz.	Tr.
(Nehi)	6 fl. oz.	11
(Patio)	6 fl. oz.	21
(Schweppes) sparkling	6 fl. oz.	17
(Shasta)	6 fl. oz.	14

Food and Description	Measure or Quantity	Sodium (milligrams)
(Slice)	6 fl. oz.	11
Peach (Nehi)	6 fl. oz.	16
Pineapple (Canada Dry)	6 fl. oz.	16
Punch (Hi-C)	6 fl. oz.	6
Purple Passion (Canada Dry)	6 fl. oz.	14
Quinine or tonic water:		
(Canada Dry)	6 fl. oz.	5
(Schweppes)	6 fl. oz.	8
Red berry (Shasta)	6 fl. oz.	10
Red Pop (Shasta)	6 fl. oz.	10
Root beer:		
Barrelhead (Canada Dry)	6 fl. oz.	13
(Dad's)	6 fl. oz.	14
(Fanta)	6 fl. oz.	10
(Nehi)	6 fl. oz.	9
On Tap	6 fl. oz.	9
(Patio)	6 fl. oz.	2
Ramblin'	6 fl. oz.	10
Rooti (Canada Dry)	6 fl. oz.	13
(Schweppes)	6 fl. oz.	17
(Shasta) draft	6 fl. oz.	15
(Spree)	6 fl. oz.	1
7-UP	6 fl. oz.	10
Slice	6 fl. oz.	5
Sprite	6 fl. oz.	22
Strawberry:		
(Canada Dry)	6 fl. oz.	16
(Nehi) can	6 fl. oz.	7
(Shasta)	6 fl. oz.	23
Tahitian Treat (Canada Dry)	6 fl. oz.	16
Teem	6 fl. oz.	16
Tom Collins or collins mix		
(Canada Dry)	6 fl. oz.	13
Tropical blend (Spree)	6 fl. oz.	1
Upper 10 (Royal Crown)	6 fl. oz.	20
Whiskey sour (Canada Dry)	6 fl. oz.	13
Wink (Canada Dry)	6 fl. oz.	14
Dietetic or low calorie:		
Apple (Slice) .	6 fl. oz.	2

Food and Description	Measure or Quantity	Sodium (milligrams)
Birch beer (Shasta)	6 fl. oz.	17
Blackberry (Schweppes) mid-calorie royal	6 fl. oz.	<5
Bubble Up:		
Diet	6 fl. oz.	16
Sugar free	6 fl. oz.	48
Cherry:		
(Diet Rite)	6 fl. oz.	0
(Shasta) black	6 fl. oz.	20
Chocolate (No-Cal)	6 fl. oz.	33
Coffee (No-Cal)	6 fl. oz.	45
Cola:		
(Canada Dry)	6 fl. oz.	20
Coca-Cola	6 fl. oz.	4
Diet Rite	6 fl. oz.	<1
Pepsi, diet, light or free	6 fl. oz.	2
RC	6 fl. oz.	<1
(Shasta) regular or cherry	6 fl. oz.	18
(Slice) cherry	6 fl. oz.	2
Cream:		
Diet Rite, caramel	6 fl. oz.	<1
(Shasta)	6 fl. oz.	21
Dr. Pepper	6 fl. oz.	Tr.
Fresca	6 fl. oz.	Tr.
Ginger ale:		
(Canada Dry)	6 fl. oz.	22
(Schweppes):		
Regular	6 fl. oz.	39
Raspberry	6 fl. oz.	55
(Shasta)	6 fl. oz.	20
Grape:		
Diet Rite, white	6 fl. oz.	<1
(Shasta)	6 fl. oz.	18
Grapefruit:		
Diet Rite, pink	6 fl. oz.	0
(Shasta)	6 fl. oz.	18
Kiwi-Passionfruit (Schweppes) mid-calorie royal	6 fl. oz.	<5

Food and Description	Measure or Quantity	Sodium (milligrams)
Lemon-lime:		
Diet Rite	6 fl. oz.	0
(Shasta)	6 fl. oz.	23
Orange:		
(Canada Dry)	6 fl. oz.	19
(Minute Maid)	6 fl. oz.	Tr.
(Shasta)	6 fl. oz.	19
(Slice)	6 fl. oz.	11
Peach, *Diet Rite*, golden	6 fl. oz.	0
Peaches 'N Cream (Schweppes) mid-calorie royal	6 fl. oz.	<5
Quinine or tonic water:		
(Canada Dry)	6 fl. oz.	18
(No-Cal)	6 fl. oz.	15
RC 100 (Royal Crown)	6 fl. oz.	19
Root beer:		
Barrelhead (Canada Dry)	6 fl. oz.	19
(Dad's):		
Diet	6 fl. oz.	14
Sugar free	6 fl. oz.	41
(Shasta) draft	6 fl. oz.	18
7-UP	6 fl. oz.	16
Slice	6 fl. oz.	5
Sprite	6 fl. oz.	Tr.
Strawberry (Shasta)	6 fl. oz.	18
Tropical citrus (Schweppes) mid-calorie royal	6 fl. oz.	<5
SOLE:		
Raw (USDA):		
Whole	1 lb. (weighed whole)	117
Meat only	4 oz.	88
Frozen:		
(Frionor) *Norway Gourmet*	4-oz. fillet	350
(Gorton's):		
Fishmarket Fresh	5 oz.	140
Light Recipe, with lemon butter sauce	1 pkg.	730

Food and Description	Measure or Quantity	Sodium (milligrams)
Microwave entree:		
with lemon butter sauce	1 pkg.	380
wine sauce	1 pkg.	770
(Healthy Choice):		
Au gratin	11-oz. dinner	470
With lemon butter sauce	8¼-oz. entree	390
(Mrs. Paul's) fillets, breaded & fried	6-oz. fillet	700
(Van de Kamp's) batter dipped, french fried	2-oz. piece	289
(Weight Watchers) stuffed	10½-oz. pkg.	940
SOUFFLE:		
(USDA) home recipe	4 oz.	413
Frozen (Stouffer's):		
Corn	4 oz.	560
Spinach	4 oz.	500
SOUP:		
Canned, regular pack:		
*Asparagus (Campbell), condensed, cream of	8-oz. serving	900
Bean (Campbell):		
Chunky, with ham, old fashioned	11-oz. can	1150
*Condensed, with bacon	8-oz. serving	860
Bean, black:		
*(Campbell) condensed	8-oz. serving	980
(Crosse & Blackwell)	6½-oz. serving	757
Beef:		
(Campbell):		
Chunky:		
Regular	10¾-oz. can	1110
Stroganoff	10¾-oz. can	1290
*Condensed:		
Regular	8-oz. serving	855
Broth	8-oz. serving	875
Consommé	8-oz. serving	785
Noodle, regular	8-oz. serving	875
(Progresso):		
Regular	10½-oz. can	1590
Regular	½ of 19-oz. can	1440

Food and Description	Measure or Quantity	Sodium (milligrams)
Hearty	½ of 19-oz. can	1210
Noodle	½ of 19-oz. can	1230
Tomato, with rotini	½ of 19-oz. can	1250
Vegetable	10½-oz. can	1260
(Swanson) broth	7¼-oz. can	750
Beef barley (Progresso)	10½-oz. can	1300
*Broccoli (Campbell) *Creamy Natural*, condensed	8-oz. serving	860
*Cauliflower (Campbell) *Creamy Natural*, condensed	8-oz. serving	850
Celery:		
*(Campbell) condensed, cream of	8-oz. serving	860
*(Rokeach):		
Prepared with milk	10-oz. serving	1020
Prepared with water	10-oz. serving	950
*Cheddar cheese (Campbell)	8-oz. serving	800
Chickarina (Progresso)	½ of 19-oz. can	820
Chicken:		
(Campbell):		
Chunky:		
Old fashioned	10¾-oz. can	1340
& rice	19-oz. can	2160
Vegetable	19-oz. can	2200
*Condensed):		
Alphabet	8-oz. serving	870
Broth:		
Plain	8-oz. serving	890
& rice	8-oz. serving	880
Cream of	8-oz. serving	850
Mushroom, creamy	8-oz. serving	940
NoodleOs	8-oz. serving	840
& rice	8-oz. serving	840
Vegetable	8-oz. serving	870
*Semi-condensed, *Soup For One*, vegetable, full flavored	11-oz. serving	1500

Food and Description	Measure or Quantity	Sodium (milligrams)
(Hain):		
Broth	8¾-oz. can	870
Noodle	9½-oz. serving	930
(Progresso):		
Barley	½ of 18½-oz. can	710
Broth	4-oz. serving	360
Cream of	½ of 19-oz. can	760
Hearty	10½-oz. can	960
Hearty	½ of 19-oz. can	900
Homestyle	½ of 19-oz. can	740
Noodle	10½-oz. can	970
Noodle	½ of 19-oz. can	920
Rice	10½-oz. can	940
Rice	½ of 19-oz. can	740
Vegetable	10½-oz. can	790
Vegetable	½ of 19-oz. can	710
(Swanson) broth	7¼-oz. can	910
Chili beef (Campbell) Chunky	11-oz. can	1150
Chowder:		
Clam:		
Manhattan style:		
(Campbell):		
Chunky	19-oz. can	2260
*Condensed	8-oz. serving	860
(Crosse & Blackwell)	6½-oz. serving	803
(Progresso)	½ of 19-oz. can	1050
*(Snow's) condensed	7½-oz. serving	630
New England style:		
*(Campbell):		
Condensed:		
Made with milk	8-oz. serving	930
Made with water	8-oz. serving	880
Semi-condensed,		
Soup For One:		
Made with milk	11-oz. serving	1410
Made with water	11-oz. serving	1360
(Crosse & Blackwell)	6½-oz. serving	637
*(Gorton's)	1 can	2960
(Hain)	9¼-oz. serving	780
(Progresso)	10½-oz. can	1050

Food and Description	Measure or Quantity	Sodium (milligrams)
*(Snow's) condensed	7½-oz. serving	670
*Corn (Snow's) New England, condensed, made with milk	7½-oz. serving	640
*Fish (Snow's) New England, condensed, made with milk	7½-oz. serving	620
*Seafood (Snow's) New England, condensed, made with milk	7½-oz. serving	690
Escarole (Progresso) in chicken broth	½ of 18½-oz. can	1100
*Gazpacho (Campbell) condensed	8-oz. serving	590
Ham'n butter bean (Campbell) *Chunky*	10¾-oz. serving	1180
Italian vegetable pasta (Hain)	9½-oz. serving	910
Lentil:		
(Hain) vegetarian	9½-oz. serving	690
(Progresso):		
Regular	10½-oz. can	1000
Regular	½ of 19-oz. can	840
With sausage	½ of 19-oz. can	940
Macaroni & bean (Progresso)	10½-oz. can	1120
*Meatball alphabet (Campbell) condensed	8-oz. serving	970
Minestrone:		
(Campbell):		
Chunky	19-oz. can	1880
*Condensed	8-oz. serving	930
(Hain)	9½-oz. serving	1060
(Progresso):		
Beef	10½-oz. can	1140
Chicken	10½-oz. can	1060
Hearty	½ of 18½-oz. can	740
Zesty	½ of 19-oz. can	1130
Mushroom:		
*(Campbell), condensed:		
Cream of	8-oz. serving	820
Golden	8-oz. serving	900

Food and Description	Measure or Quantity	Sodium (milligrams)
(Hain) creamy	9¼-oz. serving	740
(Progresso) cream of	½ of 18½-oz. can	1120
*(Rokeach) cream of,		
prepared with water	10-oz. serving	1050
Mushroom barley (Hain)	9½-oz. serving	600
*Noodle (Campbell) &		
ground beef	8-oz. serving	840
*Onion (Campbell):		
Regular	8-oz. serving	950
Cream of:		
Made with water	8-oz. serving	830
Made with water & milk	8-oz. serving	860
*Oyster stew (Campbell):		
Made with milk	8-oz. serving	900
Made with water	8-oz. serving	850
*Pea, green (Campbell)	8-oz. serving	840
Pea, split:		
(Campbell):		
Chunky, with ham	19-oz. can	1900
*Condensed, with ham		
& bacon	8-oz. serving	800
(Hain)	9½-oz. serving	970
(Progresso):		
Regular	10½-oz. can	920
With ham	10½-oz. can	1070
*Pepper pot (Campbell)	8-oz. serving	960
*Potato (Campbell) cream of:		
Made with water	8-oz. serving	930
Made with water & milk	8-oz. serving	960
Shav (Manischewitz)	1 cup	<5
Shrimp:		
*(Campbell) condensed,		
cream of:		
Made with milk	8-oz. serving	850
Made with water	8-oz. serving	790
(Crosse & Blackwell)	6½-oz. serving	1459
Steak & potato (Campbell)		
Chunky	19-oz. can	2220

Food and Description	Measure or Quantity	Sodium (milligrams)
Tomato:		
(Campbell):		
Condensed:		
Regular:		
Made with milk	8-oz. serving	770
Made with water	8-oz. serving	720
& rice, old fashioned	8-oz. serving	760
Semi-condensed, *Soup*		
For One, Royale	11-oz. serving	1080
(Progresso)	½ of 19-oz. can	1100
*(Rokeach), made with		
water	10-oz. serving	980
Tortellini (Progresso):		
Regular	½ of 19-oz. can	840
Creamy	½ of 18½-oz. can	910
Tomato	½ of 18½-oz. can	1040
Turkey (Campbell) *Chunky,*		
& vegetable	18¾-oz. can	2160
Vegetable:		
(Campbell):		
Chunky:		
Regular	19-oz. can	1940
Beef, old fashioned	19-oz. can	2140
*Condensed:		
Regular	8-oz. serving	770
Beef	8-oz. serving	820
*Semi-condensed, *Soup*		
For One, old world	11-oz. serving	1470
(Hain):		
Broth	9½-oz. serving	1180
Chicken	9½-oz. serving	930
Vegetarian	9½-oz. serving	920
(Progresso)	10½-oz. can	1100
*(Rokeach) vegetarian	10-oz. serving	1055
Vichyssoise (Crosse &		
Blackwell)	6½-oz. serving	702
*Won ton (Campbell)	8-oz. serving	870
Canned, dietetic pack:		
Bean (Pritikin) navy	½ of 14¾-oz. can	170

Food and Description	Measure or Quantity	Sodium (milligrams)
Beef (Campbell) *Chunky* & mushroom, low sodium	10¾-oz. can	65
Chicken:		
(Campbell) low sodium:		
Broth	10½-oz. can	70
Chunky	10¾-oz. can	95
(Hain) no added salt:		
Broth	8¾-oz. serving	75
Noodle	9½-oz. serving	90
(Pritikin):		
Broth, defatted	½ of 13¾-oz. can	175
Gumbo	½ of 14¾-oz. can	180
& ribbon pasta or vegetable	½ of 14½-oz. can	175
(Weight Watchers) noodle	10½-oz. can	1230
Chowder (Pritikin) any style	½ of 14¾-oz. can	170
Italian vegetable pasta (Hain) low sodium	9½-oz. serving	90
Lentil:		
(Hain) vegetarian, low sodium	9½-oz. serving	65
(Pritikin)	½ of 14¾-oz. can	170
Minestrone:		
(Estee)	7½-oz. can	45
(Hain)	9½-oz. serving	35
(Pritikin)	½ of 14¾-oz. can	130
Mushroom (Campbell) cream of, low sodium	10½-oz. can	55
Pea, split (Campbell) low sodium	10¾-oz. can	25
Tomato:		
(Campbell) low sodium, with tomato pieces	10½-oz. can	40
(Pritikin)	½ of 14½-oz. can	125
Turkey:		
(Hain) & rice	9½-oz. serving	100
(Pritikin) vegetable, & ribbon pasta	½ of 14¾-oz. can	160

Food and Description	Measure or Quantity	Sodium (milligrams)
(Weight Watchers) vegetable	10½-oz. can	1020
Vegetable:		
(Campbell) *Chunky*	10¾-oz. can	60
(Estee) & beef	7½-oz. can	130
(Pritikin)	½ of 14¾-oz. can	150
Vegetable:		
(Hain):		
Broth	9½-oz. serving	85
Vegetarian	9½-oz. serving	45
(Pritikin)	½ of 14¾-oz. can	150
(Weight Watchers) vegetarian	10½-oz. can	1250
Frozen:		
*Barley & mushroom:		
(Mother's Own)	8-oz. serving	490
(Tabatchnick)	8-oz. serving	759
Bean (Kettle Ready)	8-oz. serving	1606
Bean & barley (Tabatchnick)	8-oz. serving	493
Beef (Kettle Ready) vegetable	8-oz. serving	1034
Broccoli (Tabatchnick) cream of	7½-oz. serving	507
Cauliflower (Kettle Ready) cream of	8-oz. serving	1011
Cheddar cheese (Kettle Ready)	8-oz. serving	994
Chicken (Kettle Ready):		
Cream of	8-oz. serving	1163
Gumbo	8-oz. serving	1097
Noodle	8-oz. serving	1150
Chowder, clam:		
Boston (Kettle Ready)	8-oz. serving	1215
Manhattan (Kettle Ready)	8-oz. serving	847
New England:		
(Kettle Ready)	8-oz. serving	745
(Stouffer's)	8-oz. serving	510
Lentil (Tabatchnick)	8-oz. serving	636
Minestrone:		
(Kettle Ready)	8-oz. serving	1118
(Tabatchnick)	8-oz. serving	561

Food and Description	Measure or Quantity	Sodium (milligrams)
Mushroom (Kettle Ready) cream of	8-oz. serving	950
Onion (Kettle Ready) french	8-oz. serving	1330
Pea, split:		
(Kettle Ready) & ham	8-oz. serving	1043
*(Mother's Own)	8-oz. serving	575
(Stouffer's) & ham	8¼-oz. serving	695
Potato:		
(Kettle Ready) cream of	8-oz. serving	834
(Tabatchnick)	8-oz. serving	607
Spinach, cream of:		
(Kettle Ready)	8-oz. serving	855
(Stouffer's)	8-oz. serving	885
(Tabatchnick)	7½-oz. serving	697
Tomato (Kettle Ready)	8-oz. serving	1940
Vegetable:		
(Kettle Ready):		
Hearty	8-oz. serving	970
Nacho	8-oz. serving	981
*(Mother's Own)	8-oz. serving	560
(Tabatchnick)	8-oz. serving	514
*Won ton (La Choy)	½ of 15-oz. pkg.	1050
Mix:		
*Regular:		
Asparagus (Knorr)	8-fl. oz.	770
Barley (Knorr)	10 fl. oz.	940
Beef (Lipton)		
Cup-A-Soup:		
Regular	6 fl. oz.	746
Lots-A-Noodles	7 fl. oz.	722
Broccoli (Lipton) creamy, Cup-A-Soup:		
Regular	6 fl. oz.	610
Cheese	6 fl. oz.	595
Cauliflower (Knorr)	8 fl. oz.	750
Cheese (Hain) savory	¾ cup	890
Cheese & broccoli (Hain)	¾ cup	980
Chicken:		
(Knorr):		
Noodle	8 fl. oz.	710

Food and Description	Measure or Quantity	Sodium (milligrams)
N'pasta	8 fl. oz.	850
(Lipton):		
Cup-A-Broth	6 fl. oz.	780
Cup-A-Soup:		
Regular:		
Cream of	6 fl. oz.	840
Rice	6 fl. oz.	750
Country, supreme	6 fl. oz.	970
Hearty	8 fl. oz.	695
Lots-A-Noodles,		
regular	7 fl. oz.	755
Chowder, clam (Gorton's)		
New England	¼ of container	740
Herb (Knorr) fine	8 fl. oz.	990
Hot & sour (Knorr)		
oriental	8 fl. oz.	690
Leek (Knorr)	8 fl. oz.	800
Lentil (Hain) savory	¾ cup	810
Minestrone:		
(Hain) savory	¾ cup	870
(Knorr) hearty	10 fl. oz.	940
(Manischewitz)	6 fl. oz.	160
Mushroom:		
(Hain)	¾ cup	710
(Knorr)	8 fl. oz.	870
(Lipton):		
Regular:		
Beef	8 fl. oz.	995
Onion	8 fl. oz.	990
Cup-A-Soup, cream of	6 fl. oz.	830
Noodle (4C)	8 fl. oz.	960
Onion:		
(Hain) savory	¾ cup	900
(Knorr) french	8 fl. oz	970
(Lipton):		
Regular:		
Plain	8 fl. oz.	648
Beefy	8 fl. oz.	950
Cup-A-Soup	6 fl. oz.	870

Food and Description	Measure or Quantity	Sodium (milligrams)
Oxtail (Knorr) hearty beef	8 fl. oz.	1120
Pea, split:		
(Hain)	¾ cup	940
(Manischewitz)	6 fl. oz.	320
Potato leek (Hain) savory	¾ cup	690
Tomato:		
(Hain)	¾ cup	770
(Knorr) basil	8 fl. oz.	940
(Lipton) *Cup-A-Soup*, regular	6 fl. oz.	650
Tortellini (Knorr) in brodo	8 fl. oz.	820
Vegetable:		
(Hain) savory	¾ cup	730
(Knorr):		
Plain	8 fl. oz.	840
Spring, with herbs	8 fl. oz.	710
(Lipton):		
Regular, country	8 fl. oz.	995
Cup-A-Soup, beef	6 fl. oz	820
(Manischewitz)	6 fl. oz.	65
Dietetic:		
Beef:		
*(Estee) noodle	6 fl. oz.	140
(Weight Watchers) broth	1 packet	930
*Broccoli (Lipton) *Cup-A-Soup*, golden, lite	6 fl. oz.	427
Chicken:		
*(Estee) noodle	6 fl. oz.	135
(Weight Watchers) broth	1 packet	990
*Mushroom:		
(Estee) cream of	6 fl. oz.	115
(Hain) savory, low sodium	¾ cup	180
*Onion:		
(Estee)	6 fl. oz.	120
(4C) reduced salt	8 fl. oz.	760

Food and Description	Measure or Quantity	Sodium (milligrams)
(Hain) savory, low sodium	¾ cup	470
*Tomato (Estee)	6 fl. oz.	95
SOUP GREENS, canned (Durkee)	2½-oz. jar	408
SOURSOP, raw (USDA):		
Whole	1 lb. (weighed with skin & seeds)	43
Flesh only	4 oz.	16
SOYBEAN: (USDA):		
Young seeds, canned:		
Solids & liq.	4 oz.	268
Drained solids	4 oz.	268
Mature seeds:		
Raw	1 lb.	23
Raw	1 cup (7.4 oz.)	10
Cooked	4 oz.	2
Oil roasted:		
(Soy Ahoy) regular, barbecue or garlic	1 oz.	6
(Soytown)	1 oz.	6
SOYBEAN CURD or TOFU (USDA):		
Regular	4 oz.	8
Cake	4.2-oz. cake	8
SOYBEAN FLOUR (See **FLOUR**)		
SOYBEAN GRITS, high fat (USDA)	1 cup (4.9 oz.)	1
SOYBEAN PROTEIN (USDA)	1 oz.	60
SOYBEAN PROTEINATE (USDA)	1 oz.	340
SOYBEAN SPROUT (See **BEAN SPROUT**)		
SOY SAUCE (See **SAUCE,** Soy)		
SPAGHETTI.		
The longer the cooking, the more water is		

Food and Description	Measure or Quantity	Sodium (milligrams)
absorbed and this affects the nutritive value).		
Dry (USDA):		
Whole	1 oz.	<1
Broken	1 cup (2.5 oz.)	1
Cooked:		
8–10 minutes, "al dente"	1 cup (5.1 oz.)	1
8–10 minutes, "al dente"	4 oz.	1
14–20 minutes, tender	1 cup (4.9 oz.)	1
14–20 minutes, tender	4 oz.	1
Canned, regular pack:		
(Franco-American):		
Regular:		
With meatballs in tomato sauce	7⅜-oz. can	820
In meat sauce	7½-oz. serving	1110
In tomato sauce with cheese	7⅜-oz. serving	810
SpaghettiOs:		
With meatballs in tomato sauce	7⅜-oz. serving	910
With sliced franks in tomato sauce	7⅜-oz. serving	990
In tomato & cheese sauce	7⅜-oz. serving	910
(Hormel) & beef, *Short Orders,*	7½-oz. can	1091
(Libby's) & meatballs in tomato sauce	7½-oz. serving	1359
Canned, dietetic pack (Dia-Mel) & meatballs in tomato sauce	8-oz. can	55
Frozen:		
(Armour) *Dining Lite*, with beef	9-oz. meal	440
(Banquet) with meat sauce	8-oz. casserole	1250
(Healthy Choice)	10-oz. meal	480
(Kid Cuisine)	9¼-oz. meal	690
(Morton) dinner	10-oz. dinner	1090

Food and Description	Measure or Quantity	Sodium (milligrams)
(Stouffer's):		
Regular, & meat sauce	12⅝-oz. meal	1510
Lean Cuisine, with beef &		
mushroom sauce	11½-oz. meal	940
(Swanson) entree, in tomato		
sauce with breaded veal	8¼-oz. entree	810
(Weight Watchers) with		
meat sauce	10½-oz. meal	910
SPAGHETTI SAUCE (See also		
PASTA & SAUCE;		
SPAGHETTI SAUCE MIX):		
Regular:		
Alfredo (Progresso)		
authentic pasta sauce:		
Regular	½ cup	1080
Seafood	½ cup	360
Bolognese (Progresso)		
authentic pasta sauce	½ cup	520
Chunky (Hunt's)	4 oz.	470
Clam (Progresso):		
Red	½ cup	560
White:		
Regular	½ cup	280
Authentic pasta sauce	½ cup	460
Garden style (Ragú)		
chunky	¼ of 15½-oz. jar	400
Home style (Ragú)	4 oz.	400
Lobster (Progresso) rock	½ cup	430
Marinara:		
(Prince)	4 oz.	590
(Progresso):		
Regular	½ cup	520
Authentic pasta sauce	½ cup	250
(Ragú)	4 oz.	740
Meat flavored:		
(Hunt's)	4 oz.	570
(Prego)	4 oz.	680
(Progresso)	½ cup	660
(Ragú)	4 oz.	740

Food and Description	Measure or Quantity	Sodium (milligrams)
Meatless or plain:		
(Prego)	4 oz.	670
(Progresso)	½ cup	660
(Ragú)	4 oz.	740
Mushroom:		
(Hunt's) regular	4 oz.	560
(Prego)	4 oz.	640
(Prince)	4 oz.	580
(Progresso)	½ cup	630
(Ragú)	4 oz.	740
Primavera (Progresso) creamy	½ cup	410
Romano (Progresso) creamy	½ cup	490
Sausage & green peppers (Prego Plus)	4 oz.	480
Seafood (Progresso):		
Regular	½ cup	445
Authentic pasta sauce	½ cup	570
Sicilian (Progresso)	½ cup	660
Traditional (Hunt's)	4 oz.	530
Veal (Prego Plus) & sliced mushrooms	4 oz.	380
Dietetic:		
(Estee)	4 oz.	30
(Furman's)	½ cup	<10
(Prego) no salt added	4 oz.	25
(Pritikin) plain or mushroom	4 oz.	35
(Weight Watchers):		
Meat flavored	⅓ cup	440
Mushroom flavored	⅓ cup	430
*SPAGHETTI SAUCE MIX		
(Lawry's):		
With imported mushrooms	1.5-oz. pkg.	2015
Rich & thick	1.5-oz. pkg.	2172
SPAM (Hormel):		
Regular	1-oz. serving	432
& cheese chunks	1-oz. serving	405
Deviled	1 T.	125
Smoke flavored	1 oz.	387

Food and Description	Measure or Quantity	Sodium (milligrams)
SPANISH MACKEREL, raw (USDA):		
Whole	1 lb.	188
Meat only	4 oz.	77
SPECIAL K, cereal (Kellogg's)	1 cup (1 oz.)	230
SPINACH:		
Raw (USDA):		
Untrimmed	1 lb. (weighed with stems & roots)	232
Trimmed or packaged	1 lb.	322
Trimmed, whole leaves	1 cup (1.2 oz.)	23
Trimmed, chopped	1 cup (1.8 oz.)	37
Boiled (USDA) whole leaves, drained	1 cup (5.5 oz.)	78
Canned, regular pack: (USDA):		
Solids & liq.	½ cup (4.1 oz.)	274
Drained solids	½ cup	264
(Del Monte) solids & liq.	½ cup (4.1 oz.)	355
(Larsen) *Freshlike,* solids & liq.	½ cup	340
(Sunshine) whole leaf, solids & liq.	½ cup (4.1 oz.)	300
Canned, dietetic or low calorie: (USDA) low sodium:		
Solids & liq.	4 oz.	39
Drained solids	4 oz.	36
(Del Monte) no salt added	½ cup	57
(Larsen) *Fresh-Lite,* no salt added	½ cup	20
Frozen:		
(USDA) chopped, boiled, drained	4 oz.	59
(Birds Eye):		
Chopped or leaf	⅓ of 10-oz. pkg.	82
Creamed	⅓ of 9-oz. pkg.	277
& water chestnuts, with selected seasonings	⅓ of 10-oz. pkg.	239
(Green Giant):		
In butter sauce	5 oz.	380

Food and Description	Measure or Quantity	Sodium (milligrams)
Creamed	3.3 oz.	425
Harvest Fresh	4½ oz.	250
Polybag	½ cup	100
(Stouffer's) creamed	4½ oz.	380
SQUASH, SUMMER:		
Fresh (USDA):		
Crookneck & straightneck, yellow:		
Whole	1 lb. (weighed untrimmed)	4
Boiled, drained:		
Diced	½ cup (3.6 oz.)	1
Slices	½ cup (3.1 oz.)	<1
Scallop, white & pale green:		
Whole	1 lb. (weighed untrimmed)	4
Boiled, drained, mashed	½ cup (4.2 oz.)	1
Zucchini & cocazelle, green:		
Whole	1 lb. (weighed untrimmed)	4
Boiled, drained slices	½ cup (2.7 oz.)	<1
Canned (Progresso) zucchini, Italian style	½ cup (4.2 oz.)	540
Frozen:		
(USDA):		
Unthawed	4 oz.	3
Boiled, drained	4 oz.	3
(Birds Eye):		
Sliced	⅓ of 10-oz. pkg.	2
Zucchini	⅓ of 10-oz. pkg.	3
(Larsen)	3.3 oz.	0
(McKenzie)	3.3 oz.	19
(Mrs. Paul's) zucchini sticks, batter fried	⅓ of 9-oz. pkg.	630
(Ore-Ida) zucchini, breaded	3 oz.	445
(Southland) Crookneck	⅕ of 16-oz. pkg.	0
SQUASH, WINTER:		
Fresh (USDA):		
Acorn:		

Food and Description	Measure or Quantity	Sodium (milligrams)
Whole	1 lb. (weighed with skin & seeds)	3
Baked, flesh only, mashed	½ cup (3.6 oz.)	1
Boiled, mashed	½ cup (4.1 oz.)	1
Butternut:		
Whole	1 lb. (weighed with skin & seeds)	3
Baked, flesh only	4 oz.	1
Boiled, flesh only	4 oz.	1
Hubbard:		
Whole	1 lb. (weighed with skin & seeds)	3
Baked, flesh only	4 oz.	1
Boiled, flesh only, diced	½ cup (4.2 oz.)	1
Boiled, flesh only, mashed	½ cup (4.3 oz.)	1
Frozen:		
(USDA) heated	½ cup (4.2 oz.)	1
(Birds Eye)	⅓ of pkg.	2
(Southland) butternut	⅕ of 20-oz. pkg.	0
*START, instant breakfast drink	½ cup	7
STEAK & GREEN PEPPERS, frozen (Swanson) in oriental-style sauce	8½-oz. entree	1111
STIR-FRY SEASONING MIX (Kikkoman)	1-oz. pkg.	3
STOCK BASE (French's):		
Beef	1 tsp. (4 g.)	470
Chicken	1 tsp. (3.2 g.)	480
STRAINED FOOD (See BABY FOOD)		
STRAWBERRY:		
Fresh (USDA):		
Whole	1 lb. (weighed with caps & stems)	4
Whole, capped	1 cup (5.1 oz.)	1

Food and Description	Measure or Quantity	Sodium (milligrams)
Canned (USDA) unsweetened or low calorie, water pack, solids & liq.	4 oz.	1
Frozen (Birds Eye):		
Halves	⅓ of 16-oz. pkg.	1
Whole	¼ of 16-oz. pkg.	<1
Whole, quick thaw, in lite syrup	½ of 10-oz. pkg.	5
STRAWBERRY JELLY, sweetened (Home Brands)	1 T.	7
STRAWBERRY NECTAR, canned (Libby's)	6 fl. oz.	5
STRAWBERRY PRESERVES or JAM:		
Sweetened (Smucker's)	1 T.	0
Dietetic or low calorie:		
(Dia-Mel)	1 T.	<3
(Diet Delight)	1 T.	30
(Estee)	1 T. (.6 oz.)	Tr.
(Featherweight)	1 T.	40–50
(Louis Sherry) wild	1 T.	<3
STRAWBERRY SHORTCAKE, cereal (General Mills)	1 cup	190
STUFFING MIX:		
*Beef (Stove Top)	½ cup	582
Chicken:		
*(Bell's)	½ cup	660
(Pepperidge Farm) pan style	1 oz.	420
Cube (Pepperidge Farm) regular or unseasoned	1 oz.	430
Herb seasoned (Pepperidge Farm)	1 oz.	410
*New England style (Stove Top)	½ cup	636
*Pork (Stove Top)	½ cup	621
*With rice (Stove Top)	½ cup	505
*San Francisco style (Stove Top)	½ cup	638
*Turkey (Stove Top)	½ cup	634
White bread (Mrs. Cubbison's)	1 oz.	480

Food and Description	Measure or Quantity	Sodium (milligrams)
STURGEON (USDA) steamed	4 oz.	122
SUCCOTASH:		
Canned solids & liq.:		
(Comstock):		
Cream style	½ cup	350
Whole kernel	½ cup	500
(Larsen) *Freshlike*	½ cup (4.5 oz.)	330
(Libby's):		
Cream style	½ cup (4.6 oz.)	317
Whole kernel	¼ of 16-oz. can	262
(Stokely-Van Camp)	½ cup (4.5 oz.)	275
Frozen:		
(USDA) boiled, drained	½ cup (3.4 oz.)	36
(Birds Eye)	⅓ of 10-oz. pkg.	33
(Frosty Acres)	3.3 oz.	47
SUCKER, including **WHITE MULLET** (USDA) raw:		
Whole	1 lb. (weighed whole)	109
Meat only	4 oz.	64
SUDDENLY SALAD (Betty Crocker):		
Caesar or tortellini Italiano	⅙ of pkg.	450
Classic pasta	⅙ of pkg.	530
Creamy macaroni	⅙ of pkg.	280
Italian pasta	⅙ of pkg.	380
Pasta primavera	⅙ of pkg.	340
Ranch & bacon	⅙ of pkg.	320
SUGAR, beet or cane (USDA):		
Brown:		
Regular	1 lb.	136
Brownulated	1 cup (5.4 oz.)	46
Firm-packed	1 cup (7.5 oz.)	64
Firm-packed	1 T. (.5 oz.)	4
Confectioners':		
Unsifted	1 cup (4.3 oz.)	1
Unsifted	1 T. (8 g.)	<1
Sifted	1 cup (3.4 oz.)	<1

Food and Description	Measure or Quantity	Sodium (milligrams)
Sifted	1 T. (6 g.)	<1
Stirred	1 cup (4.2 oz.)	1
Stirred	1 T. (8 g.)	<1
Granulated	1 lb.	5
Granulated	1 cup (6.9 oz.)	2
Granulated	1 T. (.4 oz.)	<1
Granulated	1 lump (1⅛" × ¾" × ⅜", 6 g.)	<1
Maple	1 lb.	64
Maple	1¾" × 1¼" × ½" piece (1.2 oz.)	4
SUGAR, SUBSTITUTE:		
(Estee)	1 tsp.	0
Sprinkle Sweet (Pillsbury)	1 tsp.	1
Spoon for Spoon	1 tsp.	0
Sweet 'N Low:		
Brown	1 tsp.	19
Granulated	1-g. packet	3
Liquid	1 drop	0
Sweet*10 (Pillsbury)	⅛ tsp.	2
(Weight Watchers) Sweet'ner	1-g. packet	30
SUGAR APPLE, raw (USDA):		
Whole	1 lb. (weighed with skin & seeds)	22
Flesh only	4 oz.	12
SUGAR PUFFS, cereal (Malt-O-Meal)	⅞ cup (1 oz.)	23
***SUKIYAKI DINNER,** canned:		
(Chun King) stir fry	6 oz.	405
(La Choy) bi-pack	¾ cup	990
SUNFLAKES MULTI-GRAIN, cereal (Ralston-Purina)	1 cup (1 oz.)	240
SUNFLOWER SEED:		
(USDA):		
In hulls	4 oz. (weighed in hull)	18
Hulled	1 oz.	9

Food and Description	Measure or Quantity	Sodium (milligrams)
(Fisher):		
In hull, roasted, salted	1 oz.	58
Hulled, roasted:		
Dry, salted	1 oz.	160
Oil, salted	1 oz.	180
(Frito-Lay's)	1 oz.	171
(Planters):		
Dry roasted	1 oz.	260
Unsalted	1 oz.	Tr.
SUNSHINE PUNCH DRINK,		
canned, *Ssips* (Johanna Farms)	8.45-fl.-oz. container	10
SUNTOPS (Dole)	1 bar	5
SURIMI, *Crab Delights* (Louis Kemp) chunks, flakes or legs	2 oz.	550
SWEETBREADS (USDA) beef:		
Raw	1 lb.	435
Braised	4 oz.	132
SWEET POTATO:		
Raw (USDA):		
All kinds, unpared	1 lb. (weighed whole)	37
All kinds, pared	4 oz.	11
Firm-fleshed, Jersey types, pared	4 oz.	11
Soft-fleshed, Puerto Rico variety, pared	4 oz.	11
Baked (USDA) peeled after baking	3.9-oz. sweet potato (5″ × 2″)	13
Baked (USDA) peeled after boiling	5-oz. sweet potato (5″ × 2″)	15
Candied (USDA) home recipe	6.2-oz. sweet potato (3½″ × 2¼″)	74
Canned, regular pack:		
(USDA):		
In syrup, solids & liq.	4 oz.	54

Food and Description	Measure or Quantity	Sodium (milligrams)
Vacuum or solid pack	4 oz.	52
(Joan of Arc):		
Mashed	½ cup (4 oz.)	45
Whole:		
Candied	½ cup (5.2 oz.)	15
Heavy syrup	½ cup (4½ oz.)	35
Light syrup	½ cup (4 oz.)	25
In pineapple-orange sauce	½ cup (5 oz.)	35
Canned, dietetic or low calorie, without added sugar & salt (USDA)	4 oz.	14
Dehydrated flakes (USDA):		
Dry	½ cup (2 oz.)	105
*Prepared with water	½ cup (4.4 oz.)	57
Frozen (Mrs. Paul's) regular	⅓ of 12-oz. pkg.	105
SWEET POTATO PIE (USDA) home recipe, made with lard	⅙ of 9″ pie (5.4 oz.)	331
SWEET & SOUR CHICKEN (La Choy):		
*Canned	¾ cup	440
Frozen	12-oz. entree	2010
***SWEET & SOUR COCKTAIL MIX** (Holland House) liquid	1 fl. oz.	107
SWEET & SOUR ORIENTAL, canned (La Choy):		
With chicken	½ of 15-oz. can	1420
With pork	½ of 15-oz. can	1540
SWEET & SOUR PORK, frozen (La Choy)	12-oz. entree	2200
SWISS STEAK, frozen (Swanson)	10-oz. dinner	830
SYRUP:		
Sweetened:		
Blackberry (Smucker's)	1 T.	<10
Blueberry (Smucker's)	1 T.	<10
Boysenberry (Smucker's)	1 T.	<10
Chocolate:		
(USDA):		
Fudge type	1 T. (.7 oz.)	17

Food and Description	Measure or Quantity	Sodium (milligrams)
Thin type	1 T. (.7 oz.)	10
(Hersey's)	1 T. (.7 oz.)	10
(Nestlé) *Quik*	1 T. (.7 oz.)	35
Corn:		
(USDA) light & dark blend	1 T. (.7 oz.)	14
Karo:		
Dark	1 T. (.7 oz.)	40
Light	1 T. (.7 oz.)	30
Maple:		
(USDA)	1 T. (.7 oz.)	2
(Home Brands)	1 T.	13
Karo, imitation	1 T. (.7 oz.)	32
Pancake & waffle:		
(USDA) cane & maple	1 T. (.7 oz.)	<1
Golden Griddle	1 T. (.7 oz.)	15
Karo	1 T. (.7 oz.)	35
Log Cabin:		
Regular	1 T. (.7 oz.)	6
Buttered	1 T. (.7 oz.)	38
Country kitchen	1 T. (.7 oz.)	15
Mrs. Butterworth's	1 T. (.7 oz.)	24
Raspberry (Smucker's) red	1 T. (.7 oz.)	<10
Strawberry (Smucker's)	1 T. (.6 oz.)	<10
Dietetic or low calorie:		
Blueberry (Estee)	1 T.	25
Chocolate (Estee)	1 T. (.5 oz.)	5
Maple (Cary's)	1 T.	15
Pancake or waffle:		
(Estee)	1 T.	35
Log Cabin, lite	1 T.	64
Mrs. Butterworth's	1 T.	32
(Weight Watchers)	1 T.	25

Food and Description	Measure or Quantity	Sodium (milligrams)

T

*TACO (Ortega)	1 oz.	104
TACO FILLING, canned (Old El Paso)	1 T.	60
TACO SEASONING MIX:		
(Lawry's)	1 pkg.	1441
(French's)	1¼-oz. pkg.	2190
(Old El Paso)	1 pkg.	3569
TACO SHELL:		
(Gebhardt)	.4-oz. shell	0
(Old El Paso)	.4-oz. shell	50
(Ortega)	.4-oz. shell	55
(Rosarita)	.4-oz. shell	0
TACO BELL RESTAURANT:		
Burrito:		
Bean:		
Green sauce	6¾-oz. serving	763
Red sauce	6¾-oz. serving	888
Beef:		
Green sauce	6¾-oz. serving	926
Red sauce	6¾-oz. serving	1051
Supreme:		
Regular:		
Green sauce	8½-oz. serving	796
Red sauce	8½-oz. serving	921
Double beef:		
Green sauce	9-oz. serving	928
Red sauce	9-oz. serving	1053
Crispas, cinnamon	1.7-oz. serving	127
Enchirito:		
Green sauce	7½-oz. serving	993

Food and Description	Measure or Quantity	Sodium (milligrams)
Red sauce	7½-oz. serving	1242
Fajita:		
Chicken	4¾-oz. serving	619
Steak	4¾-oz. serving	485
Guacamole	¾-oz. serving	113
Meximelt	3¾-oz. serving	689
Nachos:		
Regular	3¾-oz. serving	399
Bellgrande	10.1-oz. serving	997
Pepper, jalapeño	3½-oz. serving	1370
Pico De Gallo	1 oz.	88
Pintos & cheese:		
Green sauce	4½-oz. serving	517
Red sauce	4½-oz. serving	642
Pizza, Mexican	7.9-oz. pizza	1031
Salad dressing, ranch	2.6-oz. serving	571
Salsa	.3-oz. serving	376
Taco:		
Regular	2¾-oz. serving	276
Bellgrande	5¾-oz. serving	472
Light	6-oz. serving	594
Soft:		
Regular	3¼-oz. serving	516
Supreme	4.4 oz. serving	516
Super combo	5-oz. serving	462
Taco salad:		
Without shell	18.7-oz. serving	1056
With salsa:		
Regular	21-oz. serving	1662
Without shell	18.7-oz. serving	1431
Taco sauce:		
Regular	.4-oz. packet	126
Hot	.4-oz. packet	82
Tostada:		
Green sauce	5½-oz. serving	471
Red sauce	5½-oz. serving	596
TACO JOHN'S RESTAURANT:		
Burrito:		
Bean	5-oz. serving	626

Food and Description	Measure or Quantity	Sodium (milligrams)
Beef	5-oz. serving	666
Chicken:		
Regular	5-oz. serving	639
With green chili	12¼-oz. serving	986
Combo	5-oz. serving	651
Smothered:		
With green chili	12¼-oz. serving	998
With Texas chili	12¼-oz. serving	1217
Super:		
Regular	8¼-oz. serving	856
With chicken	8¼-oz. serving	844
Chimichanga:		
Regular	12-oz. serving	1246
With chicken	12-oz. serving	1234
Mexican rice	8-oz. serving	1280
Nachos:		
Regular	5-oz. serving	444
Super	11¼-oz. serving	994
Potato Ole	6-oz. large order	1595
Taco:		
Regular	4¼-oz. serving	348
With chicken	4¼-oz. serving	334
Soft shell:		
Regular	5-oz. serving	506
With chicken	5-oz. serving	490
Taco Bravo:		
Regular	6¾-oz. serving	658
Super	8-oz. serving	826
Taco burger	6-oz. serving	660
Taco salad:		
Regular:		
Without dressing	6-oz. serving	440
With 2 oz. dressing	8-oz. serving	790
Chicken:		
Without dressing	12¼-oz. serving	882
With 2 oz. dressing	14¼-oz. serving	1232
Super:		
Without dressing	12¼-oz. serving	900
With 2 oz. dressing	14¼-oz. serving	1250

Food and Description	Measure or Quantity	Sodium (milligrams)
TAMALE:		
Canned:		
(Hormel) beef:		
Regular:		
Plain	1 tamale	275
Hot & spicy	1 tamale	306
Short Orders	7½-oz. can	1140
(Old El Paso)	1 tamale	190
(Pride of Mexico)	2-oz. tamale	310
Frozen (Patio)	13-oz. dinner	1850
TAMARIND, fresh (USDA):		
Whole	1 lb. (weighed with pods & seeds)	111
Flesh only	4 oz.	58
***TANG**, instant breakfast drink:		
Canned, *Fruit Box*:		
Cherry, grape or mixed fruit	8.45-fl.-oz. container	2
Orange:		
Regular	8.45-fl.-oz. container	1
Tropical	8.45-fl.-oz. container	3
*Mix:		
Sweetened	6 fl. oz.	1
Dietitic	6 fl. oz.	2
TANGERINE or MANDARIN ORANGE:		
Fresh (USDA):		
Whole	1 lb. (weighed with peel)	7
Whole tangerine	4.1 oz. (2⅜″ dia.)	2
Sections (without membranes)	1 cup (6.8 oz.)	4
Canned, regular pack (Del Monte) solids & liq.	5½ oz.	<10
Canned, dietetic or low calorie, solids & liq.:		
(Diet Delight) juice pack	¼ of 22-oz. can	9
	½ cup (4.3 oz.)	5

Food and Description	Measure or Quantity	Sodium (milligrams)
(Featherweight) water pack	½ cup	<10
TANGERINE DRINK, canned (Hi-C)	6 fl. oz.	<1
TANGERINE JUICE:		
Fresh (USDA)	½ cup (4.4 oz.)	1
Canned (USDA):		
Unsweetened	½ cup (4.4 oz.)	1
Sweetened	½ cup (4.4 oz.)	1
*Frozen:		
(USDA)	½ cup (4.4 oz.)	1
(Minute Maid) sweetened	6 fl. oz.	19
TAPIOCA, dry, quick cooking, granulated:		
(USDA)	1 cup (5.4 oz.)	5
(USDA)	1 T. (10 g.)	<1
(Minute)	1 T.	<1
TAQUITO, BEEF, frozen (Van de Kamp's) shredded	8 oz.	990
TARO, raw (USDA):		
Tubers, whole	1 lb. (weighed with skin)	27
Tubers, skin removed	4 oz.	8
TARRAGON (French's)	1 tsp.	1
TASTEEOS, cereal (Ralston-Purina)	1¼ cups (1 oz.)	210
TEA (See also **TEA, ICED):**		
Bag:		
(Celestial Seasonings):		
After dinner:		
Amaretto Nights, Cinnamon Vienna or *Swiss Mint*	1 bag	<1
Bavarian Chocolate Orange		
Caffeine free	1 bag	5
Fruit & tea	1 bag	<1
Herb:		
Almond Sunset, Emperor's Choice, Mandarin Orange		

Food and Description	Measure or Quantity	Sodium (milligrams)
Spice, *Red Zinger* or *Sleepy Time*	1 bag	2
Chamomile	1 bag	5
Cranberry Cove or Spearmint	1 bag	6
Mellow Mint, Mo's 24 or *Roastaroma*	1 bag	4
Premium black tea, any flavor	1 bag	<1
(Lipton)	1 bag	0
(Tender Leaf)	1 bag	0
*Nestea	1 tsp.	0
(Tender Leaf)	1 tsp.	Tr.
TEA, ICED:		
Canned, sweetened (Lipton) lemon flavored	6 fl. oz.	20
*Mix:		
Pre-sweetened, lemon flavored:		
Country Time	8 fl. oz.	Tr.
(Lipton)	8 fl. oz.	Tr.
Nestea	8 fl. oz.	<10
Unsweetened, dietetic or low calorie:		
(Crystal Light)	8 fl. oz.	<1
(Lipton) lemon flavored	1 cup (8 fl. oz.)	0
Nestea:		
Plain, sugar free	6 fl. oz.	0
Lemon flavored	8 fl. oz.	0
TEENAGE MUTANT NINJA TURTLES, cereal (Ralston-Purina)	1 cup (1 oz.)	190
TERIYAKI, frozen:		
(Chun King) beef	13-oz. entree	2200
(Stouffer's) beef	10-oz. meal	1450
TERIYAKI MARINADE & SAUCE (La Choy)	1 oz.	1640
***TEXTURED VEGETABLE PROTEIN** (Morningstar Farms):		
Breakfast links	¾-oz. link	225

Food and Description	Measure or Quantity	Sodium (milligrams)
Breakfast patties	1.3-oz. pattie	470
Breakfast strips	.3-oz. strip	124
Grillers, hamburger-like patties	2.1-oz. pattie	334
THURINGER, sausage:		
(Eckrich):		
Sliced	1-oz. slice	380
Smoky Tang	1 oz.	350
(Hormel):		
Packaged, sliced	1 slice	353
Whole:		
Regular	1 oz.	332
Beefy	1 oz.	313
Old Smokehouse	1 oz.	328
Tangy, chub	1 oz.	317
(Ohse):		
Regular	1 oz.	340
Beef	1 oz.	330
(Oscar Mayer) summer sausage:		
Regular	.8-oz. slice	269
Beef	.8-oz. slice	331
THYME, dried (French's)	1 tsp.	1
TIGER TAIL (Hostess)	2¼-oz. piece	249
TOASTER CAKE or PASTRY:		
Pop-Tarts (Kellogg's):		
Regular:		
Blueberry	1 piece (1.83 oz.)	210
Brown sugar cinnamon	1 piece (1¾ oz.)	200
Cherry	1 piece (1.83 oz.)	220
Strawberry	1 piece (1.83 oz.)	200
Frosted:		
Blueberry or raspberry	1 piece (1.83 oz.)	210
Brown sugar cinnamon	1 piece (1¾ oz.)	190
Cherry	1 piece (1.83 oz.)	220
Chocolate fudge	1 piece (1.83 oz.)	230
Chocolate-vanilla creme	1 piece (1.83 oz.)	220
Concord grape or Dutch apple	1 piece (1.83 oz.)	200

Food and Description	Measure or Quantity	Sodium (milligrams)
Toastettes (Nabisco)		
Regular:		
Apple	1 piece	170
Blueberry, cherry or strawberry	1 piece	200
Frosted:		
Brown sugar cinnamon	1 piece	170
Fudge	1 piece	220
Strawberry	1 piece	200
Toast-r-Cake (Thomas'):		
Blueberry	1.2-oz. piece	158
Bran	1.2-oz. piece	163
Corn	1.2-oz. piece	142
TOASTY O's, cereal (Malt-O-Meal) regular	1¼ cups (1 oz.)	236
TODDLER BABY FOOD (See **BABY FOOD**)		
TOFU (See **SOYBEAN CURD**)		
TOFUTTI:		
Frozen:		
Regular:		
Chocolate supreme	4 fl. oz.	130
Maple walnut or vanilla almond bark	4 fl. oz.	95
Vanilla	4 fl. oz.	90
Wildberry supreme	4 fl. oz.	100
Cuties:		
Chocolate	1 piece	130
Vanilla	1 piece	110
Lite Lite	4 fl. oz.	80
Love Drops:		
Cappuccino	4 fl. oz.	120
Chocolate vanilla	4 fl. oz.	100
Soft-serve:		
Regular	4 fl. oz.	65
Hi-Lite	4 fl. oz.	75

Food and Description	Measure or Quantity	Sodium (milligrams)
TOMATO:		
Fresh (USDA):		
Green:		
Whole, untrimmed	1 lb. (weighed with core & stem end)	12
Trimmed, unpeeled	4 oz.	3
Ripe:		
Whole:		
Eaten with skin	1 lb.	14
Peeled	1 lb. (weighed with skin, stem ends & hard core)	12
Peeled	1 med. (2″ × 2½″, 5.3 oz.)	4
Peeled	1 small (1¾″ × 2½″, 3.9 oz.)	3
Sliced, peeled	½ cup (3.2 oz.)	3
Boiled (USDA)	½ cup (4.3 oz.)	5
Canned, regular pack:		
(USDA) whole, solids & liq.	½ cup (4.2 oz.)	155
(Contadina):		
Sliced, baby	4 oz.	465
Stewed	4 oz.	405
Whole, round & pear	1 cup	390
(Del Monte) solids & liq.:		
Stewed	½ cup (4 oz.)	355
Wedges	½ cup (4 oz.)	355
Whole, peeled	½ cup (4 oz.)	220
(Hunt's):		
Crushed Italian	4 oz.	460
Cut, choice, peeled	4 oz.	460
Pear shaped, Italian	4 oz.	320
Stewed:		
Regular	4 oz.	400
Italian	4 oz.	370

Food and Description	Measure or Quantity	Sodium (milligrams)
Whole:		
Regular	4 oz.	330
Italian	4 oz.	420
(La Victoria) green, whole	1 T.	102
(Libby's)		
Stewed	½ of 16-oz. can	567
Whole, peeled, solids & liq.	½ of 16-oz. can	386
(Stokely-Van Camp) solids & liq.:		
Stewed	½ cup (4.2 oz.)	223
Whole	½ cup (4.3 oz.)	190
Canned, dietetic or low calorie:		
(USDA) low sodium	4 oz.	3
(Del Monte) no salt added	½ cup	45
(Diet Delight) whole, peeled, solids & liq.	½ cup (4.3 oz.)	15
(Furman's) crushed	½ cup	<10
(Hunt's) whole no-salt-added	4 oz.	15
(S&W) *Nutradiet*	½ cup	15
TOMATO JUICE:		
Canned, regular pack:		
(USDA)	½ cup (4.3 oz.)	244
(USDA)	6 fl. oz. (6.4 oz.)	364
(Campbell)	6 fl. oz.	570
(Hunt's)	6 fl. oz.	520
(Libby's)	6 fl. oz.	455
(Ocean Spray)	6 fl. oz.	550
Canned, dietetic or low calorie:		
(USDA)	4 oz. (by wt.)	3
(Diet Delight)	6 fl. oz. (6.4 oz.)	20
(Featherweight)	6 fl. oz.	<20
(Hunt's) no-salt-added	6 fl. oz.	25
(S&W) *Nutradiet*	6 fl. oz.	20
Concentrate (USDA):		
Canned	4 oz. (by wt.)	896
*Canned, diluted with 3 parts water by volume	4 oz. (by wt.)	237

Food and Description	Measure or Quantity	Sodium (milligrams)
*Dehydrated (USDA)	½ cup (4.3 oz.)	312
TOMATO JUICE COCKTAIL:		
(USDA)	4 oz. (by wt.)	227
(Ocean Spray) *Firehouse*		
Jubilee	6 fl. oz.	599
Snap-E-Tom	6 fl. oz. (6.5 oz.)	980
TOMATO PASTE, canned:		
Regular pack:		
(USDA) no salt added	6-oz. can	65
(USDA) no salt added	½ cup (4.6 oz.)	50
(USDA) no salt added	1 T. (.6 oz.)	6
(USDA) salt added	6-oz. can	1343
(Contadina):		
Regular	6 oz.	135
Italian	6 oz.	2130
Italian with mushroom	6 oz.	2205
(Del Monte)	6 oz.	110
(Hunt's):		
Regular	6 oz.	405
Garlic	6 oz.	1320
Italian Style	6 oz.	1290
Dietetic:		
(Del Monte)	6 oz.	110
(Featherweight) low sodium	6 oz.	70
(Hunt's) no salt added	6 oz.	25
TOMATO & PEPPERS, hot chili:		
(Old El Paso)	¼ cup	273
(Ortega) Jalapeño	1-oz. serving	22
TOMATO, PICKLED, canned		
(Claussen) Kosher, green, halves	1-oz. piece	326
TOMATO PUREE:		
Canned, regular pack:		
(USDA)	1 cup (8.8 oz.)	998
(Contadina)	1 cup (8.8 oz.)	180
(Hunt's)	1 cup (8 oz.)	300
Canned, dietetic or low calorie:		
(USDA)	8 oz. (by wt.)	14
(Featherweight)	1 cup	<20

Food and Description	Measure or Quantity	Sodium (milligrams)
TOMATO SAUCE, canned:		
Regular pack:		
(Contadina):		
Regular	½ cup	510
Italian style	½ cup	620
(Del Monte):		
Regular	½ cup (4 oz.)	665
With onions	½ cup (4 oz.)	575
(Hunt's):		
Regular	4 oz.	650
With bits	4 oz.	620
With garlic	4 oz.	480
Herb	4 oz.	470
Italian	4 oz.	460
With mushroom	4 oz.	710
With onions	4 oz.	650
Special	4 oz.	280
(Stokely-Van Camp)	½ cup (4.5 oz.)	850
Dietetic (Hunt's) no-salt-added	4 oz.	20
TOMATO SOUP (see **SOUP,** Tomato)		
TOM COLLINS (Mr. Boston)	3 fl. oz.	39
TOM COLLINS MIX:		
*(Bar-Tender's)	6 fl. oz.	32
(Holland House):		
Dry	.6-oz. packet	14
Liquid	1 fl. oz.	96
TONGUE, BEEF (USDA), medium fat, braised	4 oz.	69
TONGUE, PORK, canned, (Hormel) cured	3 oz.	966
TOOTIE FRUITIES, cereal (Malt-O-Meal)	1 cup (1 oz.)	121
TOPPING:		
Sweetened:		
Butterscotch (Smucker's) regular	1 T.	37
Caramel (Smucker's):		
Regular	1 T.	55

Food and Description	Measure or Quantity	Sodium (milligrams)
Hot	I T.	37
Chocolate:		
(Hershey's) fudge	1 T.	15
(Smucker's):		
Regular	1 T.	17
Fudge:		
Regular	1 T.	25
Hot:		
Plain or toffee	1 T.	27
Special Recipe	1 T.	30
Milk, swiss	1 T.	35
Marshmallow (see *MARSH-MALLOW FLUFF*)		
Pecan (Smucker's) in syrup	1 T.	0
Pineapple (Smucker's)	1 T.	0
Peanut butter caramel (Smucker's)	1 T.	60
Strawberry (Smucker's)	1 T.	0
Walnuts, in syrup (Smucker's)	1 T.	0
Dietetic or low calorie, chocolate (Diet Delight)	1 T. (.6 oz.)	9
TOPPING, WHIPPED:		
Canned or aerosol:		
Cool Whip (Birds Eye) frozen, non-dairy	1 T. (.2 oz.)	1
(Dover Farms) dairy	1 T.	3
(Johanna) aerosol	1 T.	2
Lucky Whip, aerosol	1 T. (.2 oz.)	4
Spoon'N Serve (Rich's) frozen, non-dairy	1 T. (.14 oz.)	9
Whip Topping (Rich's) aerosol	¼-oz. serving	5
Frozen:		
La Creme (Pet)	1 T.	5
Pet Whip	1 T.	0
*Mix:		
Regular (Dream Whip)	1 T. (.2 oz.)	4
Dietetic (Estee)	1 T.	0

Food and Description	Measure or Quantity	Sodium (milligrams)
TORTELLINI, frozen:		
(Buitoni):		
Cheese-filled entree:		
Regular	2.6-oz. serving	262
Tricolor	2.6-oz. serving	259
Verdi	2.6-oz. serving	228
Meat:		
Plain	2.4-oz. serving	297
Entree	2½-oz. serving	280
(Green Giant):		
Cheese, marinara, one serving	5½-oz. pkg.	930
Provencale, microwave Garden Gourmet	9½-oz. pkg.	720
(Stouffer's):		
Cheese:		
Alfredo sauce	8⅞-oz. meal	930
Tomato sauce	9⅝-oz. meal	860
Vinaigrette dressing	6⅞-oz. meal	540
Veal, in alfredo sauce	8⅝-oz. meal	860
TORTILLA (Old El Paso):		
Corn	1 piece	170
Flour	1 piece	360
TOSTADA, BEEF, frozen (Van de Kamp's)	8½ oz.	720
TOSTADA SHELL (Old El Paso)	1 shell	65
TOTAL, cereal (General Mills):		
Regular	1 cup (1 oz.)	140
Corn	1 cup (1 oz.)	280
Raisin bran	1 cup (1½ oz.)	190
TRIPE:		
Beef (USDA):		
Commercial	4 oz.	82
Pickled	4 oz.	52
Canned (Libby's)	¼ of 24-oz. can	147
TRIX, cereal (General Mills)	1 cup (1 oz.)	140

Food and Description	Measure or Quantity	Sodium (milligrams)
TROPICAL CITRUS DRINK,		
chilled or frozen (Five Alive)	6 fl. oz.	19
***TROPICAL QUENCHER**		
DRINK, mix, *Crystal Light*	8 fl. oz.	<1
TUNA:		
Raw (USDA) Yellowfin, meat		
only	4 oz.	42
Canned, in oil:		
(USDA) solids & liq.	6½-oz. can	1472
(Bumble Bee) undrained:		
Chunk, light	½ cup	327
Solid white	½ cup	414
(Chicken of the Sea) chunk,		
light:		
Solids & liq.	6½-oz. can	1196
Drained solids	6½-oz. can	1072
(Progresso) solid, light	⅓ cup	400
Canned in water, solids &		
liq.:		
(USDA) no salt added	6½-oz. can	75
(USDA) salt added	6½-oz. can	1610
(Featherweight) low sodium	6½-oz. can	93
(Star Kist) chunk, white	6½-oz. can	92
***TUNA HELPER** (General Mills):		
Au gratin or cheesy noodles	⅕ of pkg.	980
Buttery rice	⅕ of pkg.	1040
Creamy mushroom	⅕ of pkg.	740
Creamy noodles	⅕ of pkg.	960
Fettucini alfredo	⅕ of pkg.	1000
Tuna pot pie	⅙ of pkg.	890
Tuna salad	⅕ of pkg.	870
Tuna tetrazzini	⅕ of pkg.	780
TUNA-NOODLE CASSEROLE,		
frozen (Stouffer's)	10 oz.	1340
TUNA PIE, frozen (Banquet)	7-oz. pie	810
TUNA SALAD, canned		
(Swanson) *Spreadable*	1½-oz. serving	270
TURBOT (USDA) raw,		
meat only	4 oz.	64

Food and Description	Measure or Quantity	Sodium (milligrams)
TURF & SURF DINNER, frozen (Armour) *Classics Lite*	10-oz. meal	890
TURKEY:		
Raw (USDA):		
Dark meat	4 oz.	92
Light meat	4 oz.	58
Meat only:		
Chopped	1 cup (5 oz.)	183
Diced	1 cup (4.8 oz.)	176
Light	4 oz.	93
Light	1 slice (4″ × 2″ × ¼″, 3 oz.)	35
Dark	4 oz.	112
Dark	1 slice (2½″ × 1⅝″ × ¼″, .7 oz.)	21
Canned, boned (Swanson) chunk	2½-oz. serving	380
Packaged:		
(Carl Buddig) smoked:		
Regular	1 oz.	400
Ham	1 oz.	430
(Hebrew National) breast	1 oz.	178
(Hormel) breast:		
Regular	1 slice	242
Smoked	1 slice	270
(Ohse):		
Oven cooked	1 oz.	190
Smoked, breast	1 oz.	340
Turkey bologna	1 oz.	300
Turkey salami	1 oz.	260
(Oscar Mayer) breast, sliced:		
Oven roasted	.7-oz. slice	291
Smoked	.7-oz. slice	301
Roasted, meat only (USDA):		
Dark	4 oz.	112
Light	4 oz.	93
TURKEY DINNER or		

Food and Description	Measure or Quantity	Sodium (milligrams)
ENTREE, frozen:		
(USDA) sliced turkey, mashed potatoes & peas	12-oz. dinner	1360
(Armour) *Dinner Classics*,	11½-oz. dinner	1280
(Banquet)	10½-oz. dinner	1110
(Healthy Choice) breast of	10½-oz. meal	420
(Stouffer;s):		
Regular:		
Casserole with gravy & dressing	9¾-oz. meal	1090
Tetrazzini	10-oz. meal	1170
Lean Cuisine:		
Breast, sliced, in mushroom sauce	8-oz. meal	790
Dijon	9½-oz. meal	900
Right Course, sliced, in mild curry sauce	8¾-oz. meal	570
(Swanson):		
Dinner, 4-compartment	11½-oz. dinner	1260
Entree	8¾-oz. entree	1090
Hungry Man:		
Dinner	18½-oz. dinner	2150
Entree	13¼-oz. entree	1740
(Weight Watchers) stuffed breast	8½-oz. meal	910
TURKEY GIZZARD (USDA):		
Raw	4 oz.	66
Simmered	4 oz.	58
TURKEY PIE:		
Home recipe (USDA) baked	⅓ of 9″ pie	633
Frozen:		
(USDA) unheated	8-oz. pie	837
(Banquet)	7-oz. pie	860
(Morton)	7-oz. pie	740
(Stouffer's)	10-oz. pie	1300
(Swanson):		
Regular	8-oz. pie	800
Chunky	10-oz. pie	950
Hungry Man	16-oz. pie	1590

Food and Description	Measure or Quantity	Sodium (milligrams)
TURKEY SALAD, canned (Carnation) *Spreadable*	1-oz. serving	129
TURKEY TETRAZZINI, frozen (Stouffer's)	6 oz.	620
TURMERIC (French's)	1 tsp.	Tr.
TURNIP (USDA):		
Fresh:		
Without tops	1 lb. (weighed with skins)	191
Pared, diced	½ cup (2.4 oz.)	33
Pared, sliced	½ cup (2.3 oz.)	31
Boiled, drained:		
Diced	½ cup (2.8 oz.)	27
Mashed	½ cup (4 oz.)	39
TURNIP GREENS, leaves & stems:		
Canned:		
(USDA) solids & liq.	½ cup (4.1 oz.)	274
(Stokely-Van Camp) chopped	½ cup (4.1 oz.)	335
(Sunshine) solids & liq.:		
Chopped	½ cup (4.1 oz.)	252
& diced turnips	½ cup (4.1 oz.)	391
Frozen:		
(Birds Eye):		
Chopped	⅓ of 10-oz. pkg.	11
Chopped, with diced turnips	⅓ of 10-oz. pkg.	15
(Frosty Acres)	3.3 oz.	10
(McKenzie) chopped	3.3 oz.	66
(Southland):		
Chopped	⅕ of 16-oz. pkg.	10
With diced turnips	⅕ of 16-oz. pkg.	35
Mashed	⅓ of 11-oz. pkg.	60
TURNOVER:		
Frozen (Pepperidge Farm):		
Apple	1 turnover	220
Blueberry	1 turnover	240
Cherry	1 turnover	290
Peach	1 turnover	260

Food and Description	Measure or Quantity	Sodium (milligrams)
Raspberry	1 turnover	270
Refrigerated (Pillsbury):		
Apple	1 turnover	330
Cherry	1 turnover	320

U

UFO'S, canned (Franco-American):		
Regular	7½ oz.	790
With meteors	7½ oz.	780
ULTRA DIET QUICK (TKI Foods):		
Bar:		
Chocolate	1.2-oz. bar	90
Peanut butter	1.2-oz. bar	100
*Mix, made with low-fat milk or water:		
Dutch chocolate	8 fl. oz.	260
Strawberry or vanilla	8 fl. oz.	130

V

VEAL, medium fat (USDA):		
chunk:		
Raw	1 lb. (weighed with bone)	327
Braised, lean & fat	4 oz.	91

Food and Description	Measure or Quantity	Sodium (milligrams)
Flank:		
Raw	1 lb. (weighed with bone)	404
Stewed, lean & fat	4 oz.	91
Foreshank:		
Raw	1 lb. (weighed with bone)	212
Stewed, lean & fat	4 oz.	91
Loin:		
Raw	1 lb. (weighed with bone)	338
Broiled, medium done, chop, lean & fat	4 oz.	91
Plate:		
Raw	1 lb. (weighed with bone)	322
Stewed, lean & fat	4 oz.	91
Rib:		
Raw, lean & fat	1 lb. (weighed with bone)	314
Roasted, medium done, lean & fat	4 oz.	91
Round & rump:		
Raw	1 lb. (weighed with bone)	314
Broiled, steak or cutlet, lean & fat	4 oz.	91
VEAL DINNER or ENTREE, frozen:		
(Armour) *Dinner Classics*, parmigiana	11¼-oz. meal	1320
(Morton) dinner	10-oz. dinner	1510
(Swanson) parmigiana:		
Regular	12¾-oz. dinner	1120
Hungry Man	20-oz. dinner	2010
(Weight Watchers) parmigiana	8.44-oz. meal	760
VEGETABLE BOUILLON:		
(Herb-Ox):		
Cube	1 cube	920
Packet	1 packet	880

Food and Description	Measure or Quantity	Sodium (milligrams)
MBT	6-g. packet	780
(Wyler's) instant	1 tsp.	910
VEGETABLE FAT (See **FAT, COOKING**		
VEGETABLE FLAKES, dehydrated (French's)	1 T.	20
VEGETABLE JUICE COCKTAIL:		
Canned, regular pack:		
(USDA)	4 oz. (by wt.)	227
(Mott's)	6 fl. oz.	510
(Smucker's) hearty	8 fl. oz.	714
V-8 (Campbell):		
Regular or spicy hot	6 fl. oz.	625
Canned, low sodium:		
(S&W) *Nutradiet*	6 fl. oz.	25
V-8 (Campbell)	6 fl. oz.	50
VEGETABLES, MIXED:		
Canned, regular pack:		
(Chun King) chow mein, drained solids	½ of 8-oz. can	20
(Del Monte) solids & liq.	½ cup	355
(La Choy) Chinese style, drained	⅓ of 14-oz. can	35
(Libby's) solids & liq.	½ cup (4.2 oz.)	345
(Stokely-Van Camp) solids & liq.	½ cup (4.3 oz.)	123
(Veg-All) solids & liq.:		
Regular	½ cup	320
For stew	½ cup	380
Canned, dietetic or low calorie:		
(Featherweight)	½ cup	25
(Larsen) *Fresh-Lite*	½ cup	25
Frozen:		
(USDA) boiled, drained	½ cup (3.2 oz.)	48
(Birds Eye):		
Regular:		
Broccoli, cauliflower & carrots in cheese sauce	5 oz.	380

Food and Description	Measure or Quantity	Sodium (milligrams)
Carrots, peas & pearl onions	⅓ of 10-oz. pkg.	60
Mixed	⅓ of 10-oz. pkg.	10
With onion sauce	⅓ of 8-oz. pkg.	340
Farm Fresh:		
Broccoli, baby carrots & water chestnuts	⅕ of 16-oz. pkg.	25
Broccoli, cauliflower & carrots	⅕ of 16-oz. pkg.	25
Broccoli, corn & red pepper dices	⅕ of 16-oz. pkg.	15
Broccoli, green beans, onion & red pepper	⅕ of 16-oz. pkg.	15
Brussels sprouts, cauliflower & carrots	⅕ of 16-oz. pkg.	20
International style:		
Bavarian style beans & spaetzle	⅓ of 10-oz. pkg.	420
Chinese style	⅓ of 10-oz. pkg.	370
Italian style	⅓ of 10-oz. pkg.	570
Japanese style	⅓ of 10-oz. pkg.	490
New England style	⅓ of 10-oz. pkg.	410
San Francisco style	⅓ of 10-oz. pkg.	400
Stir fry:		
Chinese	⅓ of 10-oz. pkg.	540
Japanese	⅓ of 10-oz. pkg.	510
(Frosty Acres):		
Regular	3.3 oz.	50
Dutch style or rancho fiesta	3.2 oz.	30
Italian style	3.2 oz.	20
Oriental style	3.2 oz.	15
Soup mix	3 oz.	35
Stew	3 oz.	21
Swiss mix	3 oz.	36
(Green Giant):		
Regular:		
Broccoli, cauliflower & carrots:		

Food and Description	Measure or Quantity	Sodium (milligrams)
Butter sauce	⅓ of 9-oz. pkg.	240
Cheese sauce	⅓ of 10-oz. pkg.	408
One Serving:		
Plain	4-oz. pkg.	45
Cheese sauce	5-oz. pkg.	610
Mixed, in butter sauce	½ cup (3.9 oz.)	300
Pea, sweet, carrot & pearl onion	½ cup (4.1 oz.)	510
Harvest Fresh, mixed	½ cup	210
Polybag, mixed, plain	½ cup (2.7 oz.)	40
Valley Combination:		
Broccoli carrot fanfare	⅙ of 16-oz. pkg.	30
Broccoli cauliflower supreme	½ cup (2.7 oz.)	30
Corn broccoli bounty	½ cup (3 oz.)	15
(La Choy) stir fry	⅓ of 12-oz. pkg.	23
(Larsen):		
Regular	3.3 oz.	45
California or Italian blend	3.3 oz.	20
Chuckwagon blend	3.3 oz.	5
Midwestern or Scandinavian blend	3.3 oz.	30
Oriental blend	3.3 oz.	10
Soup or stew	3.3 oz.	40
Winter blend	3.3 oz.	25
Wisconsin blend	3.3 oz.	15
(Le Sueur) pea, onion & carrots in butter sauce	½ cup	100
(McKenzie)	3.3 oz.	56
(Ore-Ida):		
Medley, breaded	3 oz.	500
Stew	3 oz.	50
(Southland):		
Gumbo	⅕ of 16-oz. pkg.	10
Soup	⅕ of 16-oz. pkg.	40
Stew	⅕ of 20-oz. pkg.	30

VEGETABLES IN PASTRY,
frozen (Pepperidge Farm):

Asparagus with mornay sauce	½ of 7½-oz. pkg.	245

Food and Description	Measure or Quantity	Sodium (milligrams)
Broccoli with cheese	½ of 7½-oz. pkg.	455
Cauliflower & cheese sauce	½ of 7½-oz. pkg.	465
Mushrooms dijon	½ of 7½-oz. pkg.	415
Spinach almondine	½ of 7½-oz. pkg.	325
Zucchini provençal	½ of 7½-oz. pkg.	290
VEGETABLE SOUP (See **SOUP,** Vegetable)		
VEGETABLE STEW, canned, *Dinty Moore* (Hormel)	⅓ of 24-oz. can	1047
"VEGETARIAN FOODS":		
Canned or dry:		
Chicken, fried (Loma Linda) with gravy	1½-oz. piece	170
Chili (Worthington)	½ cup (4.9 oz.)	695
Choplet (Worthington)	1.6-oz. slice	263
Cutlet (Worthington)	2.2-oz. slice	434
Dinner cuts (Loma Linda):		
Regular	2.1-oz. piece	330
No salt added	1.8-oz. piece	15
Franks (Loma Linda):		
Big	1.9-oz. piece	220
Sizzle	1.2-oz. piece	170
FriChik (Worthington)	1.6-oz. piece	277
Granburger (Worthington)	6 T. (1.2 oz.)	933
Linketts (Loma Linda)	1.3-oz. link	170
Little links (Loma Linda)	.8-oz. link	105
Numete (Worthington)	½" slice (2.4 oz.)	370
Nuteena (Loma Linda)	½" slice (2.4 oz.)	120
Proteena (Loma Linda)	½" slice (2.5 oz.)	460
Protose (Worthington)	½" slice (2.7 oz.)	476
Redi-burger (Loma Linda)	½" slice (2.4 oz.)	370
Sandwich spread (Loma Linda)	1 T. (.6 oz.)	100
Saucettes (Worthington)	1 link	190
Skallops (Worthington) drained	½ cup (3 oz.)	315
Soyameat (Worthington):		
Beef-like slices	1-oz. slice	183
Chicken-like slices	1-oz. slice	167
Stew pac (Loma Linda)	2-oz.	220

Food and Description	Measure or Quantity	Sodium (milligrams)
Super links (Worthington)	1.9-oz. link	449
Swiss steak & gravy (Loma Linda)	2.6-oz. steak	350
Tender bits (Loma Linda)	.6-oz. piece	85
VegeBurger (Loma Linda):		
Regular	½ cup (3.8 oz.)	190
No salt added	½ cup (3.8 oz.)	55
Vegelona (Loma Linda)	½" slice (2.4 oz.)	210
Vegetable steak (Worthington)	1.3-oz. piece	148
Vegetarian burger (Worthington)	⅓ cup (3.3 oz.)	545
Veja-links (Worthington)	1.1-oz. link	169
Vita-Burger (Loma Linda)	1 T. (¼ oz.)	50
Worthington 209, turkey-like flavor	1.1-oz. slice	229
Frozen:		
Beef-like pie (Worthington)	8-oz. pie	1109
Bologna (Loma Linda)	1-oz. slice	245
Bolono (Worthington)	.7-oz. slice	206
Chicken, fried (Loma Linda)	2-oz. piece	510
Chicken-like pie (Worthington)	8-oz. pie	930
Chicken-like slices (Worthington)	.1-oz. slice	288
Corned beef-like, sliced (Worthington)	.5-oz. slice	155
Fillets (Worthington)	1.5-oz. piece	368
FriPats (Worthington)	2.5-oz. piece	379
Meatballs (Loma Linda)	.3-oz. piece	53
Meatless salami (Worthington)	.7-oz. slice	300
Prosage (Worthington):		
Links	.8-oz. link	140
Patties	1.3-oz. piece	297
Roll	⅜" slice (1.2 oz.)	254
Sizzle burger (Loma Linda)	2½-oz. piece	320
Smoked turkey-like slices (Worthington)	1 slice (.7-oz.)	200
Stakelets (Worthington)	3-oz. piece	604

Food and Description	Measure or Quantity	Sodium (milligrams)
Stripples (Worthington)	.3-oz. strip	123
Tuno (Worthington)	2-oz. serving	343
Wham (Worthington) sliced	.8-oz. slice	261
VERMOUTH Dry or sweet (Great Western) 16% alcohol	3 fl. oz.	20
VICHY WATER (Schweppes)	6 fl. oz.	76
VIENNA SAUSAGE (See **SAUSAGE**)		
VINEGAR:		
Cider:		
(USDA)	½ cup (4.2 oz.)	<1
(White House) apple	1 T.	2
Distilled:		
(USDA)	1 T. (.5 oz.)	<1
(USDA)	½ cup (4.2 oz.)	1
(White House) white	1 T.	5
Red wine or red wine with garlic (Regina)	1 T. (.5 oz.)	20
White wine (Regina)	1 T. (.5 oz.)	10
VODKA (See **DISTILLED LIQUOR**)		

W

WAFER (See **COOKIE; CRACKER**)

WAFFLE:

Food and Description	Measure or Quantity	Sodium (milligrams)
Home recipe (USDA)	7″ waffle (2.6 oz.)	356
Frozen:		
(USDA)	1.6-oz. waffle (8 in 13-oz. pkg.)	296
(USDA)	.8-oz. waffle (6 in 5-oz. pkg.)	155

Food and Description	Measure or Quantity	Sodium (milligrams)
(Aunt Jemima) jumbo:		
Regular	1¼-oz. waffle	261
Apple-cinnamon or		
blueberry	1¼-oz. waffle	243
Buttermilk	1¼-oz. waffle	267
(Eggo):		
Regular, any flavor	1.4-oz. waffle	250
Common Sense, oat bran,		
plain or with fruit		
& nuts	1.4-oz. waffle	220
Nutri-Grain, plain or		
raisin bran	1.4-oz. waffle	250
WAFFLE MIX (See also		
PANCAKE & WAFFLE MIX)		
(USDA):		
Complete mix:		
Dry	1 oz.	291
*Prepared with water	2.6-oz. waffle	420
Incomplete mix:		
Dry	1 oz.	406
*Prepared with egg & milk	2.6-oz. waffle	514
*Prepared with egg & milk	7.1-oz. waffle	1372
WAFFLE SYRUP (See **SYRUP)**		
WALNUT:		
(USDA):		
Black, in shell, whole	1 lb. (weighed in shell)	3
Black, shelled, whole	4 oz. (weighed whole)	3
Black, chopped	½ cup (2.1 oz.)	2
English or Persian, in shell, whole	1 lb. (weighed in shell)	4
English or Persian, shelled, whole	4 oz.	2
English or Persian chopped	½ cup (2.1 oz.)	1
English or Persian, halves	½ cup (1.8 oz.)	1
(Fisher) black or English	1 oz.	0

Food and Description	Measure or Quantity	Sodium (milligrams)
WATER CHESTNUT, CHINESE:		
Raw (USDA):		
Whole	1 lb. (weighed unpeeled)	70
Peeled	4 oz.	23
Canned:		
(Chun King) drained solids:		
Sliced	½ of 8-oz. can	22
Whole	½ of 8½-oz. can	24
(La Choy) sliced, drained solids	¼ cup	Tr.
WATERCRESS, raw (USDA):		
Untrimmed	½ lb. (weighed untrimmed)	108
Trimmed	½ cup (.6 oz.)	8
WATERMELON, fresh (USDA):		
Wedge	2-lb. wedge (4″ × 8″ measured with rind)	4
Diced	1 cup (5.6 oz.)	2
WATERMELON DRINK, canned, *Capri Sun*	6¾ fl. oz.	1
WAX GOURD, raw (USDA):		
Whole	1 lb. (weighed with skin & cavity contents)	19
Flesh only	4 oz.	7
WEAKFISH (USDA):		
Raw, whole	1 lb. (weighed whole)	163
Broiled, meat only	4 oz.	635
WELSH RAREBIT, home recipe (USDA)	1 cup (8.2 oz.)	770
WENDY'S:		
Bacon, breakfast	1 strip	223

Food and Description	Measure or Quantity	Sodium (milligrams)
Bacon cheeseburger on white bun	1 burger	860
Breakfast sandwich	1 sandwich	770
Bun:		
Wheat, multi-grain	1 bun	220
White	1 bun	266
Chicken sandwich on wheat bun	1 sandwich	500
Chili:		
Small order	8 oz.	1070
Large order	12 oz.	1605
Condiments:		
Bacon	½ strip	112
Cheese, American	1 slice	260
Ketchup	1 tsp.	65
Lettuce	1 piece	0
Mayonnaise	1 T.	80
Mustard	1 tsp.	50
Onion rings	1 piece (.3 oz.)	0
Pickle, dill	4 slices (.3 oz.)	125
Relish	.3-oz. serving	70
Tomatoes	1 slice (.5 oz.)	0
Danish	1 piece (3 oz.)	340
Drinks:		
Coffee	6 fl. oz.	0
Cola:		
Regular	12 fl. oz.	15
Dietetic or low calorie	12 fl. oz.	20
Fruit flavored drink	12 fl. oz.	10
Hot chocolate	6 fl. oz.	145
Milk:		
Regular	8 fl. oz.	120
Chocolate	8 fl. oz.	150
Non-cola soft drink	12 fl. oz.	35
Orange juice	6 fl. oz.	0
Tea:		
Hot	6 fl. oz.	15
Iced	12 fl. oz.	20
Egg, scrambled	1 order	160

Food and Description	Measure or Quantity	Sodium (milligrams)
Frosty dairy dessert:		
Small	12 fl. oz.	220
Medium	16 fl. oz.	293
Large	20 fl. oz.	367
Hamburger:		
Double on white bun	1 burger	575
Kids Meal	1 burger	265
Single:		
On wheat bun	1 burger	290
On white bun	1 burger	410
Omelets:		
Ham & cheese	1 omelet	405
Ham, cheese & mushroom	1 omelet	570
Ham, cheese, onion & green pepper	1 omelet	485
Mushroom, onion & green pepper	1 omelet	200
Potatoes:		
Baked, hot stuffed:		
Plain	1 potato	60
Bacon & cheese	1 potato	1180
Broccoli & cheese	1 potato	430
Cheese	1 potato	450
Chicken a la king	1 potato	820
Chili & cheese	1 potato	610
Sour cream & chives	1 potato	230
Stroganoff & sour cream	1 potato	910
French fries	1 regular order	95
Home fries	1 order	745
Salad bar, *Garden Spot*:		
Alfalfa sprouts	2 oz.	DNA
Bacon bits	3.5 grams	95
Blueberries, fresh	1 T. (.5 oz.)	0
Breadsticks	1 piece	DNA
Broccoli	½ cup (1.6 oz.)	10
Cantaloupe	2 pieces (2 oz.)	35
Carrot	¼ cup (1 oz.)	15
Cauliflower	½ cup (1.8 oz.)	5

Food and Description	Measure or Quantity	Sodium (milligrams)
Cheese:		
American, imitation	1 oz.	DNA
Cheddar, imitation	1 oz.	450
Cottage	½ cup	425
Mozzarella, imitation	1 oz.	320
Swiss, imitation	1 oz.	450
Chow mein noodles	¼ cup (.4 oz.)	80
Cole slaw	½ cup	70
Cracker, saltine	1 piece	37
Croutons	1 piece	5
Cucumber	1/4 cup (.9 oz.)	0
Eggs	1 T. (.3 oz.)	10
Lettuce:		
Iceberg	1 cup	5
Romaine	1 cup	5
Mushroom	¼ cup	5
Onions, red	1 T.	0
Oranges, fresh	1 piece	0
Pasta salad	½ cup	400
Pea, green	½ cup	90
Peaches, in syrup	1 piece	0
Peppers:		
Banana or milk pepperocini	1 T.	DNA
Bell	¼ cup	5
Jalapeño	1 T.	4
Pineapple chunks in juice	½ cup	0
Sunflower seeds & raisins	½ cup	10
Tomato	1 oz.	0
Watermelon, fresh	1 piece (1 oz.)	0
Salad dressings:		
Regular:		
Blue cheese	1 T.	85
Celery seed	1 T.	65
French, red	1 T.	130
Italian, golden	1 T.	260
Oil	1 T.	0
Ranch	1 T.	155
1000 Island	1 T.	115

Food and Description	Measure or Quantity	Sodium (milligrams)
Dietetic or low calorie:		
Bacon & tomato	1 T.	160
Cucumber, creamy	1 T.	140
Italian	1 T.	180
1000 Island	1 T.	125
Wine vinegar	1 T.	5
Salad, side	1 order	540
Salad, taco	1 order	1100
Sausage	1 patty (1.6 oz.)	410
Toast:		
Regular, with margarine	1 slice	205
French	1 slice	425
WESTERN DINNER, frozen:		
(Banquet)	11-oz. dinner	720
(Morton)	10-oz. dinner	1450
(Swanson):		
Regular	12¼ oz. dinner	1040
Hungry Man	17½ oz. dinner	1900
WHALE MEAT, raw (USDA)	4 oz.	88
WHEAT CEREAL (Elam's)		
cooked	1 oz.	190
WHEAT CEREAL, CRACKED		
(Elam's)	1 oz.	4
WHEATENA, dry	¼ cup (1.1 oz.)	5
WHEAT FLAKES, cereal		
(Featherweight)	1¼ cups	5
WHEAT GERM:		
(USDA) crude, commercial,		
milled	1 oz.	<1
(Kretschmer)	1 oz.	0
WHEAT GERM CEREAL:		
(USDA)	¼ cup (1 oz.)	<1
(Kretschmer):		
Regular	¼ cup (1 oz.)	<5
Brown sugar & honey	¼ cup (1 oz.)	0
*WHEAT HEARTS, cereal		
(General Mills) hot, dry	1 T.	0
WHEATIES, cereal (General		
Mills)	1 cup (1 oz.)	200

Food and Description	Measure or Quantity	Sodium (milligrams)
WHEAT PUFF, cereal		
(Post) super golden crisp	⅞ cup	44
WHEAT, ROLLED (USDA):		
Uncooked	1 cup (3.1 oz.)	2
Cooked	1 cup (7.7 oz.)	640
WHEAT, SHREDDED, cereal		
(See **SHREDDED WHEAT**)		
WHEAT, WHOLE-GRAIN		
(USDA) hard red spring	1 oz.	<1
WHEAT, WHOLE-MEAL,		
cereal (USDA):		
Dry	1 oz.	<1
Cooked	4 oz.	240
WHISKEY or WHISKY (See		
DISTILLED LIQUOR)		
WHISKEY SOUR COCKTAIL		
MIX:		
*(Bar-Tender's)	3½ fl. oz.	50
(Holland House):		
Instant	.56-oz. packet	4
Liquid	1 oz.	105
WHITE CASTLE:		
Bun only	1 bun	131
Cheese only	.3-oz. piece	154
Cheeseburger	2.3-oz. sandwich	361
Chicken sandwich	2¼-oz. sandwich	497
Fish sandwich, without tartar		
sauce	1 sandwich	201
French fries	3.4-oz. serving	193
Hamburger	2.1-oz. sandwich	266
Onion chips	3.3-oz. order	823
Onion rings	1 order	566
Sausage & egg sandwich	3.4-oz. sandwich	698
Sausage sandwich	1.7-oz. sandwich	488
WHITEFISH, LAKE (USDA):		
Raw:		
Whole	1 lb. (weighed whole)	111
Meat only	4 oz.	59

Food and Description	Measure or Quantity	Sodium (milligrams)
Baked, stuffed, made with bacon, butter, onion, celery & bread crumbs, home recipe	4 oz.	221
WHITEFISH & PIKE (See **GEFILTE FISH**)		
WIENER (See **FRANKFURTER**)		
WIENER WRAP (Pillsbury)	1 wrap	430
WILD BERRY, fruit drink (Hi-C)	6 fl. oz.	17
WILD RICE, raw (USDA)	½ cup (2.9 oz.)	6
WINE (most wines are listed throughout this guide by kind, brand, vineyard, region or grape name):		
Cooking (Holland House)	1 fl. oz.	186
Dessert (USDA) 18.8% alcohol	3 fl. oz.	4
Table (USDA) 12.2% alcohol	3 fl. oz.	4
WORCHESTERSHIRE SAUCE (See **SAUCE**)		

Y

YAM (See **SWEET POTATO**)		
YEAST:		
Baker's:		
Compressed:		
(USDA)	1 oz.	5
(Fleishmann's)	⅗-oz. cake	7
Dry:		
(USDA)	1 oz.	15
(USDA)	7-g. pkg.	4
(Fleischmann's)	¼ oz. (pkg. or jar)	10

Food and Description	Measure or Quantity	Sodium (milligrams)
Brewer's dry, debittered:		
(USDA)	1 oz.	34
(USDA)	1 T. (8 g.)	10
YOGURT:		
Regular:		
Plain:		
(Dannon)	8-oz. container	160
(Friendship)	8-oz. container	190
(Johanna)	8-oz. container	140
(La Yogurt)	6-oz. serving	140
Lite-Line (Borden)	8-oz. container	150
(Meadow Gold)	8-oz. container	160
Yoplait (General Mills):		
Regular	6-oz. container	140
Non-fat	8-oz. container	160
(Mountain High)	8-oz. container	140
Yoplait (General Mills):		
Regular	6-oz. container	140
Non-fat	8-oz. container	160
Apple:		
(Dannon) Dutch, fruit		
on the bottom	8-oz. container	120
(Sweet 'n Low) Dutch	8-oz. container	170
Banana:		
(Dannon) fruit on the		
bottom	8-oz. container	120
Yoplait General Mills):		
Regular	6-oz. container	110
Custard Style	6-oz. container	95
Berry, *Yoplait* (General		
Mills):		
Regular	6-oz. container	110
Breakfast Yogurt	6-oz. container	95
Custard Style	6-oz. container	95
Blueberry:		
(Breyer's)	8-oz. container	125
(Dannon):		
Fresh flavor	8-oz. container	160

Food and Description	Measure or Quantity	Sodium (milligrams)
Fruit on the bottom	4.4-oz. container	65
Fruit on the bottom	8-oz. container	120
(Mountain High)	8-oz. container	140
Yoplait (General Mills):		
Regular	4-oz. container	75
Custard Style	6-oz. container	95
Light	6-oz. container	100
Boysenberry:		
(Dannon) fruit on the bottom	8-oz. container	120
(Sweet'n Low)	8-oz. container	170
Yoplait (General Mills)	6-oz. container	110
Cherry:		
(Breyer's) black	8-oz. container	125
(Dannon) fruit on the bottom	8-oz. container	120
(Sweet 'n Low)	8-oz. container	170
Yoplait (General Mills):		
Regular	6-oz. container	110
Breakfast Yogurt, with almonds	6-oz. container	90
Custard Style	6-oz. container	95
Light	6-oz. container	100
Cherry vanilla, *Lite-Line* (Borden)	8-oz. container	150
Coffee:		
(Dannon) fresh flavors	8-oz. container	140
(Friendship)	8-oz. container	170
(Johanna)	8-oz. container	140
Exotic fruit (Dannon) fruit on the bottom	8-oz. container	120
Lemon:		
(Dannon) fresh flavors	8-oz. container	140
(Johanna)	8-oz. container	140
(Sweet 'n Low)	8-oz. container	170
Yoplait (General Mills):		
Regular	6-oz. container	110
Custard Style	6-oz. container	95

Food and Description	Measure or Quantity	Sodium (milligrams)
Mixed berries (Dannon):		
Extra smooth	4.4-oz. container	80
Fruit on the bottom	4.4-oz. container	65
Fruit on the bottom	8-oz. container	120
Hearty nuts & raisins	8-oz. container	120
Orange, *Yoplait* (General Mills):		
Regular	6-oz. container	110
Custard Style	6-oz. container	95
Peach:		
(Breyer's)	8-oz. container	120
(Dannon) fruit on the bottom	8-oz. container	120
Lite-Line (Borden)	8-oz. container	150
Yoplait (General Mills):		
Regular	6-oz. container	110
Light	6-oz. container	100
Pina colada:		
(Dannon) fruit on the bottom	8-oz. container	120
Yoplait (General Mills)	6-oz. container	110
Pineapple:		
(Breyer's)	8-oz. container	125
Light 'N Lively	8-oz. container	120
Yoplait (General Mills)	6-oz. container	110
Raspberry:		
(Breyer's)	8-oz. container	125
(Dannon):		
Extra smooth	4.4-oz. container	80
Fresh flavors	8-oz. container	160
Fruit on the bottom	8-oz. container	120
Light 'N Lively	8-oz. container	130
(Meadow Gold)	8-oz. container	160
(Sweet 'n Low)	8-oz. container	170
Yoplait (General Mills):		
Regular	6-oz. container	110
Custard Style	6-oz. container	95
Light	6-oz. container	100

Food and Description	Measure or Quantity	Sodium (milligrams)
Strawberry:		
(Breyer's)	8-oz. container	120
(Dannon):		
Extra smooth	4.4-oz. container	80
Fresh flavors	8-oz. container	160
Fruit on the bottom	4.4-oz. container	65
Fruit on the bottom	8-oz.container	120
Light 'N Lively	8-oz. container	130
Lite-Line (Borden)	8-oz. container	150
(Sweet 'n Low)	8-oz. container	170
Yoplait (General Mills):		
Regular	6-oz. container	110
Breakfast Yogurt, with		
almonds	6-oz. container	90
Custard Style	6-oz. container	95
Light	6-oz. container	100
Strawberry banana:		
(Dannon):		
Fresh flavors	8-oz. container	160
Fruit on the bottom	4.4-oz. container	65
Fruit on the bottom	8-oz. container	120
Light 'N Lively	8-oz. container	120
(Sweet 'n Low)	6-oz. container	170
Yoplait (General Mills):		
Regular	6-oz. container	110
Breakfast Yogurt	6-oz. container	90
Custard Style	6-oz. container	95
Light	6-oz. container	100
Strawberry-rhubarb, *Yoplait*		
(General Mills)	6-oz. container	110
Tropical fruits, *Yoplait*		
(General Mills) *Breakfast*		
Yogurt	6-oz. container	90
Vanilla:		
(Breyer's)		
(Dannon):		
Fresh flavors	4.4-oz. container	90
Hearty nuts & raisins	8-oz. container	120
Light, regular or cherry	8-oz. container	130

Food and Description	Measure or Quantity	Sodium (milligrams)
(Friendship	8-oz. container	170
Yoplait (General Mills):		
Regular	6-oz. container	120
Custard Style	6-oz. container	110
Nonfat	6-oz. container	140
Frozen, hard (Dannon):		
Boysenberry, *Danny-On-A-Stick,* carob coated	2½-fl.-oz. bar	15
Chocolate, *Danny-On-A-Stick,* chocolate coated	2½-fl.-oz. bar	15
Raspberry, red, *Danny-On-A-Stick,* chocolate coated	2½-fl.-oz. bar	15
YOGURT BAR, frozen (Dole):		
Cherry	1 bar	22
Chocolate	1 bar	50
Mixed Berry	1 bar	18
Strawberry	1 bar	16
Strawberry-banana	1 bar	15

Z

ZITI, frozen:		
(Morton) light	11-oz. dinner	790
(Weight Watchers)	11¼-oz. serving	1387
ZUCCHINI (See **SQUASH, SUMMER**)		
ZWIEBACK:		
(Gerber)	1 piece	16
(Nabisco)	1 piece	10